Diagnostic Hematology:

A Pattern Approach

Diagnostic Hematology:

A Pattern Approach

Doyen T Nguyen MD
Department of Haematology
St Bartholomew's Hospital
London, UK

Lawrence W Diamond MD
Department of Haematology
St Bartholomew's Hospital
London, UK

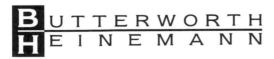

BUTTERWORTH
HEINEMANN

OXFORD AUCKLAND BOSTON JOHANNESBURG MELBOURNE
NEW DELHI

Butterworth-Heinemann
Linacre House, Jordan Hill, Oxford OX2 8DP
225 Wildwood Avenue, Woburn, MA 01801-2041
A division of Reed Educational and Professional Publishing Ltd

℞ A member of the Reed Elsevier plc group

First published 2000

©Reed Educational and Professional Publishing Ltd 2000

British Library Cataloguing in Publication Data
Nguyen, Doyen
    Diagnostic hematology : a pattern approach
    1. Hematology   2. Hematology – Technique   3. Blood – Diseases –
    Diagnosis
    I. Title   II. Diamond, Lawrence
    616'.075'61

    ISBN 07506 4247 5

Library of Congress Cataloguing in Publication Data
Nguyen, Doyen T.
    Diagnostic hematology : a pattern approach/Doyen T. Nguyen and
    Lawrence W. Diamond.
    p.   cm.
    Includes bibliographical references and index.
    ISBN 0 7506 4247 5
    1. Blood – Diseases – Diagnosis.   2. Hematology. I. Diamond
    Lawrence W.   II. Title
    [DNLM: 1. Hematologic diseases – diagnosis.   2. Blood Cells –
    pathology.   3. Bone Marrow Cells – pathology.   4. Flow Cytometry.
    WH 120 N576d]
    RC636.N48   99 – 25098
    616.1'5075 – dc21   CIP

    ISBN 0 7506 4247 5

Typeset by Keyword Typesetting Services Ltd, Wallington, Surrey SM6 9AA
Printed and bound in Spain

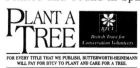

Contents

Part One: Peripheral Blood

Part Two: Flow Cytometry

Part Three: Bone Marrow

Preface

Diagnostic hematology is a problem solving process similar to detective work. For each case, a physician hopes to establish a diagnosis (or differential diagnosis) based on all of the available information. In our experience, expert hematopathologists utilize a 'pattern approach' to diagnosis. A pattern, which is formed by a constellation of relevant findings, serves as an intermediate hypothesis in diagnostic reasoning. Each pattern encompasses a set of differential diagnoses, and an experienced diagnostician uses the predominant pattern as a guide in determining which additional information needs to be gathered to render a final diagnosis.

The scope of this book is all aspects of 'liquid' hematology, including peripheral blood analysis, flow cytometry immunophenotyping, and bone marrow morphology, using an integrated multiparameter approach. The book is designed for physicians who interpret the findings in the blood and bone marrow, professionals who render interpretations of flow cytometry data, and technologists involved in the review of blood films or flow cytometry data.

In terms of organization, this book breaks away from the mold of traditional textbooks of hematopathology. As can be seen from the Contents, the chapters are devoted to patterns rather than specific diseases. Organization by patterns reflects the real-life problem solving methods applied daily in the diagnostic evaluation of hematological disorders. It is our hope that this approach will help the reader incorporate patterns into their diagnostic armamentarium. In addition, we point out diagnostic clues and offer practical advice on how to avoid potential errors caused by both technical artifacts and morphologic 'look-alikes'.

After scanning the Contents, the reader will immediately recognize that more than one pattern can be present in the same case. The goal of the pattern approach is to arrive at a single predominant pattern that indicates a list of differential diagnoses based on common features. Therefore, a hierarchical classification of the patterns must be established. This hierarchical classification is based on two principles: (1) if WBC abnormalities are present, associated RBC and platelet abnormalities tend to be secondary to the WBC disease; and (2) the predominant pattern is that pattern which suggests a more specific (i.e. shorter) list of differential diagnoses. The latter rule can be inferred from a commonly accepted heuristic criterion of diagnostic reasoning known as Occam's razor, which states that the simpler of competing hypotheses is more likely to depict reality than the more complex hypothesis. The 'abnormal mononuclear cell' pattern (peripheral blood) and 'mononuclear cell infiltration' pattern (bone marrow) are at the top of their respective hierarchies.

Organizing this book based on patterns necessitates that certain groups of diseases, such as the myelodysplastic syndromes, are discussed over several chapters. In order not to carry this approach to the extreme, we have arbitrarily grouped the discussion of many of the protean bone marrow findings in AIDS along with the concomitant infections that can occur in this disease.

The list of suggested reading near the end of the book is not meant to be exhaustive. The references were chosen mainly for the reader to gain more depth on certain topics, e.g. the pathogenesis and molecular genetics of diseases.

The patterns used in this book form the basis of diagnostic reasoning in three knowledge-based computer systems for hematology diagnosis developed by the authors: 'Professor Petrushka' for peripheral blood analysis, 'Professor Fidelio' for flow cytometry immunophenotyping of leukemias and lymphomas, and 'Professor Belmonte' for bone marrow diagnosis. These systems have been used daily to generate over 2500 diagnostic bone marrow reports at St. Bartholomew's Hospital, London, UK, since June 1996. Educational versions of these programs are included with this book on the accompanying CD-ROM. Throughout the book, there are icons pointing the reader to example cases that have been entered into the knowledge-based systems. The reader can view real case data, the interpretations generated by the knowledge-based systems, and additional images such as photomicrographs of the peripheral blood and bone marrow, or flow cytometry graphics.

Each example case is given a title as well as a case number so that the reader can browse the educational programs independent of the textbook. These titles are specific to the educational version of the programs and are provided for the reader's convenience. It should be kept in mind that the case titles are derived from final diagnoses based on all available information (such as hemoglobin electrophoresis and cytogenetics, where appropriate). Therefore, the titles do not necessarily reflect the interpretation based on the more limited information available to Professor Petrushka or Professor Fidelio.

Doyen T. Nguyen
Lawrence W. Diamond
October 1998

Acknowledgments

The authors would like to thank the Coulter Corporation (now Beckman-Coulter) for sponsoring the research that has made this project possible. We wish to express our sincere appreciation to Sandy Piepho and Peter Frost, our principal contacts at Beckman-Coulter in the United States and the United Kingdom. We would also like to acknowledge the support of the Dr Mildred Scheel Foundation for Cancer Research (Germany).

The work on knowledge-based systems in diagnostic hematology was started at Hospital Henri Mondor (Paris, France) in the laboratory of the late Professor Claude Sultan, and we are very grateful for the support and encouragement that he provided.

We are particularly grateful to Dr John Amess for helpful discussions, Dr Raul Braylan, who reviewed the flow cytometry (FCM) section of this book and provided FCM list mode data, Neal Benson, who assisted in mastering the CD-ROM, and Donna Wong for contributing slides of rare congenital disorders.

We would also like to acknowledge the generous help of the technical staff in the hematology department, St. Bartholomew's Hospital (London, UK), and the FCM Laboratory at Shands Hospital, University of Florida (Gainesville, FL, USA).

We are indebted to the editorial and technical staff at Butterworth-Heinemann, especially Melanie Tait, Myriam Brearley, Alex Hollingsworth, Chris Jarvis, Jess Dawe, Angela Davies and Jane Campbell.

List of abbreviations

ACD	Anemia of chronic disease
AIDS	Acquired immunodeficiency syndrome
AIHA(s)	Autoimmune hemolytic anemia(s)
ALCL	Anaplastic large cell lymphoma
ALL(s)	Acute lymphoblastic leukemia(s)
AML(s)	Acute myeloid leukemia(s)
AMM	Agnogenic myeloid metaplasia
ANAE	α-Naphthyl acetate esterase
ANBE	α-Naphthyl butyrate esterase
APAAP	Alkaline phosphatase anti-alkaline phosphatase
APL	Acute promyelocytic leukemia
ATLL	Adult T-cell leukemia-lymphoma
BUN	Blood urea nitrogen
CAE	Chloroacetate esterase
CBC	Complete blood count
CD	Cluster designation
CDA(s)	Congenital dyserythropoietic anemia(s)
cIg	Cytoplasmic immunoglobulin
CLL	Chronic lymphocytic leukemia
CLL/PL	Chronic lymphocytic leukemia with increased prolymphocytes
CML	Chronic myeloid leukemia
CMMoL	Chronic myelomonocytic leukemia
CMV	Cytomegalovirus
DAT	Direct antiglobulin test
DIC	Disseminated intravascular coagulopathy
DLCL	Diffuse large cell lymphoma
DNA	Deoxyribonucleic acid
EBV	Epstein-Barr virus
EDTA	Ethylenediamine tetra-acetic acid
ET	Essential thrombocythemia
FAB	French-American-British
FCC	Follicular center cell
FCM	Flow cytometry
FISH	Fluorescence *in-situ* hybridization
FITC	Fluorescein isothiocyanate
FSC	Forward scatter
G6PD	Glucose-6-phosphate dehydrogenase
G-CSF	Granulocyte colony stimulating factor
HCL	Hairy cell leukemia
Hct	Hematocrit
HDN	Hemolytic disease of the newborn

HE	Hereditary elliptocytosis
H&E	Hematoxylin and eosin
Hgb	Hemoglobin
HIV	Human immunodeficiency virus
HPFH	Hereditary persistence of fetal hemoglobin
HS	Hereditary spherocytosis
HTLV	Human T-cell lymphotropic virus
HUS	Hemolytic uremic syndrome
IM	Infectious mononucleosis
ITP	Idiopathic thrombocytopenic purpura
JCMMoL	Juvenile chronic myelomonocytic leukemia
kb	kilobases
kd	kilodaltons
LCL(s)	Large cell lymphoma(s)
LDH	Lactate dehydrogenase
LGL(s)	Large granular lymphocyte(s)
LPC	Lymphoplasmacytoid
LPD(s)	Lymphoproliferative disorder(s)
MAHA	Microangiopathic hemolytic anemia
M-bcr	Major breakpoint cluster region
m-bcr	Minor breakpoint cluster region
MCH	Mean corpuscular hemoglobin
MCHC	Mean corpuscular hemoglobin concentration
MCL	Mantle cell lymphoma
MCV	Mean corpuscular volume
MDS(s)	Myelodysplastic syndrome(s)
M:E ratio	Myeloid/erythroid ratio
MF	Mycosis fungoides
MGUS	Monoclonal gammopathy of undetermined significance
MNC(s)	Mononuclear cell(s)
MPD(s)	Myeloproliferative disorder(s)
MPO	Myeloperoxidase
MRD	Minimal residual disease
mRNA	Messenger ribonucleic acid
N/C	Nuclear/cytoplasmic
NCNC	Normochromic, normocytic
NEC	Nonerythroid cells
NHL(s)	Non-Hodgkin's lymphoma(s)
NK	Natural killer
NRBC(s)	Nucleated red blood cell(s)
NSE	Nonspecific esterase
OMNC	Other mononuclear cells
PAS	Periodic acid Schiff
PCL	Plasma cell leukemia
PCR	Polymerase chain reaction
PE	Phycoerythrin
PerCP	Peridinium-chlorophyll-protein complex
PLL	Prolymphocytic leukemia

PNH	Paroxysmal nocturnal hemoglobinuria
PPMM	Post-polycythemic myeloid metaplasia
PRV	Polycythemia rubra vera
PTCL(s)	Peripheral T-cell lymphoma(s)
RAEB	Refractory anemia with excess blasts
RAEB-T	Refractory anemia with excess blasts in transformation
RARS	Refractory anemia with ring sideroblasts
RBC(s)	Red blood cell(s)
RCA	Red cell aplasia
RDW	Red cell distribution width
RT-PCR	Reverse transcriptase polymerase chain reaction
sIg	Surface immunoglobulin
SLE	Systemic lupus erythematosus
SLL	Small lymphocytic lymphoma
SSC	Side scatter
TCR	T-cell receptor
TIBC	Total iron binding capacity
TP	Touch preparation (imprint)
TRAP	Tartrate-resistant acid phosphatase
TTP	Thrombotic thrombocytopenic purpura
WBC(s)	White blood cell(s)

Peripheral Blood

Approach to the peripheral blood

A CBC and examination of the peripheral blood film are the first steps in the work-up of most hematological disorders, both benign and malignant. The preparation of good quality films (i.e. well spread and properly stained) is crucial to the proper interpretation of the peripheral blood findings.

1.1 Blood film preparation

The preferred specimen for preparing blood films is EDTA anticoagulated blood. The EDTA tube should be well filled. If the tube is only partially filled, the relative excess of EDTA can result in artifacts even if a film is prepared promptly. Prolonged storage is another significant source of blood film artifacts despite the fact that modern automated analyzers can process stored blood with only minimal fluctuations in the counts. Therefore, the film should always be made within 2–4 hours after the blood is drawn. It is important to ensure that the specimen tube is gently rocked back and forth for adequate mixing before making the smear.

The glass slides should be clean and free of grease. Fat globules on a greasy slide disrupt the distribution of cells during the spreading process. The glass should not be too porous, since overly porous material can lead to excessive uptake of the stains resulting in a dark background and overstained leukocyte nuclei.

A well spread blood film should have the following characteristics (Figure 1.1): (1) lateral edges; (2) an adequate zone of morphology; (3) a straight feather-edge; and (4) adequate length.

Large cells (e.g. blasts) are preferentially distributed to the lateral edges of the slide. Therefore, the spreader must be narrower than the width of the slide. It should also be narrower than the width of the coverslip to allow for proper examination of the lateral edges. This is especially important in the context of a low WBC count with few circulating abnormal cells.

> There are two ways to make a spreader:
> 1. A hemocytometer coverslip attached to an alligator clip. The edge of the coverslip should be smooth. If necessary, polish the edge with sandpaper.
> 2. Incise the corner of a glass slide with a diamond pen, and then break off the corner.

The zone of morphology is the area of the film where the RBCs barely touch each other (Figure 1.2a). This is the appropriate area for carrying out blood film examination. The film should be thin to have an adequate zone of morphology.

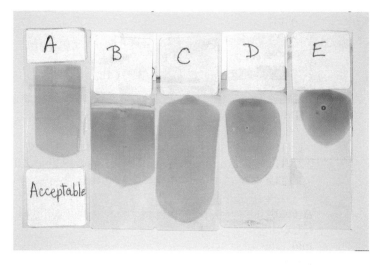

Figure 1.1 Examples of blood films. The optimal blood film (A) is thin and of medium length. It has a quasi-straight feather-edge and good lateral edges. The other blood films are suboptimal because of the lack of lateral edges (B, C), excessive length (C), a curved zone of morphology (D) or excessive thickness (E)

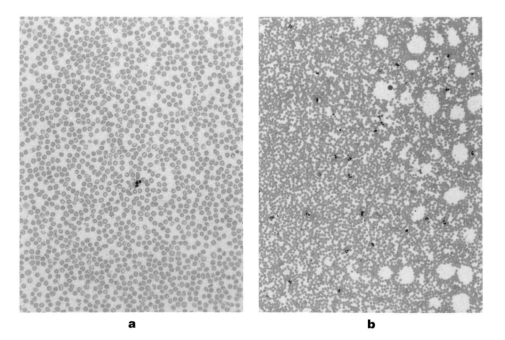

a   b

Figure 1.2 (a) Zone of morphology. The RBCs are well separated from each other or barely touch each other. (b) Thick film with no zone of morphology. The RBCs are crowded even at the feather-edge where they are flattened (far right of the figure)

A blood film with a straight feather-edge also has a straight zone of morphology. As the film is scanned and examined from one lateral edge to the other across the width of the slide, the fields under view remain uniformly thin. In contrast, if this maneuver is performed on a blood film with curved edges (i.e. a 'thumbprint' blood film), the microscopist crosses from thin, well-spread areas to thick areas that are not appropriate for examination.

Preparing a good quality smear depends on three main factors (Figure 1.3):

1. The size of the drop of blood.
2. The angle applied to the spreader.
3. The speed and steadiness in pushing the spreader.

A small drop of blood is preferred. Invariably, too much blood will result in a thick film even if the spreader is pushed at a low angle. In most cases, the optimal angle for spreading is 25–30 degrees. If the speed is too fast or the angle too high, the film will be short and thick, without an adequate zone of morphology. A long blood film cannot be examined properly, since the tail of the slide will be located at the gap on the microscope stage.

The angle of spreading must be modified in cases of severe anemia or polycythemia. A lower Hgb requires a higher angle of spreading. Conversely, a very low angle is necessary for cases with an increased Hgb. An alternative for preparing a blood film from a polycythemic specimen is to take a sample from the EDTA tube, dilute it 1:1 with either saline or AB plasma, and make the films from the diluted sample.

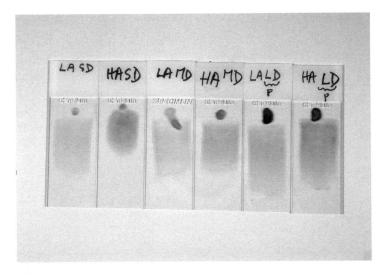

Figure 1.3 Six blood films prepared from the same blood tube (normal individual) by varying the angle of spreading and the size of the blood drop. Only the films using a low angle of spreading and a small or medium-size drop (LASD, LAMD) are satisfactory. A high spreading angle and/or a large drop of blood (even when not fully used) result in thick blood films without an adequate zone of morphology. LA, low angle; HA, high angle; SD, small drop; MD, medium drop; LD, large drop

1.1.1 Manual technique for preparing a proper wedge-spread blood film

A capillary tube is used to draw some blood from the EDTA specimen. A small drop of blood is applied from the capillary tube onto the glass slide near the edge. The edge can be either the free edge of the slide or that near the frosted end (this is the preferred practice), depending on the preference of the laboratory. The spreader is applied at an appropriate angle in front of the drop, and pulled back to it. As soon as the blood has run along the edge of the spreader, it is pushed forward in a smooth and steady manner. The film should be fan-dried immediately, and then labeled with the patient's name and/or identification number. If a fan is not available then dry the film vigorously by arm and hand motion. The edge of the spreader must be cleaned after each use.

Quick drying of the blood film is extremely important to prevent slow-drying artifacts. Slow drying occurs if the slide is not fan-dried or the technologist stops to label the slide in between making the smear and fan drying.

The blood film should be fixed as soon as possible in water-free methanol. Adequate fixation is necessary, since underfixation leads to dissolution of nuclear chromatin. If a slide is left unfixed for more than 24–48 hours, the breakdown of plasma proteins will alter the quality of staining. It is important that the methanol is completely free of water contamination to prevent the formation of water artifacts that may be misinterpreted as hypochromia. When the ambient humidity is high, it is often necessary to change the methanol bath several times a day.

1.1.2 Automated methods of preparing blood films

1. **Centrifugation method** using a specialized centrifuge. A small drop of blood is placed on the center of a glass slide set flat on the centrifuge. The spinning process results in a uniform monolayer blood film. Since the film produced has no lateral edges, this method is not recommended.
2. **Automated slide maker** to prepare wedge-spread blood films. Several slide makers are commercially available. The characteristics of an ideal slide maker are shown in Table 1.1.

Table 1.1 Characteristics of an ideal automated slide maker

- The ability to prepare blood films of optimal quality irrespective of the Hgb level.
- Quick drying and automated bar-code labeling of the slides.
- The possibility to make multiple blood films from the same specimen for special stains or teaching.
- An associated automated stainer.
- Compact in size and interfaced to the hematology analyzer.

1.2 Blood film staining

A suboptimal stain will defeat the purpose of preparing a well-spread film. Current staining procedures are variations of the Romanovsky stain, based on a combination of basic and acidic dyes. While one staining procedure may be more commonly used in a certain geographical area (e.g. the Wright stain in North America and the May-Grünwald-Giemsa stain in Europe), an optimally stained blood film should have the following features:

- The film must be free of stain deposits. Aesthetic considerations aside, the presence of stain deposits interferes with the identification of Howell-Jolly bodies and parasites. Therefore, the preparation of the stain mixture must include a filtering step.
- RBCs should appear tan and WBCs should not be overstained or understained. The correct pH of the staining buffer is critical. A high pH buffer results in gray RBCs and overstaining of nuclei and cytoplasmic granules in WBCs. Too low a pH results in pale leukocytes and vermilion red eosinophilic granules.

Although the Wright stain is quicker to carry out, the nuclei often stain too pink. Therefore, either a May-Grünwald-Giemsa or a Wright-Giemsa procedure is preferred. The type of stainer also affects the quality of staining. A 'dipping' stainer is superior to a 'flatbed' type, since it allows the glass slides to be well immersed in the staining baths and therefore uniformly stained. To protect blood films from dust and scratches, it is good practice to use a coverslip. For patient care (e.g. follow-up) and medical education, blood films should be stored for an appreciable length of time, at least 6–12 months, if not longer.

1.3 Summary of blood film artifacts from suboptimal preparation and staining

One or a combination of several factors can cause the main artifacts encountered on blood films. Even if blood films are spread by a skilled hand, and therefore devoid of streaks and ridges, artifacts may still occur because of any of the following:

- A delay in blood film preparation.
- Improper drying of the film.
- Inadequate or delayed fixation.
- Methanol that is contaminated with water.
- Incorrect pH of the staining buffer or a 'poor' batch of staining reagents.

The artifacts are grouped below according to key steps in preparation and staining.

1. **Storage (EDTA) artifacts.** The longer the delays in blood film preparation, the greater the extent of 'storage' artifacts. The artifacts can include:

- Cytoplasmic vacuolation in WBCs, especially neutrophils (Figure 1.4), mimicking that seen in infection/sepsis.
- Nuclear lobulation, especially in lymphoid cells (Figure 1.5), which can lead to the misinterpretation of benign cells as malignant.

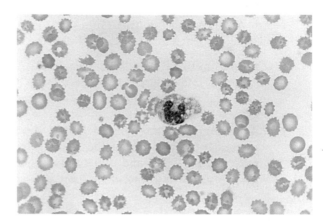

Figure 1.4 Delayed blood film preparation resulting in echinocytes and cytoplasmic vacuoles in neutrophils

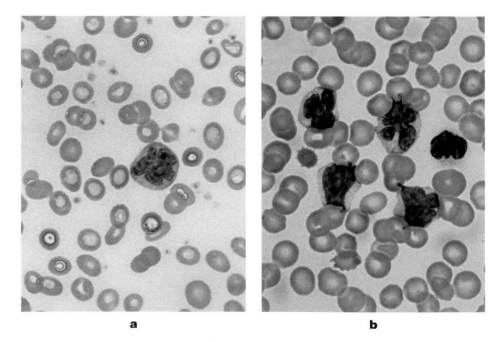

a   b

Figure 1.5 (a) Artifactual nuclear lobulations in a reactive lymphoid cell from a child. The appearance simulates that of a lymphoma cell. (b) The lymphocytes in a case of CLL were misinterpreted as 'cleaved' lymphoma cells because of the artifactual nuclear irregularities. These artifacts, which primarily affect lymphoid cells, appear before other artifacts (e.g. crenated RBCs)

- Loss of central pallor in RBCs (Figure 1.6), which can cause misidentification of normal erythrocytes as spherocytes.
- Crenated RBCs (Figure 1.4).

2. **Slow-drying artifacts.** Slow drying leads to shrinkage artifacts. The artifacts manifest as villi, hairs and blebs (Figure 1.7), which are seen predominantly in lymphoid cells, especially plasmacytoid lymphocytes. Because of shrinkage (however slight it may be) nuclei appear darker and nucleoli become indistinct (Figure 1.8).
3. **Fixation artifacts.** The most common fixation artifacts are caused by water contamination of the methanol bath (Figure 1.9). Water artifacts interfere with adequate assessment of RBC morphology.
4. **Staining artifacts.** As mentioned above, staining artifacts are most often caused by an incorrect pH of the staining buffer. They can also be due to delayed fixation of the blood film, a film prepared from heparin anticoagulated blood, a poor batch of staining reagents, or excessive porosity of a particular brand of glass slides (lower quality than the standard).

The features of suboptimal staining include:

- Altered RBC color. Mature RBCs appear gray simulating polychromatophilic RBCs.
- Washed out WBC cytoplasm (Figure 1.10).
- Vermilion red eosinophilic granules.
- Gray eosinophilic granules.
- Darkly stained secondary granules in neutrophils, simulating toxic granulation (Figure 1.11) .
- Darkly stained nuclei with loss of nuclear chromatin detail.

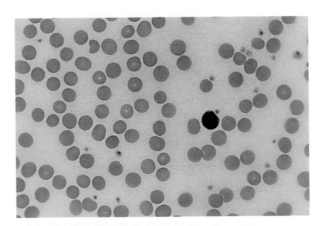

Figure 1.6   Loss of central pallor in RBCs secondary to delayed processing

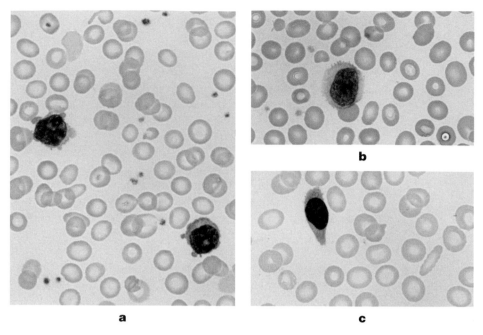

Figure 1.7 Blood films from three different children. Slow drying has resulted in the formation of cytoplasmic blebs (a) and hairy/villous projections (b) which can impart a bipolar appearance to lymphocytes (c). On the blood film of this child, all of the lymphocytes, including LGLs, appear bipolar

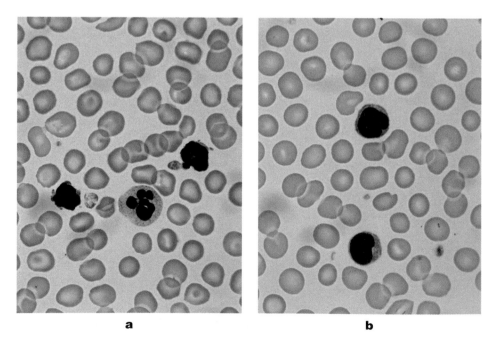

Figure 1.8 Blood films from the same patient. (a) Shrinkage artifacts with cytoplasmic blebs and darkening of the nuclear chromatin. (b) The result of quick drying of the blood film. The cytologic details can be better appreciated

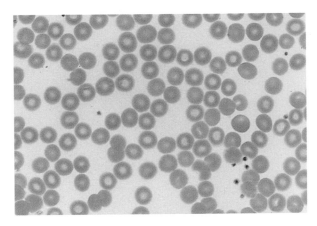

Figure 1.9 Water artifacts in RBCs, giving a false appearance of hypochromia

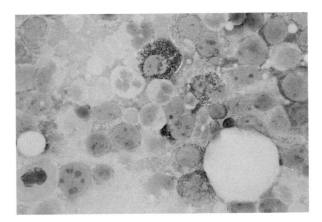

Figure 1.10 Suboptimal stain of a bone marrow smear. The eosinophils are bright red. Other cells are understained and appear washed out. The cytoplasmic and nuclear details cannot be adequately evaluated

1.4 Blood film examination

A systematic approach to the examination of the blood film is important.

1. Check that the patient identification on the slide agrees with that on the hemogram.
2. Examine the film with the unaided eye looking for unusual staining (e.g. deep blue in multiple myeloma) or unusual spreading (e.g. a serrated or streaked pattern in agglutination).
3. If the slide does not have a coverslip, smear a thin film of immersion oil on the slide. Scan the film (including the lateral edges and tail) at low-power magnification using a 20–25× objective. Low-power scanning of the blood film is an essential step for the following reasons:

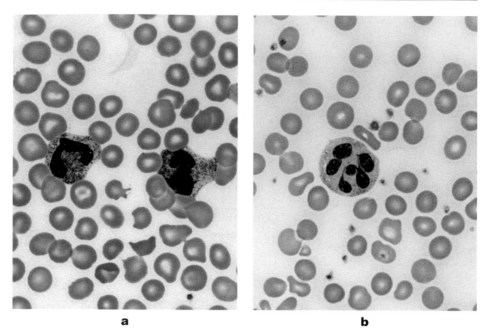

a   b

Figure 1.11 Blood films from the same patient. (a) Overstaining secondary to the high pH of the staining buffer. The neutrophilic granules are heavily stained, simulating toxic granulation. (b) The result of staining at the correct pH

- To estimate whether the RBC and WBC counts, and the WBC differential match those reported by the automated analyzer. In many instances, a quick 'scan differential' can be performed in lieu of a standard manual differential. The scan differential is most useful when the overall WBC distribution is essentially normal and similar to the automated differential, but a small number of other cell types are present. Vague descriptions, such as 'metamyelocytes/myelocytes seen on scan' or 'occasional blast on scan' should be avoided.

The 'scan differential' is based on a number of principles, as outlined below.

Current blood cell counters categorize nucleated cells other than NRBCs into the five categories of leukocytes that normally circulate in the peripheral blood (neutrophils, lymphocytes, monocytes, eosinophils and basophils). Some analyzers, e.g. the Technicon H series which incorporates a peroxidase cytochemical reaction in the automated differential, use six categories including 'large unstained cells' (referring to peroxidase-negative cells). Therefore, most instruments count large abnormal mononuclear cells (e.g. blasts, large lymphoma cells, hairy cells and prolymphocytes) as 'monocytes', resulting in an apparent monocytosis. Small blasts and small circulating lymphoma cells are classified as 'lymphocytes' by the analyzer.

When abnormal cells are present, their percentage can be estimated mentally while scanning with a 20–25× objective. Subtract this percentage from the automated per cent monocytes or per cent lymphocytes, whichever is appropriate, to obtain the manual percentages of monocytes and lymphocytes. Round off the automated per cent neutrophils to make 100.

Hypogranular neutrophils may be counted as monocytes by the analyzer. This is a common phenomenon with specimens from AIDS patients, especially if the specimen is analyzed the day after it was drawn. Consequently, the relative percentages of neutrophils and monocytes are reversed from those seen on the blood film. In addition, the automated analyzer may count hypogranular eosinophils as neutrophils.

Example. Analyzer data: WBC 3.2 × 10^9/l, neutrophils 11.3%, lymphocytes 6.7%, monocytes 80.0%, eosinophils 1.6%, and basophils 0.4%. Scanning of the blood smear revealed that the predominant population is granulocytic in the range of 80% including 5–6% myelocytes and metamyelocytes. Monocytes were approximately 10%. The scan differential was therefore reported as follows: neutrophils 75%, myelocytes 2%, metamyelocytes 4%, lymphocytes 7%, monocytes 10%, and eosinophils 2%.

- Although scanning with a 10× objective picks up rouleaux (Figure 1.12), RBC agglutination (Figure 1.13), and platelet clumps, the resolution at 10× is not sufficient to determine whether or not RBC and WBC morphology need to be evaluated at higher magnification. Despite the high quality of current state-of-the-art analyzers, flagging for various abnormalities does not reach 100% specificity and sensitivity. Therefore, scanning at 20–25× is necessary to confirm any important suspect flags (e.g. the blast flag) which can indicate the presence of large abnormal mononuclear cells. False-positive WBC flags are usually caused by delayed processing. A low number of circulating abnormal mononuclear cells can result in false negatives.
  Based on the findings at scanning magnification, a decision is made whether or not to examine the blood film at higher magnification and perform a manual differential. Note that certain morphologic differences (e.g. spherocytes vs. irregularly contracted cells, or plasmacytoid lymphocytes vs. large granular lymphocytes) cannot be evaluated properly at low power.
- To choose the 'zone of morphology' for evaluation of RBC and WBC morphology at higher magnification. The 50–65× oil immersion objective is the 'workhorse' of the hematology laboratory since the manual WBC differential

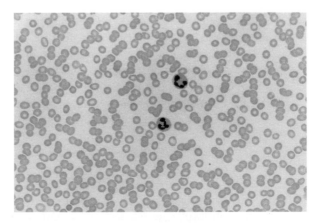

Figure 1.12 Rouleaux in a case of multiple myeloma

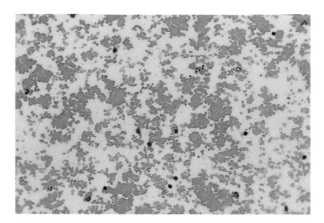

Figure 1.13   RBC agglutination secondary to cryoglobulins in a case of lymphoplasmacytoid lymphoma-leukemia

count and morphologic evaluation of white cells and red cells should be performed at this power. The 100× objective is only necessary for observation of fine or subtle details such as sparse, minute cytoplasmic granules or faint basophilic stippling. A well-spread film contains an appreciable zone of morphology (Figure 1.2a). A poorly prepared, thick film contains no zone of morphology (Figure 1.2b).

In the assessment of RBC abnormalities, variations in size and shape need to be specified instead of being reported under the generic terms 'anisocytosis' and 'poikilocytosis'. Grading of anisocytosis without specifying microcytes or macrocytes adds no information to that already provided by the RDW. Similarly, reporting poikilocytosis without indicating the specific poikilocytes that are present in significant numbers (e.g. 2+ schistocytes) does not provide adequate diagnostic information.

It is also important to keep in mind that the value of a finding for diagnostic purposes is dependent on:

1. The inherent specificity of the finding. The longer the list of differential diagnoses corresponding to a feature, the less specific and less diagnostically useful it is. The two most specific RBC findings are sickle cells and Howell-Jolly bodies, since each feature indicates one corresponding group of disorders. In contrast, RBC abnormalities such as target cells, elliptocytes and stomatocytes are much less specific, being present in a wide range of different diseases. An informative semiquantitative assessment (e.g. 1+, 2+ or 3+) should take into account the inherent specificity as well. The less specific a feature is, the higher must be the number of affected RBCs to qualify as 2+.
2. Whether the abnormality occurs in large numbers (2+/3+) or is found in rare/occasional cells (1+). An abnormality of relatively low specificity can be a helpful clue when it is present as the sole predominant finding. For example, elliptocytes are a nonspecific finding, since a moderate number

$(2+)$ of elliptocytes can be found in several disorders including iron deficiency, macrocytic anemia (B_{12}/folate deficiency) and bone marrow infiltration. When there are $3+$ elliptocytes on the peripheral blood film, however, it is virtually diagnostic of hereditary elliptocytosis. With the exception of sickle cells and Howell-Jolly bodies, any other $1+$ RBC abnormality is not helpful in identifying the underlying disorder.

3. The context in which the abnormality occurs. The presence of basophilic stippling, in combination with a hypochromic and/or microcytic anemia, essentially excludes iron deficiency and suggests thalassemia or congenital sideroblastic anemia. Basophilic stippling is of less value when present in the context of a macrocytic anemia, however. The combination of macrocytosis and basophilic stippling simply indicates dyserythropoiesis, which can occur in a variety of disease states including severe B_{12}/folate deficiency, congenital dyserythropoietic anemia, bone marrow infiltration, or a myelodysplastic syndrome (MDS).

For certain hematological malignancies, the diagnostic specimen of choice is the peripheral blood, which can also be used for adjunctive studies (e.g. immunophenotyping and cytogenetics). This group includes the following:

- Lymphoproliferative disorders such as CLL, CLL/PL, lymphoplasmacytoid (LPC) lymphoma-leukemia, prolymphocytic leukemia (PLL), large granular lymphocytosis, adult T-cell leukemia-lymphoma (ATLL) and Sezary syndrome.
- Myeloproliferative disorders, especially CML and CMMoL, as well as polycythemia vera (PRV) and essential thrombocythemia (ET), if the clinical causes of a reactive polycythemia and/or thrombocytosis have been excluded.

1.4.1 Approach to the manual differential

As mentioned above, large cells are preferentially distributed toward the lateral edges of the blood film. Furthermore, most microscopists perform the manual differential on consecutive high-power fields starting from an area in the body of the blood film. Therefore, it is not uncommon to miss a low number of circulating abnormal cells (e.g. blasts, hairy cells). A more sensitive approach is to perform the differential on nonconsecutive fields from one lateral edge to the other. This facilitates finding rare abnormal cells and reduces the incidence of false negatives.

1.5 Reporting CBC results and correlation with laboratory and clinical data

Assessment of the CBC and peripheral blood film should not be done in a vacuum. The repertoire of quantitative and qualitative changes in the hemogram and blood film is limited, in contrast to the multitude of hematological and nonhematological conditions that can cause changes in the blood. Similar findings can be observed in unrelated disorders and several diseases can simulate each other. This can lead to the potential for misinterpretation and erroneous diagnosis unless pertinent clinical information and/or additional laboratory data are available when evaluating the findings.

1.5.1 Approach to reporting CBC results

How meaningful to clinicians is the current format of peripheral blood reports? In many laboratories, so-called blood smear 'comments' consist mainly of a list of morphologic observations (e.g. 2+ target cells, 1+ elliptocytes) or a repeat of the abnormalities already apparent on the hemogram (e.g. lymphocytosis, anemia), often without suggestions as to what the findings mean. One of the functions of the hematology laboratory should be to provide a consultative service. Therefore, if blood film comments are judged to be necessary in nonroutine cases, then an interpretive format, with a differential diagnosis and suggestions about pertinent additional laboratory studies, would seem to be appropriate.

CHAPTER 2

Normal peripheral blood morphology

In most instances, review of the blood film is not necessary when the hemogram, including the automated WBC differential, is reported as normal. Exceptions can occur, however, depending on the clinical history provided with the CBC requisition. For example, patients with mycosis fungoides (MF)/Sezary syndrome can have a normal WBC count and a 'normal' automated differential if there are too few circulating cerebriform cells to elicit a WBC suspect flag.

This chapter is primarily concerned with normal peripheral blood morphology. For completeness, descriptions of some abnormal morphologic features are also included.

2.1 Normal erythrocytes

The normal RBC is a biconcave disc with a diameter of about 7.5 μm, approximately the size of the nucleus of a small lymphocyte (Figure 2.1a). A well-stained normal erythrocyte appears tan-pink with an area of central pallor merging gradually with the more deeply staining periphery. Water artifacts, which can be seen when condensation occurs on the slide prior to fixation, or when water is present in the methanol fixative, cause the area of central pallor to appear as a clear, colorless center, sharply demarcated from the ring of hemoglobin (Figure 2.1b).

2.2 White blood cells

Neutrophils, lymphocytes and monocytes are the three major cell types seen in a normal blood film. A few eosinophils may be present. Basophils are rare.

2.2.1 Neutrophils

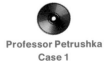

**Professor Petrushka
Case 1**

In normal neutrophils, nuclear segmentation ranges from two to five lobes. Most cells possess three nuclear lobes (Figure 2.2a). Hypersegmentation is defined as more than 5% of peripheral blood neutrophils with five nuclear lobes, or any neutrophils with six or more lobes (Figure 2.2b). Hypersegmentation suggests B_{12}/folate deficiency, but it is also a frequent feature associated with hydroxyurea therapy. The occurrence of hypersegmentation in iron deficiency, or as a hereditary abnormality is uncommon. An increase in the number

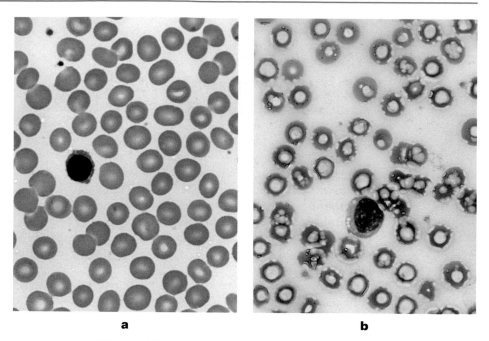

Figure 2.1 (a) Normal RBCs and a normal small lymphocyte. (b) In this preparation, severe water artifacts preclude any assessment of RBC morphology

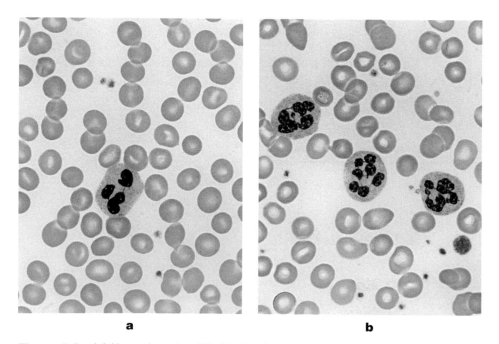

Figure 2.2 (a) Normal neutrophil. (b) One hypersegmented neutrophil in a patient on hydroxyurea therapy

of hyposegmented (monolobed or bilobed) neutrophils with a characteristic 'spectacle' or 'pince nez' appearance (Figure 2.3) can be seen in Pelger-Huët anomaly (an inherited condition) or as an acquired dysplastic feature (pseudo-Pelger-Huët anomaly). Hyposegmented neutrophils need to be distinguished from bands (see Section 3.1).

In assessing the granularity of neutrophils, beware of artifacts caused by prolonged storage and/or suboptimal staining. In the normal neutrophil, the cytoplasm is acidophilic with finely dispersed granules. Decreased or absent granulation is nearly always an acquired abnormality. It is also seen in the rare neutrophil lactoferrin deficiency that results in altered formation of secondary granules. Increased granulation ('toxic granulation') can be found in infection/inflammation and may be accompanied by Döhle bodies (Figure 2.4) and/or cytoplasmic vacuoles. Both toxic granulation and Döhle bodies are normal findings in pregnancy, however. Intense hypergranulation is characteristically seen in G-CSF therapy, invariably associated with circulating immature myeloid precursors.

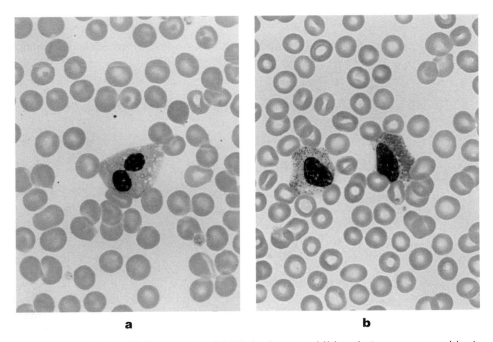

a   b

Figure 2.3 Pelger-Huët anomaly. (a) Bilobed neutrophil in a heterozygous subject. (b) Monolobed neutrophil and eosinophil in a homozygous individual

2.2.2 Eosinophils

Normal eosinophils have bilobed nuclei. A small number may be trilobed. The cytoplasm is packed with large, reddish-orange granules (Figure 2.5a). Abnormalities in eosinophils, such as hypersegmentation, nonsegmentation, hypogranulation, or the presence of basophilic granules, can be observed in

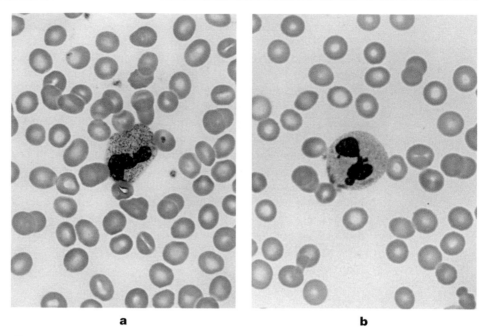

a   b

Figure 2.4   Blood films from two different HIV-positive patients. (a) Toxic granulation in a band granulocyte. (b) Döhle bodies

myeloproliferative disorders (MPDs), myelodysplastic syndromes, and the hypereosinophilic syndrome.

2.2.3 Basophils

Large, purplish metachromatic granules obscure the nucleus of a normal basophil (Figure 2.5b). Hypogranulation of basophils can be observed in MPDs or during an acute allergic attack. Hypogranulation can be an artifact, however, due to the water solubility of the granules.

2.2.4 Lymphocytes

Normal peripheral blood lymphocytes vary in size and shape. They can be arbitrarily divided into small and large lymphocytes. Functional and immunological subsets cannot be reliably distinguished by morphology, however.

Small lymphocytes can be divided into the following categories:

1. Small round lymphocytes with regular nuclear contours and condensed chromatin (Figure 2.6a). The 'mature-appearing' nucleus is slightly larger than the size of a normocytic RBC and is surrounded by a thin rim of cytoplasm. In children, normal small lymphocytes may have nuclear clefts (Figure 2.6b).

2. A variant of the small lymphocyte is the plasmacytoid lymphocyte (Figure 2.7a). The eccentric nucleus is usually larger than that in small round lym-

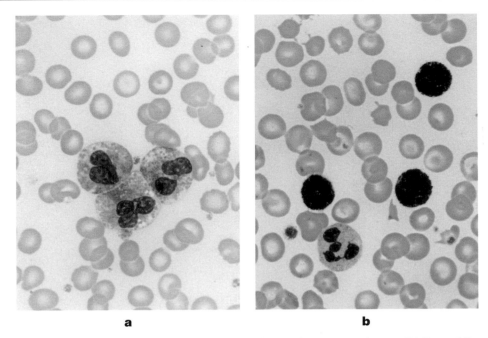

a   b

Figure 2.5   (a) Eosinophils from a case of Churg-Strauss syndrome. (b) Basophils from a case of CML

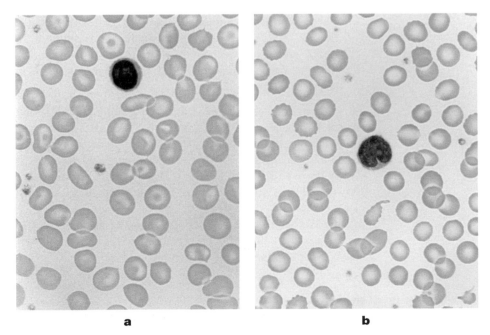

a   b

Figure 2.6   (a) Normal small round lymphocyte from a case of thalassemia minor. (b) Nuclear indentation in a normal small lymphocyte from a child

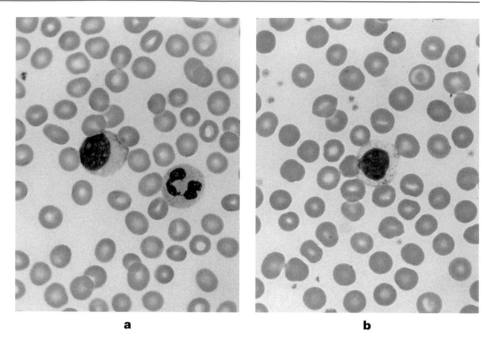

a   b

Figure 2.7 (a) Plasmacytoid lymphocyte from a child with pulmonary artery stenosis. (b) Large granular lymphocyte from a patient on chemotherapy

phocytes (up to 2.5 times the size of an RBC). A small distinct nucleolus is invariably present.

3. Large granular lymphocytes (LGLs). So-called LGLs also have eccentric nuclei and contain scattered small, azurophilic granules (Figure 2.7b). Large granular lymphocytes normally comprise 10–20% of the total lymphocyte population. Note that neither the cell size nor the granules are large.

Large lymphocytes (Figure 2.8) have pale blue moderate to abundant cytoplasm, with a less condensed nuclear chromatin than small lymphocytes, small indistinct nucleoli, and round to slightly irregular nuclear contours. The so-called Downey I and Downey II cells are large lymphocytes. Downey I cells, which are smaller than Downey II cells, can be found in healthy individuals. Downey II cells are typically seen in viral infections such as infectious mononucleosis (IM).

Rare storage disorders which are clinically apparent in infants and young children (failure to thrive, hepatosplenomegaly) can manifest with prominent and sharp cytoplasmic vacuoles in lymphocytes (Figure 2.9).

2.2.5 Monocytes

The largest normal cell in the peripheral blood is the monocyte, characterized by a reniform or multilobulated nucleus with reticulated chromatin, abundant gray cytoplasm with small vacuoles and fine azurophilic granules (Figure 2.10).

2.3 Platelets

Platelet morphology is often of limited usefulness in the differential diagnosis of hematological disorders. Normal platelets are 1–3 μm in diameter (Figure 2.11a). The size usually varies inversely with the platelet count (Figure 2.11b).

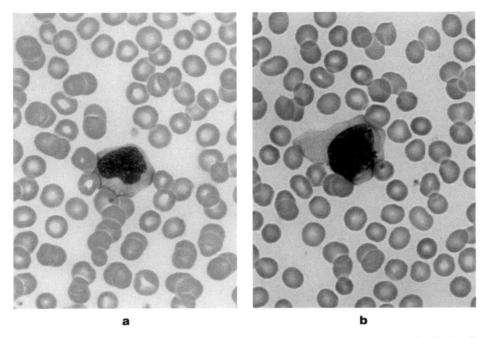

a   b

Figure 2.8 (a) and (b) Reactive lymphoid cells in infectious mononucleosis. Nucleoli are visible

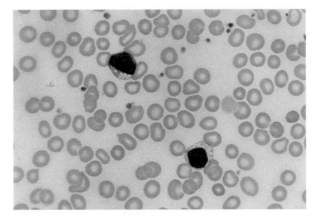

Figure 2.9 Prominent cytoplasmic vacuoles in the lymphocytes of a Mexican infant with β-galactosidase deficiency

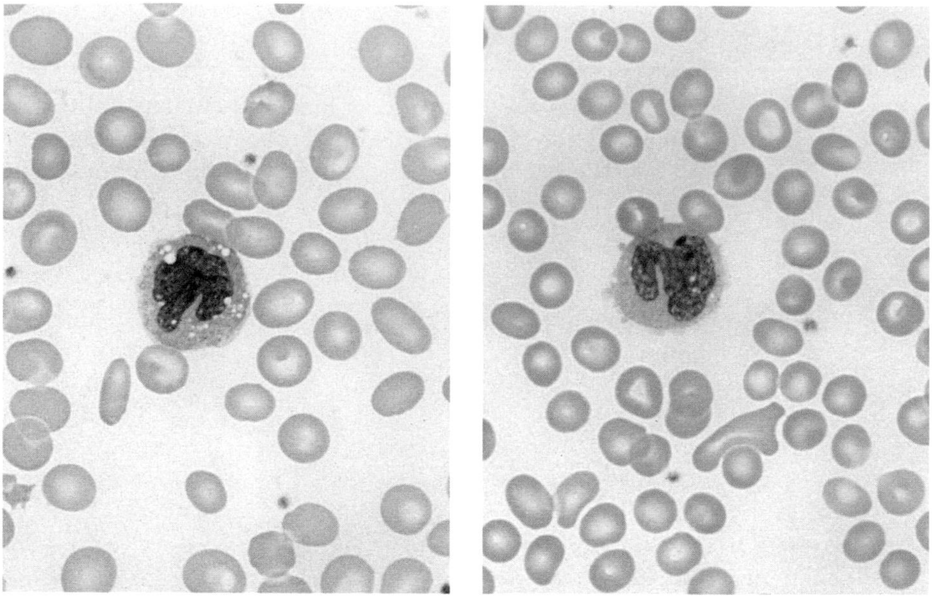

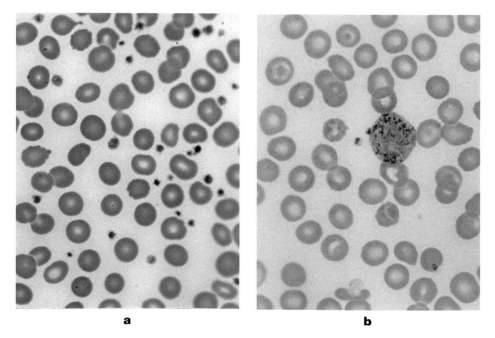

a   b

Figure 2.10 (a), (b) Blood films from the same subject. Normal monocytes. Note one with cytoplasmic blebs in (b) as the blood film was not fan-dried

a   b

Figure 2.11 (a) Normal-size platelets from a case of neoplastic thrombocytosis. (b) Giant platelet in a patient with mild thrombocytopenia

CHAPTER 3

Neutrophilia pattern

The neutrophilia pattern is defined as a mild to moderate increase in the WBC count (i.e. $< 50 \times 10^9/l$) along with an absolute granulocytosis. Circulating intermediate myeloid precursors (myelocytes, metamyelocytes, and promyelocytes) may be present. A 'leukocytosis with an absolute neutrophilia' is normal during the first few days after birth.

Four possible mechanisms (acting alone or in combination) can result in peripheral blood neutrophilia:

1. Demargination.
2. Decreased transit to solid tissues.
3. Mobilization from the maturation-storage pool of the bone marrow.
4. Increased production (as in G-CSF therapy).

Peripheral blood neutrophils are divided into two equal and freely exchangeable compartments: the circulating pool and the marginated pool. Stressful conditions (accompanied by endogenous adrenaline release) cause neutrophils to be mobilized from the marginated pool into the circulation. The resulting neutrophilia (up to twice the normal count) occurs rapidly but is of short duration. It is not associated with a left shift.

Neutrophils normally remain in the blood for about 12 hours before leaving the circulation and entering solid tissues. Administration of corticosteroids can delay the transit and produce a mild to moderate neutrophilia.

Mobilization of granulocytes from the maturation-storage compartment of the bone marrow (metamyelocytes, bands, and segmented neutrophils) may cause a mild left shift. Infections and other inflammatory processes are the most common causes of cell mobilization from this pool. Neutrophilia in the third trimester of pregnancy is presumably secondary to endogenous glucocorticoids. Since the morphologic changes are similar to those seen in infections, knowledge of the clinical history is vital to avoid misinterpretation.

Inflammation secondary to infections is one of the most common causes of neutrophilia. Neutrophilia can be secondary to bacterial, fungal and parasitic infections. Viral infections, rickettsial infections, and certain bacterial infections such as salmonella, shigella, brucellosis and tularemia do not cause neutrophilia.

Noninfectious causes of neutrophilia include tissue injury due to surgery, myocardial infarctions, tumor necrosis, acute gout, autoimmune diseases and burns. Neutrophilia may also be secondary to drug effects (e.g. corticosteroids, catecholamines, lithium, growth factors and chemical poisons) or metabolic disorders (e.g. diabetic ketoacidosis, eclampsia and thyrotoxic crisis).

Physiologic causes of neutrophilia include pregnancy and physical stress. Other miscellaneous causes of neutrophilia include cigarette smoking, post-neutropenia rebound, acute hemorrhage/hemolysis and treated CML.

Treated CML can present with either a normal WBC count or a neutrophilia. When neutrophilia is present, the features suggestive of treated CML include a high percentage of circulating intermediate myeloid precursors, basophilia (the strongest clue), and hypersegmented neutrophils (usually due to hydroxyurea therapy). It is important to know about a prior history of CML, since therapy can mask the left shift and basophilia.

3.1 Morphologic findings in neutrophilia

Prominent azurophilic granules (toxic granulation) are frequent in infectious conditions (Figure 3.1a). The hypergranulation induced by G-CSF therapy may be distinguished from toxic granulation by its higher density of granules, which stain redder and often obscure the nucleus (Figure 3.1b).

To untrained eyes, the rare Alder-Reilly anomaly, when present in granulocytes (Figure 3.2), can be confused with toxic granulation. Alder-Reilly anomaly is commonly seen in subgroups of the mucopolysaccharidoses (i.e. Hurler's syndrome and Hunter's syndrome). Alder-Reilly bodies are larger than normal azurophilic and basophilic granules. They can also be seen in lymphocytes (Figure 3.3) and monocytes (Figure 3.4). In eosinophils, the anomaly is expressed as abnor-

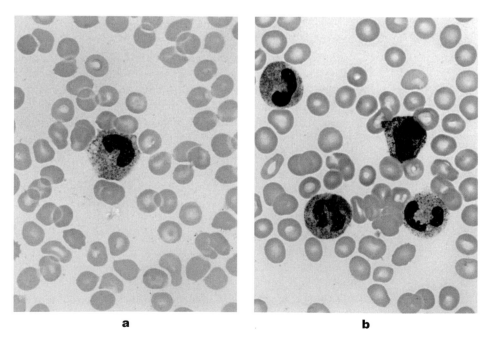

a b

Figure 3.1 (a) Toxic granulation in a band granulocyte from an elderly female with pneumonia. (b) Heavy granulation associated with G-CSF therapy

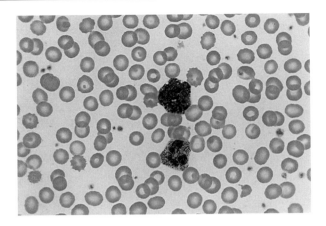

Figure 3.2 Alder-Reilly anomaly from a case of Hurler's syndrome. The abnormal granules in neutrophils simulate toxic granulation. The abnormal granules are more easily appreciated in eosinophils (upper cell)

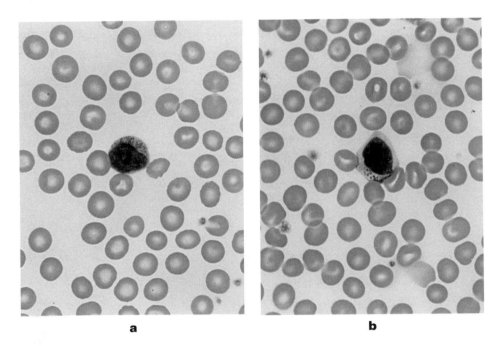

a   b

Figure 3.3 (a) Alder-Reilly bodies in a lymphocyte. The appearance may be overlooked as a large granular lymphocyte on a normal blood film (b)

mally stained granules that may appear dark gray to purple (Figure 3.2). The abnormality is easier to detect in the bone marrow. It is present inconsistently in the peripheral blood.

Döhle bodies are pale cytoplasmic inclusions that are often found together with toxic granulation. By electron microscopy, they are parallel stacks of rough endoplasmic reticulum. Although toxic granulation and Döhle bodies are commonly

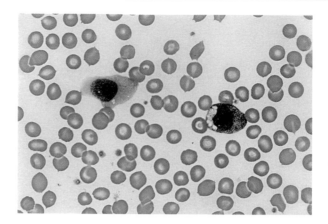

Figure 3.4 The monocyte on the right contains Alder-Reilly bodies

associated with infection, they can also occur in MPDs such as CML and AMM (Figure 3.5).

The inclusions of May-Hegglin anomaly (a rare, benign, autosomal dominant disorder characterized by thrombocytopenia, giant platelets and large granulocytic inclusions) resemble Döhle bodies but are larger, more sharply defined, and stain more intensely (Figure 3.6). Under the electron microscope, they correspond to amorphous cytoplasmic areas devoid of organelles.

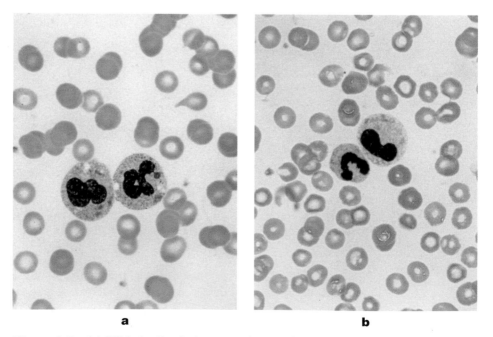

a   b

Figure 3.5 (a) Döhle bodies in two granulocytes from a patient with systemic infection. (b) Döhle bodies in one granulocyte from a case of CML

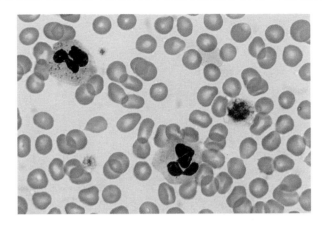

Figure 3.6 May–Hegglin anomaly: Döhle-like inclusions in granulocytes, large platelets and thrombocytopenia

Vacuoles in neutrophils are associated with sepsis. Vacuoles can also be an artifact if the blood has been subjected to prolonged storage (Figure 1.4).

Chronic inflammatory conditions, e.g. rheumatoid arthritis and systemic lupus erythematosus (SLE), are often accompanied by a mild increase in polyclonal immunoglobulins. Increased immunoglobulins in the serum, like other high molecular weight proteins (e.g. fibrinogen, alpha-2 macroglobulin), can cause rouleaux.

Circulating immature granulocytes, referred to as a 'left shift', can be a feature of both benign and malignant conditions. In reactive neutrophilia, the left shift is composed mostly of bands and a lesser number of metamyelocytes. Occasional myelocytes and rare promyelocytes may be present. Unless the patient is receiving G-CSF, circulating blasts are almost never seen in reactive neutrophilia.

An increased number of bands (Figure 3.7a) often coexists with neutrophilia. Bands normally constitute 1–5% of the leukocyte differential. The authors consider a band percentage of 20% or more to be a left shift. There has been little uniformity in the definition of the band between various laboratories. A band is a nonsegmented neutrophil with curved nuclear contours (i.e. horseshoe shape). The sides of the nuclear curvature are parallel over most of the length of the nucleus (Figure 3.7a). When bands occur together with neutrophilia and other reactive changes, it is not necessary to enumerate them. When the WBC count is normal or low, however, the proper identification of bands may be the only clue to a serious infection.

An apparent increase in the number of bands may be caused by the Pelger-Huët anomaly which is characterized in the peripheral blood by an increased number of hyposegmented neutrophils (Figure 3.7b). The neutrophils can be single-lobed, dumbbell-shaped, or bilobed with a spectacle-like appearance. In Pelger-Huët anomaly, usually 69–93% of the neutrophils are hyposegmented and less than 10% have three lobes. Despite this band-like appearance, the nuclear chromatin in Pelger-Huët cells is inappropriately coarse for the band stage. In this autosomal dominant condition, the granulocytes are functionally normal. The presence of the same anomaly in family members confirms the diagnosis.

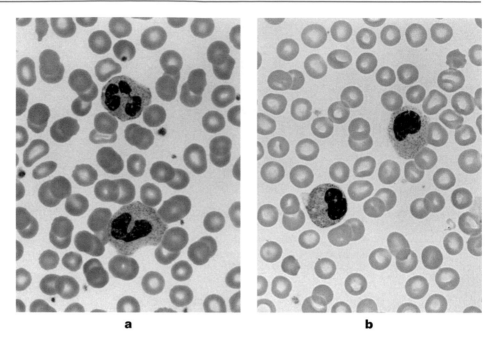

a   b

Figure 3.7 (a) A neutrophil and a band. (b) Hyposegmented neutrophils in Pelger-Huët anomaly

Metamyelocytes have a reniform nucleus, with pale orange-pink, finely granular cytoplasm. The orange-pink hue is conferred by the secondary granules. To avoid overcalling bands as metamyelocytes or vice versa, consider the cell to be a circle with an imaginary diameter drawn across it. The concavity of the nuclear contour of a metamyelocyte should fall in front of the diameter (Figure 3.8). Myelocytes and promyelocytes are discussed in Section 4.1.

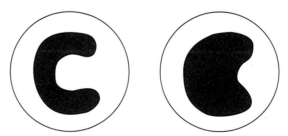

Figure 3.8 A band versus a metamyelocyte (schematic drawing)

CHAPTER 4

Leukoerythroblastic pattern

The leukoerythroblastic pattern is characterized by circulating NRBCs and immature myeloid precursors, often with RBC anisopoikilocytosis. The WBC count can be normal or high. In most cases, this pattern is associated with anemia. A high RDW and analyzer flags for NRBCs and immature granulocytes are often present.

Two major mechanisms, acting alone or in concert, have been proposed to account for the peripheral blood changes characteristic of a leukoerythroblastic reaction:

1. Altered marrow–blood barrier (i.e. disrupted marrow sinusoids) due to bone marrow infiltration. Bone marrow infiltrative disorders include hematological malignancies, metastatic carcinomas and non-neoplastic conditions such as granulomata and storage disorders (e.g. Gaucher's disease). Any of these disorders can elicit a variable degree of reticulin fibrosis that may progress to collagen fibrosis and new bone formation. This evolution is typically encountered in agnogenic myeloid metaplasia (AMM), also known as idiopathic myelofibrosis. Noninfiltrative marrow fibrosis can also occur as the result of injury to the bone marrow microenvironment (e.g. radiation therapy).
2. Extramedullary hematopoiesis as a compensatory response to either marrow infiltration/fibrosis or the bone marrow stress caused by severe chronic hemolytic anemias.

4.1 Morphologic findings in the leukoerythroblastic pattern

Circulating NRBCs are abnormal except in the neonatal period (Figure 4.1). A few NRBCs may be observed in the peripheral blood of term, healthy newborns up to 5 days of age. In premature infants or those with hypoxic stress, the number of NRBCs is higher.

The number of circulating NRBCs in leukoerythroblastic reactions varies depending on the severity of the underlying pathology. All of the different stages of erythroid maturation may be represented and NRBCs may exhibit qualitative abnormalities (Table 4.1) reflecting dyserythropoiesis (Figure 4.2). In the enumeration of circulating NRBCs, it is not necessary to separate the large early erythroid precursors (proerythroblasts and basophilic erythroblasts) from the late precursors (polychromatophilic and orthochromatic erythroblasts). Early erythroid precursors have deeply basophilic cytoplasm (Figure 4.3). The late pre-

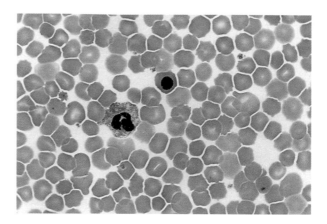

Figure 4.1 Normal blood film from a 1-day-old neonate. There are a few circulating NRBCs along with some intermediate myeloid precursors (not in this field) on the blood film

Table 4.1 Qualitative abnormalities in erythroid precursors

- Binucleation, multinucleation, nuclear lobulation.
- Nuclear fragmentation (karyorrhexis).
- Nuclear/cytoplasmic asynchrony.
- Ragged cytoplasm or hypochromia, indicating defective hemoglobinization.
- Basophilic stippling.
- An increase in the number of siderotic granules (more than four per cell) as seen on a Prussian blue (iron) stain. When visible on routine Romanovsky stains, this finding is termed 'Pappenheimer bodies'.

**Professor Petrushka
Case 2**

cursors are smaller, with increased nuclear condensation and gray-blue to gray-brown cytoplasm indicating an accumulation of hemoglobin.

The extent of anisopoikilocytosis in leukoerythroblastic reactions depends on the underlying pathology. Marked poikilocytosis with many teardrop cells usually indicates bone marrow infiltration. If the underlying etiology is stressed hematopoiesis (e.g. severe hemolysis, hemorrhage or severe infection), poikilocytosis is often less severe, except in thalassemia major or sickle cell anemia.

The following RBC changes are frequently observed in the leukoerythroblastic pattern:

- Teardrop cells (Figure 4.4) are an acquired abnormality caused by one of two mechanisms: (1) normal RBCs may be damaged in transit through marrow sinuses that are distorted by fibrosis; or (2) erythrocytes with hemoglobin precipitates become too rigid to pass through the microvasculature. The precipitates may be secondary to denatured hemoglobin (e.g. Heinz bodies, unstable Hgb) or can arise from an excess of globin chains (as seen in thalassemia).
- Macrocytes and ovalocytes/elliptocytes are relatively nonspecific changes reflecting disturbed erythropoiesis in both benign conditions (e.g. B_{12}/folate deficiency) and malignant diseases such as AMM (Figure 4.5).

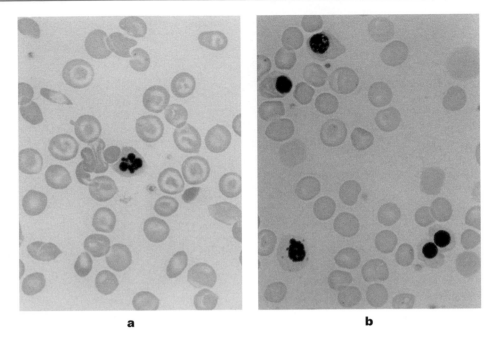

a   b

Figure 4.2 Circulating abnormal erythroid precursors. (a) An NRBC with nuclear lobulation from a case of sickle cell anemia. (b) NRBCs with karyorrhexis, nuclear lobulation and poorly hemoglobinized cytoplasm from a case of transfusion-dependent thalassemia major

- Schistocytes (i.e. fragmented erythrocytes) are acquired when RBCs squeeze through fibrin strands (as in microangiopathic anemia) or an altered (rigidified) bone marrow (or splenic) microvasculature damaged by infiltration with accompanying fibrosis (Figure 4.6).
- Basophilic stippling represents aggregates of ribosomes and degenerating mitochondria. It is found in dyserythropoiesis (e.g. B_{12}/folate deficiency or

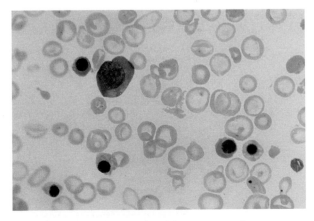

Figure 4.3 One early and five late erythroid precursors from a case of hydrops fetalis (hemoglobin Bart's). Note the severe hypochromia

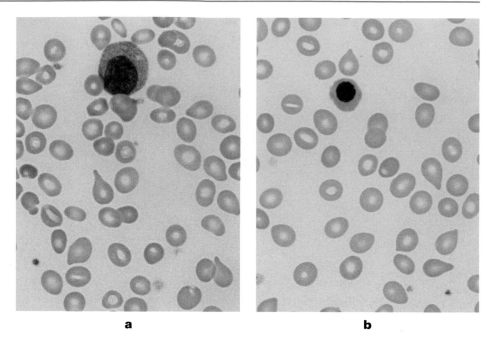

a   b

Figure 4.4   Frequent teardrop cells with circulating intermediate myeloid precursors (a) and an NRBC (b) from a case of AMM

myelodysplastic syndromes) and abnormal Hgb formation (e.g. thalassemias, unstable Hgb and heavy metal poisoning) (Figure 4.7a).

● Polychromatophilic RBCs, which correspond to young reticulocytes with a high RNA content. The younger the cell, the more basophilic the appearance. Late reticulocytes are indistinguishable from mature RBCs on Romanovsky films, except by virtue of their larger size. Supravital staining with methylene blue allows better visualization of reticulocytes at various stages. Polychromatophilic RBCs may have the teardrop deformity and can be abnormally large, indicating dyserythropoiesis (Figure 4.7b).

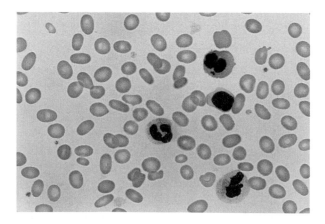

Figure 4.5   Abundant elliptocytes and ovalocytes from another case of AMM

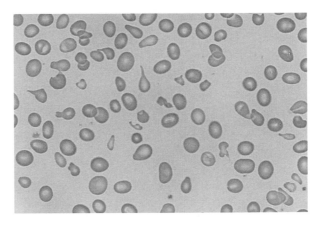

Figure 4.6 Frequent schistocytes along with teardrop cells, ovalocytes and macrocytes in breast carcinoma metastatic to the bone marrow

- Microcytosis and/or hypochromia, which when present in a leukoerythroblastic pattern strongly suggests thalassemia intermedia or thalassemia major. If sickle cells are also present, consideration must be given to S β-thalassemia, or, less commonly, Hgb S with superimposed iron deficiency (Figure 4.8).

Other RBC abnormalities, for example spherocytes, often indicate the specific cause of the leukoerythroblastic pattern (see Chapter 17). Giant platelets, mega-

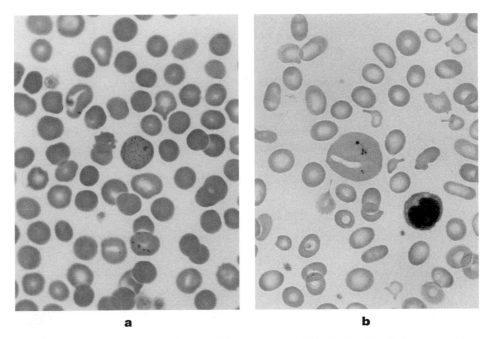

a   b

Figure 4.7   (a) Basophilic stippling from a case of AMM. (b) Giant polychromatophilic RBC with multiple Howell-Jolly bodies (there was no splenectomy) from a child in the recovery phase after induction chemotherapy for ALL. Note other RBC abnormalities including schistocytes, macrocytes, oval macrocytes and elliptocytes

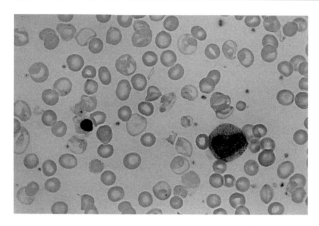

Figure 4.8 Leukoerythroblastic picture with microcytic and hypochromic RBCs from a case of thalassemia major

karyocyte fragments and circulating micromegakaryocytes may be encountered in a leukoerythroblastic pattern.

Intermediate myeloid precursors include promyelocytes, myelocytes and metamyelocytes. Myelocytes and metamyelocytes are usually present in higher numbers than promyelocytes. The promyelocyte has nuclear features that resemble those of a blast (high nuclear/cytoplasmic ratio, fine chromatin, and conspicuous nucleoli) along with basophilic cytoplasm that contains an appreciable number of azurophilic (primary) granules. The myelocyte, the last myeloid precursor capable of cell division, acquires secondary (specific) granules that eventually outnumber the primary granules as the cell matures. Specific granules can barely be seen by light microscopy. Their presence confers a pale, pink, acidophilic blush to the cytoplasm. The nucleus, which is located off-center next to a prominent pale Golgi hof, appears flattened on one side.

A leukoerythroblastic picture may be accompanied by qualitative abnormalities in granulocytes such as hypogranulation, hyposegmentation, and/or giant forms (Figure 4.9a). These may, but do not necessarily, indicate that the underlying pathology is a stem cell disorder (MDS, leukemia or an MPD). Marked hypergranulation is a telltale feature of G-CSF therapy (Figure 4.9b).

4.2 Features suggestive of agnogenic myeloid metaplasia (AMM)

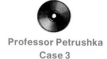

Professor Petrushka
Case 3

The presence of basophilia in a leukoerythroblastic pattern is highly suggestive of an underlying MPD, namely CML, AMM and the spent phase of PRV, also known as post-polycythemic myeloid metaplasia (PPMM). All three disorders can present with variable hemoglobin levels and platelet counts, as well as frequent giant platelets. In general, the WBC count is usually higher ($> 50 \times 10^9/$l) and the number of circulating NRBCs is often lower in CML than in the other two conditions. Any of the above disorders may have some circulating

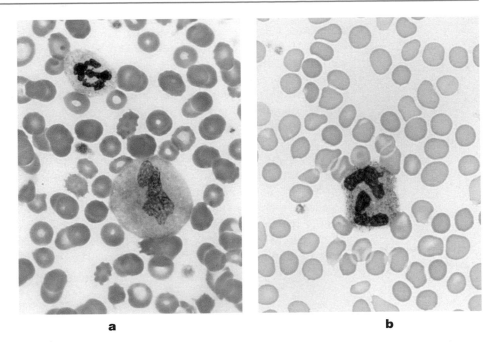

a   b

Figure 4.9   (a) Giant granulocyte from a case of AMM. (b) Binucleated granulocyte associated with G-CSF therapy

blasts (usually less than 10%). The presence of blasts will change the predominant pattern to the abnormal mononuclear cell pattern.

Similar to other MPDs, the peripheral blood findings in AMM are often more informative than the bone marrow morphology, especially since many patients present late in the course of the disease. In most instances, the peripheral blood demonstrates a mild normochromic, normocytic (NCNC) anemia that is due to a combination of ineffective erythropoiesis and shortened RBC survival secondary to splenomegaly. The other peripheral blood features that are highly suggestive of AMM are listed in Table 4.2.

The following situations, which occur mainly in the early stage of AMM, can raise diagnostic difficulties:

Table 4.2 Peripheral blood findings suggestive of agnogenic myeloid metaplasia (idiopathic myelofibrosis)

- Marked poikilocytosis with abundant teardrop cells and elliptocytes/ovalocytes. Teardrop cells are not always present at diagnosis. Reduction of splenomegaly by chemotherapy can also result in the disappearance of teardrop cells.
- Circulating micromegakaryocytes and giant platelets. Both of these features are present in CML, however.
- Basophilia.
- Circulating blasts in variable proportions (usually in the 1–10% range), which may exceed the number of myelocytes and metamyelocytes or may be missed on blood film examination.
- Qualitative abnormalities in circulating erythroid precursors, myeloid precursors and neutrophils.
- An increased WBC count, but not in the leukemoid range (i.e. $< 50 \times 10^9/l$).
- Platelets increased but not exceeding $1000 \times 10^9/l$. The platelet count is within the normal range in a substantial number of cases, however.

- A marked leukocytosis in the leukemoid range, similar to that associated with CML. The differential diagnosis can best be resolved by testing for *bcr-abl* rearrangements.
- Increased hemoglobin or a marked thrombocytosis, with a minimal or absent leukoerythroblastic reaction, simulating PRV and ET, respectively. Laboratory investigations for PRV (such as the determination of RBC mass) can facilitate the distinction between early AMM and PRV (see Chapter 6).

If basophilia and circulating blasts are not present, other processes including recovery from chemotherapy, inflammation/sepsis and carcinomatosis need to be considered.

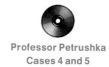

Professor Petrushka
Cases 4 and 5

In general, there is a higher proportion of NRBCs to circulating intermediate myeloid precursors in chronic, congenital hemolytic anemias. The reverse is usually true in MPDs. Since there is considerable overlap in WBC counts between these two groups, the degree of leukocytosis is less helpful as a differentiating feature.

4.3 Recommended work-up for a leukoerythroblastic pattern

A history of malignant neoplasm, exposure to radiation, chemotherapy (including G-CSF), sepsis, severe thermal injury, severe bleeding, or congenital/hereditary hemolytic anemia may indicate the cause of a leukoerythroblastic pattern.

If the peripheral blood findings, or the clinical and laboratory data, suggest an underlying hemolytic anemia, the following additional studies may be helpful:

- Supravital stains for Heinz bodies and/or a search for Hgb H inclusions.
- Hemoglobin electrophoresis with quantitation of globin chain synthesis.
- An osmotic fragility test and/or a direct Coombs test, if spherocytes are present.
- Heat denaturation or isopropanol precipitation tests, if RBC abnormalities are minimal or bite cells are seen.
- Enzyme screening.
- Determination of plasma or urine Hgb.

If the peripheral blood findings and clinical history do not clearly indicate a benign etiology for the leukoerythroblastosis, a bone marrow aspirate and biopsy are usually indicated. It is important that enough bone marrow is obtained for FCM immunophenotyping, cytogenetics and fungal/mycobacterial cultures, since these studies may be necessary to confirm the diagnosis.

Abnormal mononuclear
cell pattern

The abnormal mononuclear cell pattern encompasses malignant conditions (leukemias, lymphomas) and reactive processes with a cytology that may be mistaken for malignancy. Because of a lower density of nucleated cells, the morphology of abnormal mononuclear cells is better appreciated on blood films than on bone marrow smears. Mononuclear cells considered abnormal in the peripheral blood include:

- Cells that do not normally circulate (e.g. blasts).
- Cells for which there is no known benign counterpart in the blood (e.g. hairy cells, follicular center cells).
- Reactive lymphoid cells of the type seen in infectious mononucleosis, CMV infection, or the acute phase of HIV infection. Since these cells can simulate neoplastic cells morphologically, they are considered abnormal mononuclear cells.

Abnormal mononuclear cells often trigger analyzer flags for blasts, variant lymphocytes or large unstained cells. Since these flags may be false positives, they need to be confirmed by examination of the blood film.

Knowledge of the patient's clinical history and laboratory data are extremely helpful in classifying abnormal cells, since different types of large cells may mimic each other (e.g. lymphoma cells and blasts). Note that the morphology of neoplastic cells may change during the course of the disease, especially with protracted disease and exposure to multiple chemotherapy regimens.

5.1 General approach to recognizing abnormal mononuclear cells morphologically

1. **Small cells with sharp nuclear indentation.** In this category are lymphoma cells, Sezary cells and the 'flower' cells seen in ATLL. Ensure that the nuclear irregularities are not artifacts caused by a delay in blood film processing.
2. **Medium or large cells with a relatively high nuclear/cytoplasmic ratio.** In this group are blasts, large lymphoma cells, prolymphocytes and some reactive lymphocytes.
3. **Cells with a characteristic cytology.** In this group are hairy cells, plasmablasts and promonocytes.

When trying to deduce the identity of critical cells, the concept of 'the company the cell keeps' often provides clues to help distinguish between morphologic look-alikes (see Sections 5.2 and 5.11).

Additional details on the different abnormal mononuclear cells are presented below, along with a brief description, where appropriate, of the phenotypic profile. Before making a diagnosis, it is important to obtain corroborating clinical and laboratory data, especially FCM immunophenotyping. If available, previous specimens (e.g. peripheral blood, bone marrow and lymph node) should also be reviewed.

5.2 Blasts

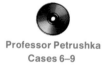

**Professor Petrushka
Cases 6–9**

The authors use the term blast to designate the immature cells which can be seen in a variety of disorders including acute leukemias, myelodysplastic syndromes, and MPDs. The morphologic features of blasts are: (1) large cell size; (2) high nuclear/cytoplasmic ratio; (3) scant to moderate pale blue cytoplasm (which may contain rare small granules and/or vacuoles); (4) round to irregular nuclei; (5) conspicuous nucleoli; and (6) fine chromatin (Figure 5.1a). Slight variations in film preparation and staining can alter the appearance of nuclear chromatin, making it appear coarser and obscuring the nucleolus.

The typical morphologic appearance described above is 'nondescript', since it can be shared by prolymphocytes, large lymphoma cells (Figure 5.1b) and some

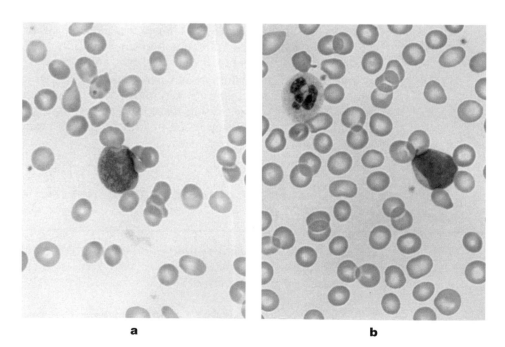

a

b

Figure 5.1 Morphologic similarities between the blast from a case of AML-M6 (a) and the circulating large lymphoma cell from a case of high-grade B-cell lymphoma (b)

reactive lymphoid cells. For this reason, immaturity and cell lineage are best established by immunophenotyping. The terms 'L3 blast', 'plasmablast', and 'immunoblast' are engrained in the literature, and are used even though these cells are not immature. These three terms, introduced to describe large cells with visible nucleoli, antedate the use of immunophenotyping and our current understanding of lymphoid cell maturation.

The presence of Auer rods, which result from the fusion of primary granules, is a feature virtually pathognomonic of myeloid differentiation (Figure 5.2). Using the concept of 'the company the cell keeps', the myeloid origin of the blasts can also be inferred from the presence of abundant monocytes/promonocytes, as seen in CMMoL or AML with monocytic differentiation (Figure 5.3). In the absence of these features, however, the lineage cannot be reliably determined without cytochemical stains and/or FCM immunophenotyping.

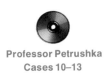
Professor Petrushka
Cases 10–13

With extreme stressed hematopoiesis in sickle cell anemia or thalassemia major, a small percentage of circulating blasts ($<5\%$) may be present, invariably accompanied by an overwhelming number of NRBCs (>100 NRBCs/100 WBCs) (Figure 5.4). Similarly, a vigorous response to G-CSF therapy can manifest with a small number of circulating blasts (usually in the range of 3–5%, rarely exceeding 10%) accompanied by intermediate myeloid precursors. The blood picture may be indistinguishable from acute leukemia or CML. An important clue is the presence of hypergranulation in myeloid cells. Follow-up reveals that the manifestations are transient, subsiding within 1–2 weeks.

Professor Petrushka
Case 14

In neonates with Down's syndrome, a high WBC count with abundant blasts can be a manifestation of a 'transient proliferation of hematopoietic precursors'. The differential diagnosis between this benign condition and acute leukemia can be difficult. In the benign disease, the blasts are of heterogeneous lineage (myeloid, lymphoid, megakaryocytic, erythroid). The process spontaneously regresses in several weeks.

The cytochemical stains most useful for identifying the myeloid lineage are myeloperoxidase (MPO) and α-naphthyl butyrate esterase (ANBE), also discussed in Section 40.5.1 (Figure 5.5). In large mononuclear cells, ANBE reactivity

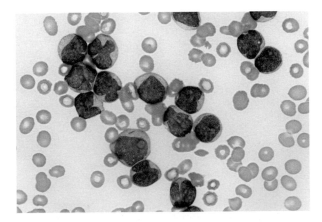

Figure 5.2 Distinct Auer rod in one myeloblast. The nuclear irregularities in blasts do not imply monocytic differentiation. This patient had AML-M1

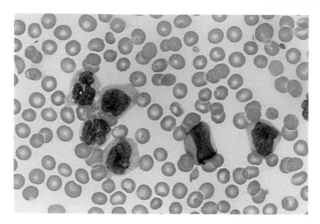

Figure 5.3   A myeloblast in the company of several promonocytes and monocytes

implies monocytic differentiation. A useful internal control is the dot-positivity in T lymphocytes. AML-M0 and AML-M7 (acute megakaryoblastic leukemia) are both MPO-negative by light microscopy. Peroxidase-positive granules are present in AML-M0 ultrastructurally (Figure 5.6). Immunophenotyping is necessary for identifying AML-M0 and AML-M7 (see Chapters 22 and 24).

With the exception of AML-M3, which can be diagnosed in the peripheral blood, the identification of the other French-American-British (FAB) subtypes of AML is based primarily on bone marrow aspirates (see Section 40.5). The presence of at least 30% circulating blasts is an accepted criterion for acute leukemia, irrespective of the blast proportion in the marrow.

The constellation of significant basophilia, high numbers of circulating intermediate myeloid precursors and less than 10% circulating blasts is the typical blood picture seen in CML. Since blasts are preferentially distributed toward the lateral sides of the slide, and the manual differential usually includes only 100 cells, small numbers of blasts are sometimes missed on the manual differential

Professor Petrushka
Cases 15 and 16

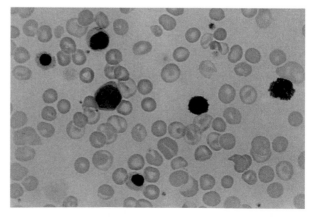

Figure 5.4   A rare circulating blast in a case of transfusion-dependent thalassemia major

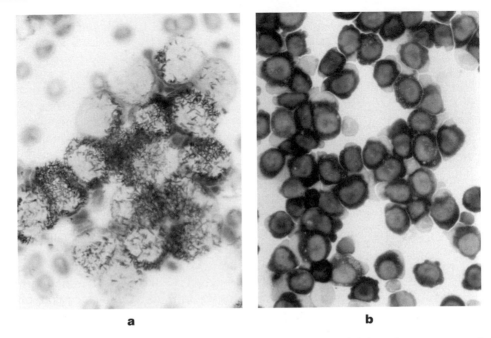

a   b

Figure 5.5 (a) Positive myeloperoxidase reaction, highlighting the presence of numerous Auer rods from a case of AML-M3. (b) Positive ANBE reaction in AML-M5a

resulting in an apparent leukemoid pattern (see chapter 18 for a discussion of CML). A blast crisis of an underlying or unsuspected MPD/CML can be diagnosed if there is basophilia and the blast count exceeds 20%.

In some instances, the morphology of the blasts may be distinctive enough to suggest certain diagnoses (which should always be confirmed with cytochemical stains and FCM immunophenotyping):

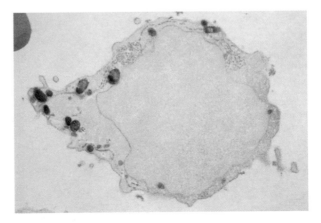

Figure 5.6 Peroxidase granules at the electron microscopy level, from a case of AML-M0. In this instance, the blasts were peroxidase-negative by light microscopy and did not express any lineage-associated markers. Only TdT and CD34 were expressed

Professor Petrushka
Cases 17 and 18

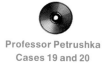

Professor Petrushka
Cases 19 and 20

- The typical lymphoblasts of ALL ('L1' subtype by FAB criteria) are small to medium, with a homogeneously dense nucleus, inconspicuous nucleoli and scant cytoplasm (Figure 5.7a). When sizable cytoplasmic vacuoles occur in L1 blasts, it is important not to confuse the blasts with Burkitt's cells. Small lymphoblasts can often be overlooked and counted as benign lymphocytes in a manual differential (Figure 5.7b). Be aware of this possibility in the presence of an unexplained bicytopenia (anemia and thrombocytopenia) associated with an apparent mild lymphocytosis. Lymphoblastic leukemias are now classified immunologically. Therefore, the distinction between ALL-L1 and ALL-L2, based on the scoring of nuclear and cytoplasmic features, is no longer necessary (see Section 40.6.2.2).

- The finding of blasts with abundant coarse azurophilic granules and/or bundles of Auer rods obscuring the nucleus (Figure 5.8) is diagnostic of acute promyelocytic leukemia (APL, AML-M3). A prompt diagnosis is critical to initiate preventive measures against the associated coagulopathy. In the microgranular variant (AML-M3v), the size of the granules is below the resolution of light microscopy. The blasts exhibit reniform, bilobed, or twisted nuclei and dusty purple to agranular cytoplasm (Figure 5.9a). The morphology may be mistaken for monocytic differentiation (Figure 5.10). Cases of AML-M3v with agranular blasts that are devoid of nuclear lobulation can be easily misinterpreted as AML-M1 (Figure 5.9b). Careful review of the blood film in such cases will invariably reveal a small proportion of blasts with the more typical AML-M3v morphology. The diagnosis of AML-M3 can be confirmed by the characteristic myeloid phenotype: CD34⁻,

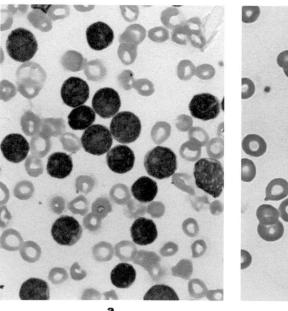
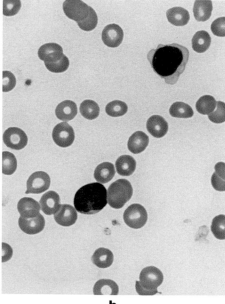

a   b

Figure 5.7 (a) Numerous ALL blasts with minimal cytoplasm, round nuclei and inconspicuous nucleoli. (b) A small lymphoblast and a large lymphocyte. The nuclei are similar in size. The malignant cell has an inappropriately high nuclear/cytoplasmic ratio

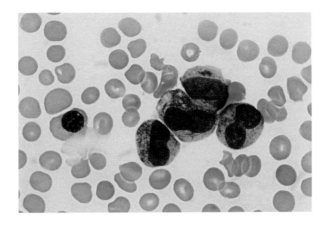

Figure 5.8 AML-M3 blasts with abundant Auer rods

CD13$^+$, CD33$^+$, HLA-DR$^-$, the uniformly intense MPO reaction, and the (15;17) translocation (see Sections 40.5.1.1 and 40.5.1.2).

- Typical monoblasts are very large cells with round nuclei, prominent 'owl-eye' nucleoli, ample basophilic cytoplasm and frequent vacuoles (Figure 5.11). A few scattered minute azurophilic granules may be present. Slightly more 'mature-appearing' variants have lobulated nuclei, smaller (but still conspicuous) nucleoli, and less basophilic cytoplasm. Monocytic differentia-

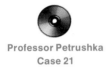

Professor Petrushka
Case 21

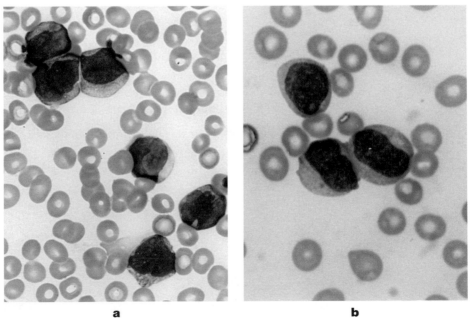

a   b

Figure 5.9 (a) AML-M3v blast with twisted nuclear irregularities and finely dusty cytoplasm. (b) AML-M3v blast with regular nuclear contours and virtually agranular cytoplasm. This case was initially misinterpreted as AML-M1. The blasts were CD13$^+$, CD33$^+$ and HLA-DR negative. Cytogenetic studies revealed t(15;17)

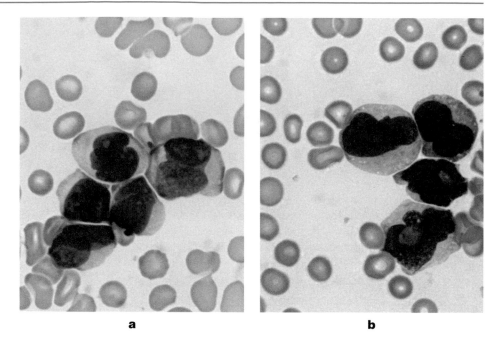

a   b

Figure 5.10 Morphologic similarities between the markedly hypogranular blasts of AML-M3v (a) and the neoplastic cells in AML-M5b (b)

tion must be confirmed by ANBE reactivity or the determination of serum/urine lysozyme levels. Large cell lymphoma in leukemic phase and 'undifferentiated' blasts of other types (megakaryoblasts, erythroblasts) can simulate the morphology of monoblasts.

The following systematic work-up is recommended for all acute leukemias:

1. FCM immunophenotyping.
2. Cytochemical stains on peripheral blood and/or bone marrow.
3. A bone marrow aspirate/biopsy including cytogenetics.

In acute non-myeloid leukemia, DNA content analysis by FCM is helpful.

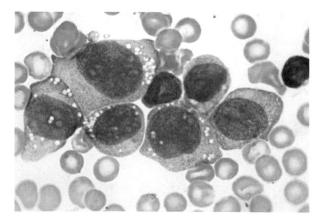

Figure 5.11 Monoblasts in AML-M5a

5.3 Promonocytes

**Professor Petrushka
Cases 10, 13 and 22**

**Professor Petrushka
Case 23**

Promonocytes (Figure 5.12) represent an intermediate stage between monoblasts and monocytes. Typically, promonocytes demonstrate reniform nuclei,
reticulated chromatin, small nucleoli and abundant blue-gray cytoplasm with
fine azurophilic granules. It is acknowledged that it can be difficult to distinguish promonocytes from monocytes. In promonocytes, the nucleus is less
lobulated, the chromatin finer and the cytoplasm not as gray as in monocytes.
The term 'atypical monocytes' should be avoided. When present, promonocytes are a helpful clue to distinguish a neoplastic process from a reactive
monocytosis.

In the peripheral blood, promonocytes can be seen in either CMMoL or AML
with monocytic differentiation, i.e. AML-M4, AML-M5a or AML-M5b. The
morphology of AML-M5b may be mimicked by AML-M3v.

By current criteria, CMMoL requires an absolute peripheral monocytosis
(monocytes $> 1.0 \times 10^9$/l) and less than 5% circulating blasts. Bone marrow
studies are helpful to differentiate CMMoL from AML with monocytic
differentiation and other myeloproliferative/myelodysplastic disorders. Qualitative abnormalities (e.g. hypogranulation, hypersegmentation and hyposegmentation in granulocytes) are frequently present in all of these disorders
(Figure 5.13).

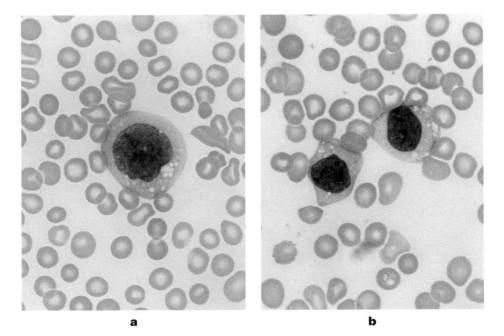

a   b

Figure 5.12   (a), (b) Promonocytes from two different cases of CMMoL

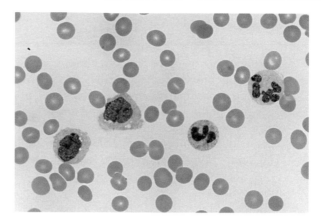

Figure 5.13 From a case of CMMoL: the neutrophil on the far right is enlarged and hypogranulated

5.4 Hairy cells

Proper identification of hairy cells is the key to the identification of HCL. Typically, hairy cells in a well-spread film have a 'fried egg' appearance (Figure 5.14) with abundant pale, translucent cytoplasm. The nucleus is ovoid, reniform or dumbbell-shaped with a reticulated chromatin pattern reminiscent of that in

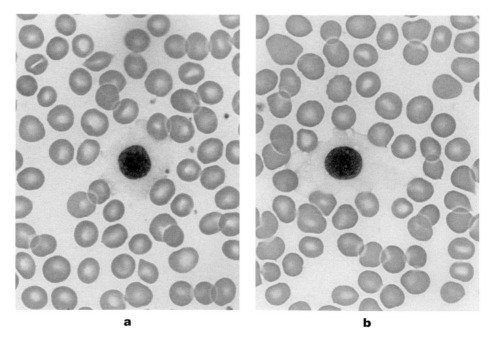

a   b

Figure 5.14 (a), (b) Hairy cells from the zone of morphology of a well-prepared blood film. The abundant pale cytoplasm extends to the border of the neighboring RBCs

monocytes. Nucleoli are virtually absent. In the thick end of the film, or in poorly prepared films that have not been quickly air-dried, the cells become shrunken with cytoplasmic 'hairy' projections, condensed chromatin, and spongy-appearing cytoplasm (Figure 5.15).

'Hairy' projections, by light microscopy, are not the pathognomonic features of hairy cells. Osmotic hypertonicity in slowly dried blood films can cause cytoplasmic projections in any lymphocyte (see Section 1.3).

Hairy cell leukemia is more common in males older than 50 years. The typical clinical presentation is pancytopenia with splenomegaly and a low number of circulating hairy cells (1–5% range) that can easily be missed on a manual differential if the blood smear is not scanned thoroughly. A helpful alternative is examination of a well-spread buffy coat preparation. A frank leukemic picture with mild to moderate leukocytosis and abundant circulating cells can be seen in hyposplenic states. The characteristic diffuse tartrate-resistant acid phosphatase (TRAP) reactivity is a useful diagnostic marker for HCL, especially if FCM was not performed (Figure 5.16). Note that the reactivity must be diffuse to be considered positive.

Multiparameter FCM immunophenotyping is an exquisitely sensitive technique for detecting low numbers of circulating hairy cells because of their characteristic antigenic expression, strong CD20 and CD11c, and positive CD25 and CD103 (see Section 27.7).

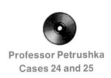

Professor Petrushka
Cases 24 and 25

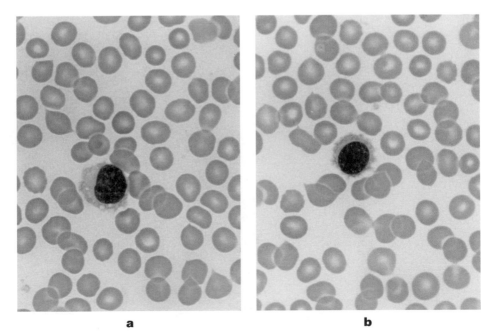

a   b

Figure 5.15 (a), (b) Hairy cells (same patient as in Figure 5.14) from the zone of morphology of a poorly prepared blood film which was left to air-dry slowly. The cytoplasm and the nuclei are shrunken and the nuclear chromatin appears more condensed

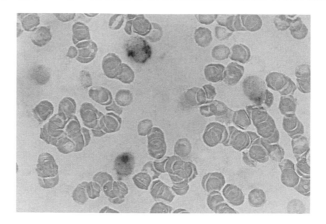

Figure 5.16   Diffuse TRAP positivity in hairy cell leukemia

5.5 Prolymphocytes

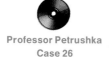

Professor Petrushka
Case 26

Immunologically, there are two types of prolymphocytes: (1) B prolymphocytes, as found in B-PLL (Figure 5.17), CLL and related disorders (Figure 5.18); and (2) T prolymphocytes (found in T-PLL).

According to the FAB criteria, the number of circulating B prolymphocytes is up to 10% in typical CLL. Cases with between 10 and 55% prolymphocytes at presentation are classified as CLL with an increased number of prolymphocytes (CLL/PL). Cases presenting with more than 55% of B prolymphocytes are desig-

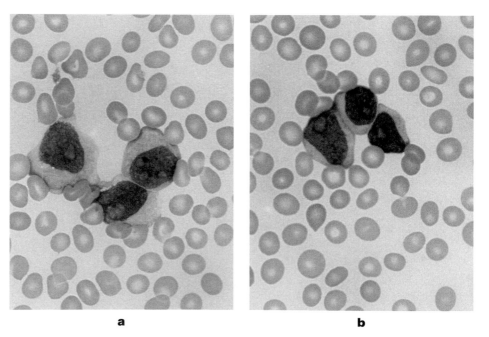

a   b

Figure 5.17   (a), (b) Prolymphocytes from two different fields, in a case of B-prolymphocytic leukemia

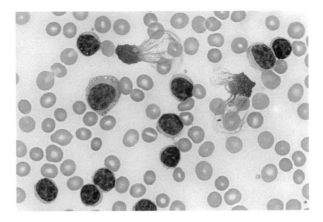

Figure 5.18   A prolymphocyte in a case of CLL

nated B-PLL. With chemotherapy, the blood picture in CLL can be altered, with a decrease or clearing of lymphocytosis but a relative increase in the proportion of residual prolymphocytes (> 10%) resulting in a CLL/PL picture. Prolymphocytes seen following chemotherapy often have altered morphology. When the nuclear/ cytoplasmic ratio is increased, the cells may become indistinguishable from blasts (Figure 5.19).

Slow drying of blood films or bone marrow aspirate smears can easily result in 'hairs', 'villi' (Figure 5.20) or 'blebs'. These artifacts disappear if the slides are

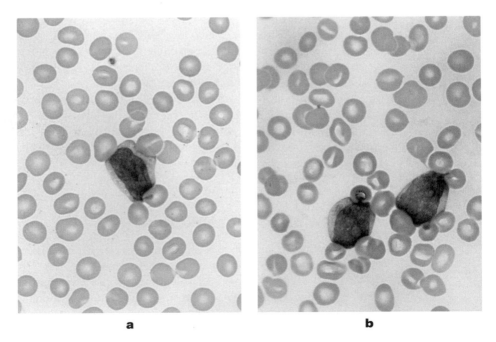

a   b

Figure 5.19 Morphologic similarities between the prolymphocyte from a case of treated CLL (a) and the blasts in AML (b)

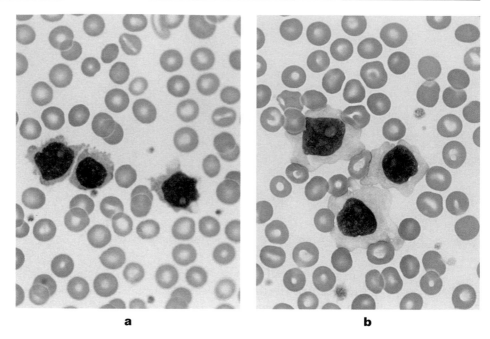

a   b

Figure 5.20   Blood films from the same patient with B-prolymphocytic leukemia. (a) The slowly dried smear results in shrunken neoplastic cells with artifactual hairy projections. (b) The cytology of the prolymphocytes (abundant cytoplasm, prominent nucleolus and reticulated chromatin) can be better appreciated on the quickly dried film

immediately fan-dried. When the WBC count or the surrounding humidity is high, the propensity for such artifacts is higher. Since hairs, villi, and blebs can be induced by suboptimal blood film preparation, it is important not to attach diagnostic significance to these features.

The morphology of a prolymphocyte (especially a B prolymphocyte) can also simulate a reactive lymphocyte (Figure 5.21). The subtle differences are a lower nuclear/cytoplasmic ratio and coarser chromatin in reactive lymphocytes (Downey II cells). The company they keep and the proper clinical context best identify large cells of this type.

5.5.1 Prolymphocytic leukemia

Prolymphocytic leukemia is a disease of older patients (peak incidence between ages 70 and 80). Marked leukocytosis (usually in the $100 \times 10^9/l$ range with >55% prolymphocytes) and splenomegaly are two constant features of PLL. The peripheral leukocytosis mirrors the extensive bone marrow infiltration. Anemia and thrombocytopenia are common.

The diagnosis of PLL is primarily a peripheral blood diagnosis. The leukemic population is uniform in most instances. The subtype of PLL, B-cell or T-cell can sometimes be suspected based on the cytology of the leukemic population:

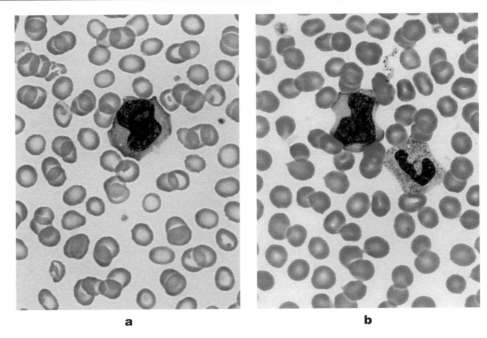

a   b

Figure 5.21   Morphologic similarities between the prolymphocyte from a case of CLL (a) and a reactive lymphoid cell in a case of infectious mononucleosis (b)

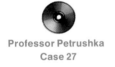

Professor Petrushka
Case 27

- Large cells with a round nucleus, a prominent nucleolus surrounded by moderately condensed, reticulated chromatin (an appearance suggesting that the cells are mature) and ample pale blue cytoplasm suggest B-PLL, which accounts for about 80% of PLL.
- Medium to large cells (smaller than the B prolymphocytes described above) with a high nuclear/cytoplasmic ratio, a small distinct nucleolus, coarse chromatin and nuclear irregularities suggest T-PLL (Figure 5.22). This morphol-

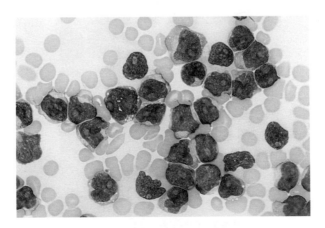

Figure 5.22   T-prolymphocytic leukemia: the neoplastic population in this case is composed of medium to large cells with prominent nucleoli and frequent nuclear indentations

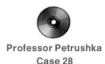

ogy, seen in 50–60% of T-PLL, may be mimicked by cases of ATLL presenting with a relatively uniform leukemic population. Less frequently, T-PLL may present with a heterogeneous leukemic population in which the nuclei can have deep indentations or multiple lobulations simulating either the cerebriform cells of Sezary syndrome or the 'flower' cells of ATLL. A substantial number of T-PLL cases demonstrate the same cytology as B-PLL and can only be identified by FCM immunophenotyping. Most T-PLL cases demonstrate a normal T-helper phenotype and dot-positivity for NSE. Cytoplasmic blebs should not be considered morphologic evidence of T-PLL cells (Figure 5.23).

The following clinical features differentiate T-PLL from B-PLL:

1. Lymphadenopathy is virtually absent in B-PLL except at the terminal stage. In contrast, generalized lymphadenopathy and cutaneous involvement occur in a substantial number of patients with T-PLL.
2. T-PLL pursues a more aggressive clinical course than B-PLL with a median survival of 24 months.

The work-up of PLL should include peripheral blood FCM immunophenotyping. A bone marrow aspirate/biopsy can be performed if determination of the baseline tumor burden is deemed necessary.

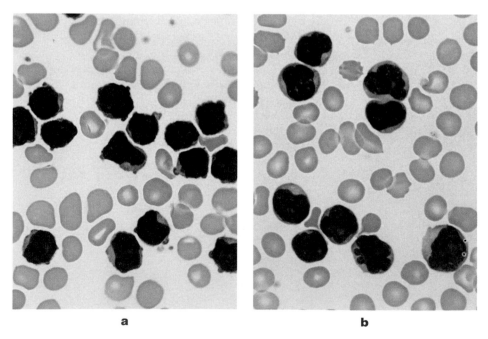

a   b

Figure 5.23 Blood films from the same patient with T-prolymphocytic leukemia. (a) The slowly dried film results in shrunken neoplastic cells with artifactual cytoplasmic blebs and excessive darkening of the nuclear chromatin. (b) The blebs disappear and the cytologic details are more apparent on the fan-dried smear

5.5.2 Chronic lymphocytic leukemia with an increased number of prolymphocytes (CLL/PL)

According to FAB criteria, CLL/PL has features halfway between CLL and PLL. Given the potential fluctuations in the proportion of prolymphocytes during the course of CLL, the diagnosis of CLL/PL is reserved for those cases with a sustained high proportion of prolymphocytes. Morphologically, the WBC count is invariably elevated, with an increased proportion of prolymphocytes (10–55%) and a variable number of plasmacytoid lymphocytes (Figure 5.24).

The cell size, nuclear size, prominence of the nucleolus, and quality of the chromatin are features that allow the separation of plasmacytoid lymphocytes from prolymphocytes (Figure 5.25). Prolymphocytes are larger than plasmacytoid

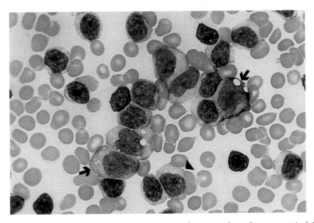

Figure 5.24 A mixture of prolymphocytes (arrows), plasmacytoid lymphocytes (arrowhead) and small lymphocytes in a case of CLL/PL. Prolymphocytes constitute 35% of the differential

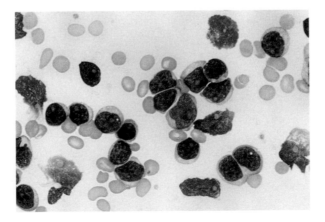

Figure 5.25 Numerous plasmacytoid lymphocytes from a case of lymphoplasmacytoid lymphoma-leukemia. Compared to the prolymphocyte in the center, the plasmacytoid lymphocytes have smaller nuclei, more condensed chromatin and a less prominent nucleolus

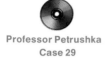

lymphocytes, with a more prominent nucleolus and more open chromatin. In the authors' experience, cases of CLL/PL are immunologically similar to CLL, i.e. with coexpression of CD5 and CD23 and monoclonal sIg that is weakly expressed. In some cases, the sIg intensity may be stronger, i.e. intermediate between that of CLL and PLL.

5.6 Burkitt's cells (ALL-L3)

Burkitt's cells are encountered in ALL, L3 subtype. The disease is more appropriately referred to as Burkitt's lymphoma in leukemic phase (see Section 40.5.2.3). Burkitt's lymphoma-leukemia is not composed of immature cells (blasts). It is a mature B-cell disorder with strong monoclonal sIg expression. The diagnostic work-up recommended in section 5.2 is applicable to this disease.

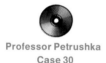

In Burkitt's lymphoma-leukemia, the number of circulating cells is usually low compared to the overwhelming involvement in the marrow. Neoplastic cells are medium to large, with moderate amounts of deeply basophilic cytoplasm, round nuclei, stippled chromatin, and visible nucleoli (Figure 5.26a). This morphology can be closely mimicked by large lymphoma cells (of either B-cell or T-cell lineage) as well as the reactive Downey III cells seen in IM (Figure 5.26b). Sharply defined cytoplasmic vacuoles are frequently present. This feature is more obvious in the bone marrow than in the peripheral blood (Figure 5.27a). Cytoplasmic

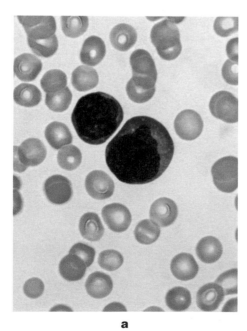
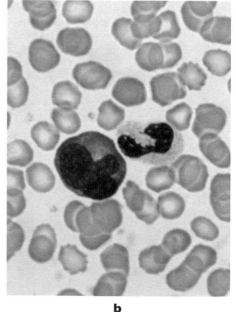

a   b

Figure 5.26 (a) Two Burkitt's cells with deeply basophilic cytoplasm. Note the lack of cytoplasmic vacuoles. (b) A reactive lymphoid cell (Downey III) for comparison

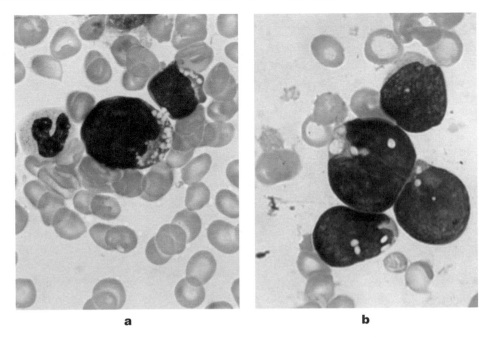

a   b

Figure 5.27   (a) Two Burkitt's cells with cytoplasmic vacuoles. (b) Precursor B-cell ALL with cytoplasmic vacuoles

vacuoles also feature in other neoplastic mononuclear cells however, e.g. B pro-lymphocytes, large lymphoma cells, the nondescript blasts of AML (especially after chemotherapy), the blasts of AML-M5, and, less commonly, the blasts in ALL (Figure 5.27b).

5.7 Plasma cells and plasmablasts

Circulating mature-appearing plasma cells raise the differential diagnosis of reactive processes versus plasma cell dyscrasias. Autoimmune diseases, infections (bacterial, viral), immunizations and drug hypersensitivity can all cause a reactive plasmacytosis (Figure 5.28a). The proportion of plasma cells in reactive conditions is low (< 10%) and other reactive features (e.g. reactive lymphocytes, eosinophilia or neutrophilia) are present.

The accepted criteria for plasma cell leukemia (PCL) include: (1) greater than 20% plasma cells in the peripheral blood differential count; (2) an absolute plasma cell count of greater than 2×10^9/l; and (3) evidence of monoclonality. The leukemic manifestation may be seen at presentation or as a terminal phase of multiple myeloma. In comparison to multiple myeloma, the following clinical characteristics are associated with PCL: younger age group, fewer lytic lesions, higher incidence of organomegaly/lymphadenopathy, and poorer prognosis (median survival of 2 months).

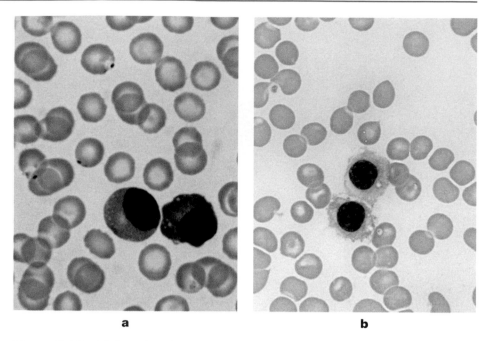

a   b

Figure 5.28 (a) Reactive plasma cells in a case of Plasmodium falciparum infestation. (b) Circulating neoplastic plasma cells with hairy projections secondary to slow drying of the blood film

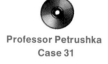

**Professor Petrushka
Case 31**

    The leukemic population often consists of a mixture of plasma cells and plasmablasts (i.e. immature-appearing plasma cells). Slow drying or ruptured cytoplasm can impart a 'hairy' appearance to the neoplastic cells (Figure 5.28b). Compared to plasma cells, plasmablasts are larger cells with conspicuous nucleoli, reticulated to finely dispersed chromatin (in contrast to the clumped cartwheel chromatin of plasma cells), and a variable degree of cytoplasmic basophilia (Figure 5.29).

    The morphology of plasmablasts may be indistinguishable from that of Downey III cells (Figure 5.30). It may also be difficult to discriminate plasmablasts from large lymphoma cells with plasmacytoid differentiation (i.e. immunoblastic lymphoma), both morphologically and phenotypically.

    If the serum immunoglobulin level is high, rouleaux can be present. Rouleaux may not be a feature if the disease produces mostly free light chains that are easily lost in the urine.

    An appropriate diagnostic work-up for plasma cell dyscrasias includes:

1. Serum protein electrophoresis and immunoelectrophoresis (or immunofixation) to identify the monoclonal immunoglobulin (M protein). The M protein can be composed of complete immunoglobulin molecules, free light chains (usually in addition to complete molecules), or fragments of heavy chains only. On serum protein electrophoresis, the location of the M protein peak generally corresponds to its immunoglobulin composition. IgG often has γ mobility. IgA has predominantly β mobility. An IgM peak is often found in the γ to β region. Free light chains have α2 mobility.

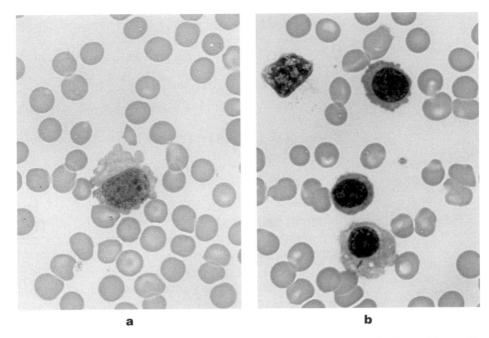

Figure 5.29 Plasma cell leukemia in two different patients. (a) A plasmablast with reticulated chromatin and a visible nucleolus. (b) Mature- and immature-appearing neoplastic plasma cells with more basophilic cytoplasm. One neoplastic cell contains an immunoglobulin rod

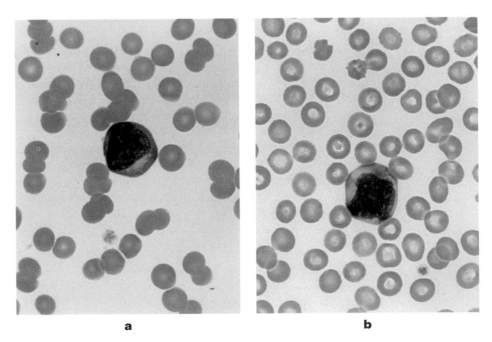

Figure 5.30 Rouleaux and a plasmablast (a) morphologically reminiscent of a reactive Downey cell (b)

2. Detection of free light chains in the urine. Heat or acid precipitation detects free light chains in the urine (referred to as Bence-Jones protein). Urine immunoelectrophoresis can be used to determine the nature of the light chains.
3. A bone marrow aspirate/biopsy.
4. Immunophenotyping on cells isolated from peripheral blood and/or a bone marrow aspirate.
5. Review of skeletal X-rays for lytic lesions.

5.8 Circulating lymphoma cells

Non-Hodgkin's lymphoma (NHL) cells may circulate in the peripheral blood. The cytological features of circulating lymphoma cells (e.g. coarse chromatin, distinct nuclear indentations, visible nucleoli) indicate mature neoplastic cells.

Cells with cytological characteristics that allow a more specific subclassification (e.g. hairy cells, prolymphocytes and plasmablasts) are not considered circulating lymphoma cells. In addition, cells with a known benign counterpart in the blood (e.g. plasmacytoid lymphocytes) are not designated by this term.

When the clinical context is known, it is appropriate to refer to certain NHL cells by the morphologic terms that indicate a specific clinicopathological entity. For example, the cells of Sezary syndrome are known as cerebriform cells and the circulating cells in ATLL are referred to as 'flower' cells. In absence of the clinical information, cerebriform and flower cells can be designated by the less specific term 'lymphoma cells'.

Lymphoma cells may circulate when the WBC count is normal, particularly in low-grade NHL of the small cell type. The term 'leukemic phase' of NHL is used when circulating lymphoma cells are sufficiently numerous for an automated analyzer to indicate an apparent absolute lymphocytosis, often with flagging for blasts and/or variant lymphocytes.

Circulating lymphoma cells can be grouped as small or large. In general, lymphomas of the small cell type, e.g. follicular center cell (FCC) lymphoma and mantle cell lymphoma (MCL), have a higher likelihood of developing a leukemic phase during the course of the disease. In diffuse large cell lymphoma (DLCL), a leukemic phase is often a pre-terminal event. Automated analyzers often classify large lymphoma cells as 'monocytes' resulting in an apparent monocytosis.

5.8.1 Small lymphoma cells

Rare circulating lymphoma cells are not uncommon in low-grade lymphoma. In the leukemic phase of the disease, the distribution of the neoplastic population may suggest the subtype of the lymphoma.

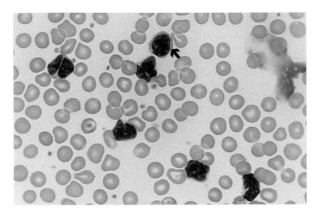

Figure 5.31 Circulating small lymphoma cells with nuclear indentations ('cleaved' cells) from a case of FCC lymphoma in leukemic phase. Compared to the benign lymphocyte (arrow), the neoplastic cells also have an inappropriately high nuclear/cytoplasmic ratio

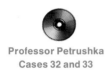

Professor Petrushka
Cases 32 and 33

A relatively uniform population of small cells with a high nuclear/cytoplasmic ratio, scant cytoplasm, smooth, dense chromatin, no visible nucleoli, and irregular nuclei with one to two deep, narrow clefts, is very suggestive of an FCC lymphoma (Figure 5.31). Up to 5% of lymphocytes in CLL can have nuclear clefts, however (Figure 5.32). The differential diagnosis also includes cases of MCL and rare forms of ATLL which demonstrate a uniform leukemic population (Figure 5.33). The diagnosis of FCC lymphoma in leukemic phase should be corroborated by immunophenotyping, i.e. positive B-cell markers, positive CD10, and strong monoclonal sIg (see Section 27.6).

The morphology of MCL in leukemic phase is highly variable, ranging from a uniform population of small cells with infrequent nuclear indentations (Figure 5.34b) to a heterogeneous population of small, medium, and large cells with a variable degree of nuclear irregularity (Figure 5.35). In the heterogeneous variant, distinct nucleoli are visible in the medium and large cells. A heterogeneous

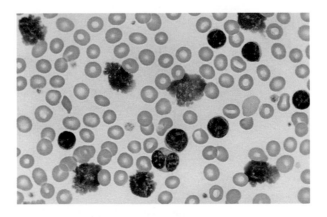

Figure 5.32 A 'cleaved' cell in CLL. This patient had long-standing disease and was given several chemotherapy regimens over the years

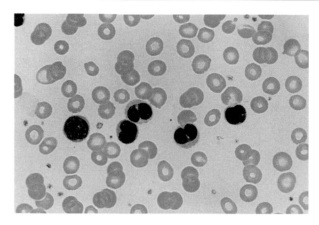

Figure 5.33 ATLL with a uniform neoplastic population composed mostly of 'cleaved' cells

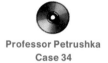

Professor Petrushka
Case 34

population can also be a feature of FCC in transformation and ALL-L2. Conversely, a monotonous population of small lymphoma cells with round nuclei can be easily overlooked as lymphocytes (Figure 5.34b).

Although MCL can be suspected based on the heterogeneity of the lymphoid cells, the diagnosis rests on the immunophenotype (mature B-cell profile, CD5$^+$, CD23$^-$, bright monoclonal sIg), molecular genetics (*bcl*-1 rearrangement) and the lymph node biopsy findings (see Sections 27.5.3 and 40.4.2).

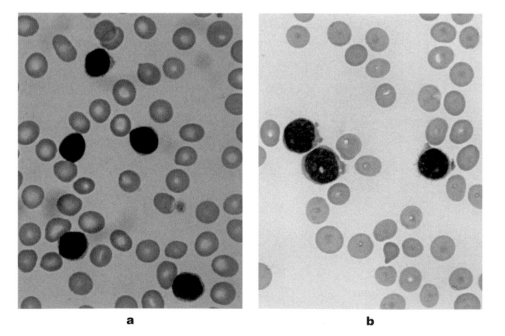

a   b

Figure 5.34 Follicular center cell lymphoma (a) and mantle cell lymphoma (b) in leukemic phase. The neoplastic populations in these two cases are composed mostly of cells with round nuclei, which may be overlooked as lymphocytes. The inappropriately high nuclear/cytoplasmic ratio is a subtle clue for identifying these small lymphoma cells

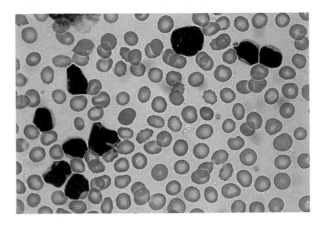

Figure 5.35   Mantle cell lymphoma with a heterogeneous neoplastic population

5.8.2 Large lymphoma cells

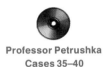

**Professor Petrushka
Cases 35–40**

Circulating large lymphoma cells can easily be confused with blasts or reactive lymphoid cells (Downey cells) when they exhibit either a 'nondescript' morphology (moderate to ample cytoplasm, round to irregular nuclei, prominent nucleoli and 'open' chromatin) or a plasmacytoid/immunoblastic morphology (Figure 5.36). Cytoplasmic vacuoles or small azurophilic granules may be present (Figure 5.37a). The morphologic identification of large lymphoma cells is more straightforward when the nuclei are hyperchromatic (Figure 5.37b).

When circulating lymphoma cells are identified, a careful review of the clinical history and any prior lymph node biopsies should be performed. The recommended work-up of NHL in leukemic phase is shown in Table 5.1.

Table 5.1 Work-up of non-Hodgkin's lymphoma in leukemic phase

1. A bone marrow aspirate/biopsy.
2. Immunophenotyping on blood, bone marrow, or a lymph node suspension.
3. A repeat lymph node biopsy to rule out histologic progression. Fresh tissue should be saved for FCM cell cycle analysis (determination of the percentage of cells in the S-phase), which may provide objective information for grading the tumor.

5.9 Flower cells

Typical flower cells found in ATLL are medium-sized cells with 'cloverleaf' nuclei, basophilic cytoplasm, and a high nuclear/cytoplasmic ratio (Figure 5.38). It is important to ensure that the cloverleaf appearance is not an artifact due to prolonged storage or centrifugation. The nuclear indentations are more readily identifiable than those of Sezary (cerebriform) cells. A small percentage of ATLL cells are large with prominent nucleoli, less condensed nuclear chromatin, scant to moderate amounts of deep blue cytoplasm and minimal nuclear irregularities. The nuclear features in some cases mimic those of small Sezary

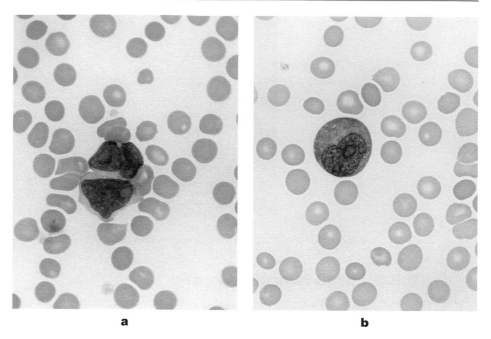

Figure 5.36 (a) Large lymphoma cells with a 'nondescript' morphology. (b) A large lymphoma cell with immunoblastic/plasmacytoid morphology

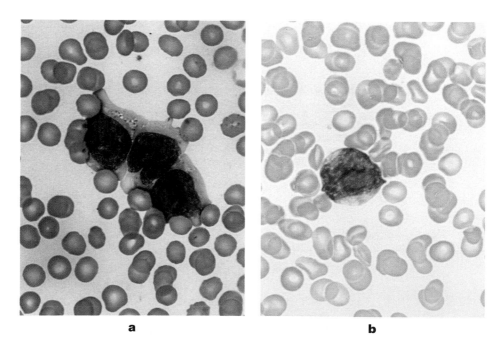

Figure 5.37 (a) Circulating large lymphoma cells with cytoplasmic azurophilic granules from a case of high-grade B-cell lymphoma. (b) A large lymphoma cell with a hyperchromatic nucleus

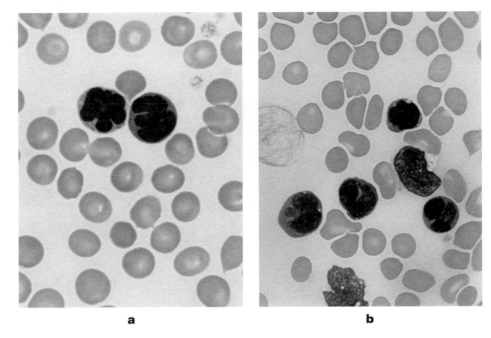

a   b

Figure 5.38   (a), (b) ATLL: neoplastic cells from two different patients

cells. Rare cases of ATLL present with a monomorphous population of small lymphoid cells with deep clefting (Figure 5.33), simulating FCC in leukemic phase.

Adult T-cell leukemia-lymphoma should be differentiated from other mature B-cell and T-cell malignancies including T-PLL (Figure 5.22) and Sezary syndrome with a high number of circulating cells (Figure 5.39). Distinct CD25 expression is characteristic of ATLL, however (see Section 28.5). Most cases demonstrate an aberrant helper T-cell phenotype, usually with down-regulated production or loss of CD7.

Adult T-cell leukemia-lymphoma is endemic in south-west Japan, the Caribbean and Africa. The etiologic agent is the HTLV-I virus. Only 2–5% of individuals infected with HTLV-I develop full-blown ATLL. The long latency period after HTLV-I infection (estimated at 20–30 years) suggests that additional events, including immunosuppression (e.g. infection by *Strongyloides*), are necessary for development of leukemia. Infection by HTLV-I leads to T-cell proliferation, which can slowly progress from polyclonal to monoclonal. This results in the progression from the HTLV-I carrier stage to the smoldering ATLL phase with a few circulating 'flower' cells. The disease can subsequently progress to chronic ATLL, acute ATLL or the lymphoma type of ATLL.

The most common form of the disease is acute ATLL (60% of cases), characterized by an aggressive clinical course and a rapidly progressive leukocytosis composed of a heterogeneous population of 'flower' cells. Other common clinical features include hypercalcemia, an elevated LDH, opportunistic infections and widespread systemic involvement (lymph nodes, liver, spleen, lung and skin).

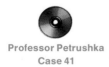

Professor Petrushka
Case 41

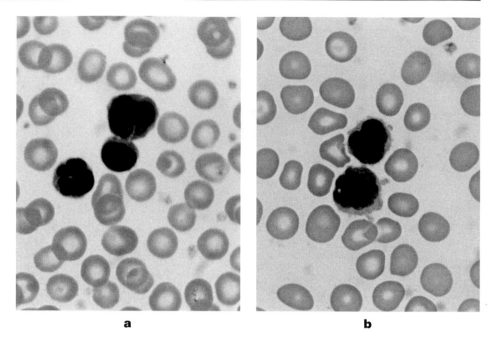

a   b

Figure 5.39 Morphologic similarities between the neoplastic cells in ATLL (a) and Sezary syndrome (b). Both patients presented with similar WBC counts of $12 \times 10^9/l$

In chronic ATLL, the absolute lymphocytosis is stable, less severe and composed predominantly of small lymphoid cells (at least 5% of which are 'flower' cells). Features that differentiate chronic ATLL from the acute form include an absence of hypercalcemia, lack of serous effusions, and an LDH level that does not exceed twice the upper limit of normal.

Patients with smoldering ATLL have no lymphadenopathy, and a normal lymphocyte count with at least 5% abnormal lymphocytes. Extranodal involvement, if present, is limited to cutaneous and/or pulmonary infiltrates. In the absence of these lesions, it may be difficult to differentiate smoldering ATLL from the 'healthy' HTLV-I carrier state. Molecular analysis for HTLV-I proviral DNA integration may be helpful in such cases. Skin lesions in smoldering ATLL usually consist of dermal infiltrates causing a nodular or maculopapular rash. Occasionally the skin lesions can mimic MF both clinically and histologically.

The recommended work-up for ATLL is shown in Table 5.2.

Table 5.2 Work-up of ATLL

1. Immunophenotyping of peripheral blood and involved lymph nodes (a mature T-helper phenotype with CD25 expression in most cases).
2. A chemistry profile to document hypercalcemia, a high LDH, and abnormal liver function tests.
3. HTLV-I status assessed by one or more of the currently available techniques (enzyme assay and/or Western blot).
4. Detection of monoclonality in integration of HTLV-I proviral DNA in lymphocytes.
5. Histologic examination of involved tissues (e.g. skin, lymph nodes, bone marrow).

5.10 Cerebriform cells

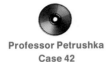

**Professor Petrushka
Case 42**

The term 'cerebriform cell' refers to the abnormal mononuclear cell characteristic of MF/Sezary syndrome. The following triad defines Sezary syndrome: (1) erythroderma with histologically proven MF, (2) lymphadenopathy, and (3) circulating cerebriform cells (i.e. Sezary cells).

The diagnosis of MF/Sezary syndrome requires correlation of the clinical presentation, skin biopsy findings and the cerebriform cytology of the neoplastic cells, especially since other NHLs, including ATLL and various peripheral T-cell lymphomas, can involve the skin. Because the disease is confined to the skin for many years, the patients often carry a diagnosis of long-standing chronic dermatitis.

There are two types of cerebriform cells, a small cell variant about the same size as a normal small lymphocyte, and a large cell variant (Figure 5.40). Both variants demonstrate a high nuclear/cytoplasmic ratio and hyperchromatic nuclei with marked nuclear folding. Fine focusing is often required to appreciate the cerebriform cytology. The presence of PAS-positive cytoplasmic vacuoles, arranged in a 'pearl necklace' pattern, is a helpful diagnostic clue (Figure 5.41).

In the early stage of peripheral blood involvement, the hemogram may be normal with few circulating Sezary cells, most of which are small. The involvement can be easily missed unless the clinical history of MF/Sezary syndrome was provided to prompt a careful search for Sezary cells. In some cases, the only hemogram abnormality may be eosinophilia or macrocytic anemia. Buffy coat preparations may be necessary to detect low numbers of circulating cerebriform cells. Similarly, the FCM results may be apparently normal. Subtle clues are usually present, however, including up-regulated expression of a T-cell marker

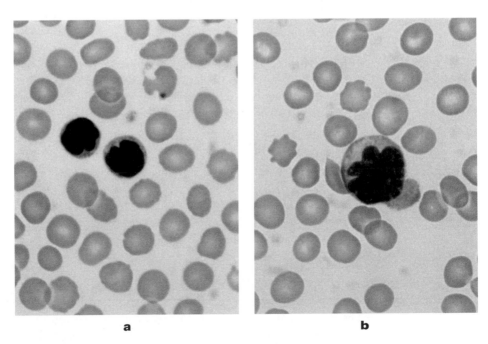

a   b

Figure 5.40   Small (a) and large (b) Sezary cells from the same patient

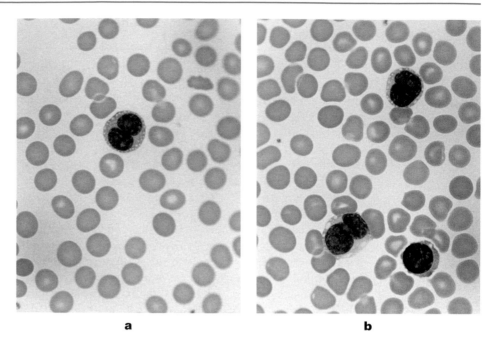

a   b

Figure 5.41 (a), (b) Sezary cells with cytoplasmic vacuoles arranged in a ' pearl necklace' pattern. Note that one of the cells also has a 'cleaved' appearance

or a marked increase in the proportion of CD4-positive helper T-cells (see Section 28.7). In cases where the FCM data are noninformative, molecular analysis of the *TCRβ* gene can reveal clonal rearrangement.

With disease progression, Sezary cells in the peripheral blood and bone marrow become more easily detectable because of an increase in large cells with marked nuclear irregularities and dense chromatin. At this stage, the cytologic features and heterogeneity of the neoplastic population overlap with those observed in ATLL and other leukemic non-Hodgkin's lymphomas.

Additional work-up that may help to establish a diagnosis of Sezary syndrome is shown in Table 5.3.

Table 5.3 Ancillary tests helpful in the diagnosis of Sezary syndrome

- A history of MF, documented by skin biopsies.
- Immunophenotyping by FCM if there is a high number of circulating abnormal cells.
- Electron microscopy.
- Determination of the patient's HTLV-I status to distinguish Sezary syndrome from ATLL. Sezary syndrome patients are HTLV-I negative. Patients with ATLL are HTLV-I positive.

5.11 Reactive lymphocytes (Downey II and Downey III cells)

The presence of large reactive lymphocytes in certain viral infections (e.g. IM) can trigger automated analyzers to generate suspect flags for blasts, variant/ reactive lymphocytes, and/or large unstained cells. Morphologically, the large lymphocytes may simulate a lymphoma cell (Figure 5.42) or blasts. Downey II and Downey III cells are the two main types of reactive lymphocytes. In practice, all intermediate stages between the small lymphocyte and the Downey III cell can be seen on the film. This reflects the spectrum of reactive changes in lymphocytes in response to antigenic stimuli, manifesting as enlarged cell size, increased cytoplasmic basophilia, less condensed nuclear chromatin and the appearance of nucleoli.

Downey II cells, typically associated with IM, have abundant pale blue cytoplasm with scalloped borders (Figure 5.43a). This morphology can be mimicked by the neoplastic plasmacytoid lymphocytes in LPC lymphoma-leukemia (Figure 5.43b). In IM, the reactive lymphocytes represent the proliferation of cytotoxic/suppressor CD8$^+$ T-cells reacting against EBV-infected B-cells. Although the morphologic findings in IM are highly characteristic, they are not pathognomonic. Similar features can be found in IM-like syndromes (e.g. CMV, toxoplasmosis, adenovirus, acute HIV infection, human herpes virus 6), other viral infections (e.g. viral hepatitis, rubella, roseola, mumps, chickenpox), and allergic reactions to drugs.

Downey III cells (also referred to as immunoblasts) demonstrate deeply basophilic cytoplasm, ovoid nuclei, reticulated chromatin and visible nucleoli (Figure 5.44a). Cytoplasmic vacuoles may be present. The nucleus may appear in a cloverleaf form because of delayed processing (Figure 5.44b). Downey III cells may simulate large lymphoma cells or Burkitt's cells. Therefore, it helps to examine any mononuclear cell against 'the company it keeps'.

Professor Petrushka
Cases 43 and 44

Professor Petrushka
Case 45

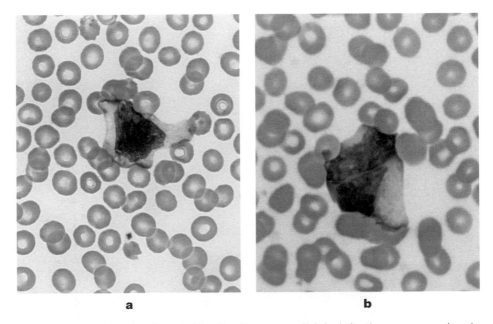

a   b

Figure 5.42 Reactive lymphoid cells (Downey cells) in infectious mononucleosis (a) and in an HIV-positive patient (b). Note the deep nuclear cleft in the Downey cell of the second patient, simulating the morphology of a large lymphoma cell. Subsequent work-up and follow-up disclosed no evidence of malignant lymphoma

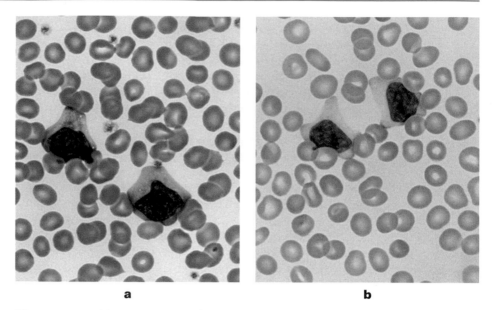

Figure 5.43 (a) Downey cells in an 18-year-old male with infectious mononucleosis (IM). (b) Neoplastic plasmacytoid lymphocytes in a 55-year-old male with lymphoplasmacytoid lymphoma-leukemia. The neoplastic cells were initially misinterpreted as reactive lymphocytes. Furthermore, the monospot test yielded a false-positive result. The patient's age and the persistent lymphocytosis were the only clues to warn against the diagnosis of IM. The correct diagnosis was established by FCM immunophenotyping. Serum IEP demonstrated a small monoclonal IgM spike

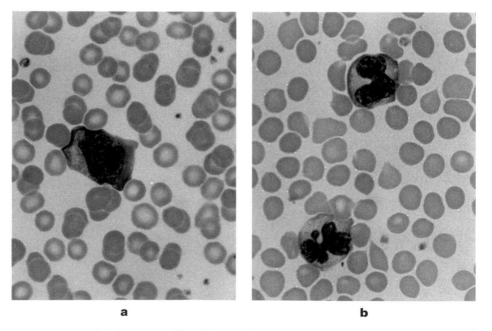

Figure 5.44 (a) A Downey III cell in a child with viral infection. Note the prominent nucleolus (compare with Figure 5.36b). (b) Artifactual 'cloverleaf' nuclear irregularities in one Downey cell caused by delayed processing

In reactive conditions, large basophilic lymphocytes are few in number and are accompanied by many other reactive lymphocytes including Downey II cells and intermediate forms. The Hgb level and platelet count are normal. These features point to the large basophilic cells being Downey III cells (immunoblasts). In a malignant process (e.g. ALL-L3), large basophilic cells predominate, and are accompanied by anemia and thrombocytopenia. In addition, the spectrum of reactive changes is lacking, i.e. there are too many large basophilic lymphocytes without accompanying Downey II cells. In difficult cases, the diagnosis should not rest on morphology alone. Additional studies (e.g. EBV serology and FCM immunophenotyping) should be performed.

The term 'atypical lymphocyte' has been used to mean either a benign reactive cell or a malignant lymphoid cell by different individuals or by the same individual at different times. The authors' have seen the following cell types referred to as atypical lymphocytes: (1) Sezary cells, (2) blasts, (3) hairy cells, (4) large granular lymphocytes, (5) prolymphocytes, (6) Burkitt's cells, (7) circulating lymphoma cells, and (8) reactive lymphocytes. Therefore, it is best to avoid the terminology 'atypical lymphocyte'. Distinctive lymphocytes should be classified precisely, and the term 'variant lymphocyte' or 'reactive lymphocyte' can be used for Downey cells.

Infectious mononucleosis is an acute viral illness caused by Epstein-Barr virus (EBV) infection. It is prevalent in affluent societies, since under lower socio-economic conditions immunity to EBV is acquired during childhood, often without any clinical manifestations. The infection is most frequent in young adults and rare above the age of 40. The most common clinical manifestations include sore throat, cervical lymphadenopathy (resolving within 4 weeks) and splenomegaly. During the acute illness, the WBC count is mildly increased with an absolute lymphocytosis composed of a spectrum of reactive/variant lymphocytes. Strict criteria for IM have been proposed as follows: in addition to the absolute lymphocytosis, the percentage of lymphocytes should be greater than 50% with at least 10% reactive/variant lymphocytes. At the time of diagnosis, many patients do not fulfill these criteria, however. A mild thrombocytopenia (i.e. a platelet count of $100–150 \times 10^9$/l) or a mild autoimmune hemolytic anemia (associated with a cold agglutinin having anti-i specificity) may be present.

Confirmation of IM can be carried out by testing for the presence of heterophil antibodies (Paul-Bunnell test) or with EBV serologies based on the detection of antibodies produced against various viral components during the course of IM. The first antibody to appear is an IgM anti-VCA (viral capsid antigen) which peaks around the second week and then declines rapidly. It is closely followed by IgG anti-VCA (peak around third to fourth week) which persists for life and represents permanent immunity to EBV. Antibodies to EA (early antigen) represent another marker of acute infection. The pattern here parallels that of IgM anti-VCA but these antibodies are not usually tested for. IgG anti-EBNA (Epstein-Barr nuclear antigen) appears only after resolution of symptoms and is a useful marker for remote EBV infection. The combination of a positive IgM anti-VCA and a negative IgG anti-EBNA is diagnostic of acute IM.

A rapid slide test (i.e. Monospot) is the most common method for detecting heterophil antibodies. In the proper clinical context, if the peripheral blood morphology meets the above criteria and the rapid slide test is positive, then the diagnosis of IM is confirmed. It is important to keep in mind the possibility of a false-positive rapid slide test in the context of a lymphoproliferative disorder. In patients with a persistent lymphocytosis above the age of 40, the diagnosis of IM warrants caution. In this setting, EBV serology is indicated to confirm a positive Monospot test.

If the blood film does not meet the diagnostic criteria, and the slide test is negative, IM is excluded. If the blood film criteria are met, but the slide test is negative, then the differential diagnosis is IM (with low heterophil antibodies which are not yet detectable) versus an IM-like syndrome such as CMV infection. A serologic test for EBV may be necessary. If the blood film is negative, but the slide test is positive, then a quantitative Paul-Bunnell tube test to rule out early IM should be performed.

The titer of the heterophil antibody can be determined by the quantitative Paul-Bunnell tube test. If the tube test is negative, the rapid slide test is presumed to be a false positive (which can occur in lymphomas and rubella). If the tube test is positive, the patient should be followed up with another peripheral blood sample since the appearance of the reactive lymphocytes may be lagging behind. Alternatively, the patient may be in the recovery phase of IM. Note that a few Downey cells may be present without an absolute lymphocytosis in either the early stage or resolution phase of a viral infection.

5.12 Mast cells

Similar to basophils, mast cells contain metachromatic granules. The larger cell size and abundance of granules distinguish mast cells from basophils (Figure 5.45). Mast cells are not detectable in the peripheral blood under normal circumstances. The presence of circulating mast cells is therefore indicative of systemic mastocytosis/mast cell leukemia. Mast cell leukemia is rare, usually presenting with mild leukocytosis and a variable proportion of circulating mast cells.

5.13 Unclassified cells

The vague, catch-all term 'unclassified cells' should be used only as a last resort when low numbers of abnormal cells are present (too few for adequate assessment and classification) and no additional clinical and laboratory information is available.

The phrases 'atypical cells present' or 'atypical mononuclear cells present' should be avoided because they can cause confusion with the reactive lymphocytes seen in viral disorders and do not help in the differential diagnosis between benign and malignant diseases.

When small numbers of unclassifiable cells are present, the following possibilities should be considered:

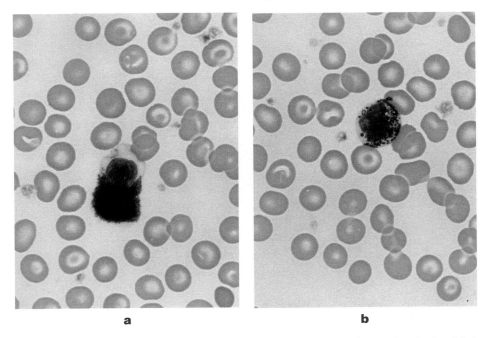

a   b

Figure 5.45   (a) A circulating mast cell in a case of systemic mastocytosis. (b) A basophil for comparison

1. Reactive lymphocytes, mainly Downey III cells, which can be pleomorphic enough to mimic malignant cells (blasts or circulating lymphoma cells). As noted above, the key to identifying Downey III cells is to pay attention to 'the company they keep'. In viral diseases, the absolute lymphocytosis is composed of a spectrum of reactive cells.
2. Hematogones, which are bone marrow stem cells seen primarily in children. It is extremely unusual to find hematogones on the peripheral blood film. The immunophenotype of hematogones is discussed in Section 25.4.
3. Blasts, usually in the setting of bicytopenia or pancytopenia. Rare blasts may circulate in myelodysplastic syndromes, acute leukemia, and during or following recent administration of multiagent chemotherapy.
4. Circulating lymphoma cells, which may be difficult to classify when the WBC count and the remainder of the hemogram are otherwise normal.
5. Solid tumor cells, which may rarely circulate in disseminated carcinomatosis (e.g. breast carcinoma) or small round cell sarcomas such as rhabdomyosarcoma (Figure 5.46). When present as single cells, they can be confused with blasts or Burkitt's cells.

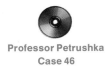

Professor Petrushka
Case 46

The clinical data, especially a history of known malignancies, and examination of follow-up blood films can help to determine the nature of 'unclassifiable' cells. If the unusual cells persist or increase, bone marrow studies and immunophenotyping may be indicated.

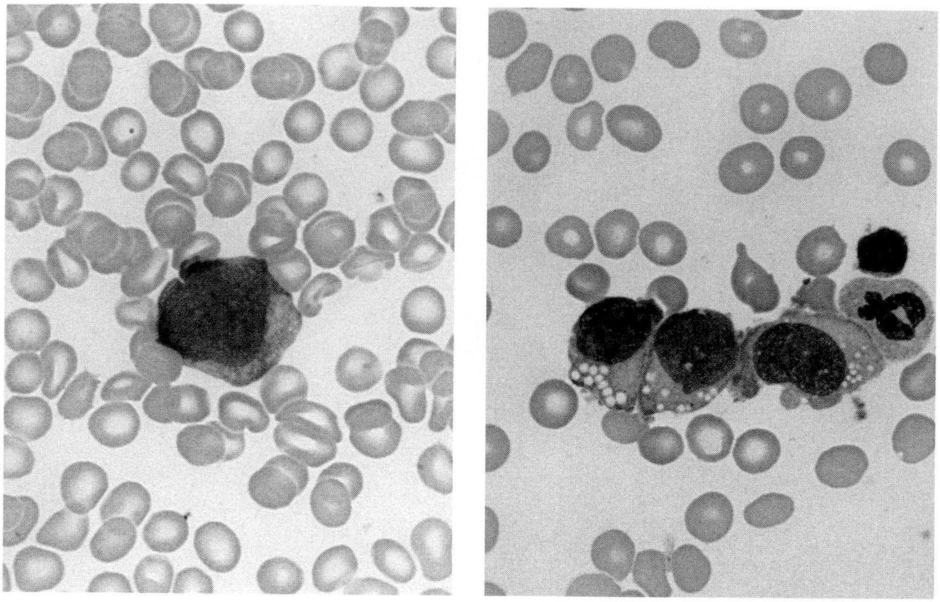

a   b

Figure 5.46   Two different cases of rhabdomyosarcoma with a low number (3–5%) of circulating malignant cells. (a) The neoplastic cell simulates the morphology of a blast. (b) Neoplastic cells with cytoplasmic vacuoles, simulating the morphology of Burkitt's cells

Erythrocytosis pattern

The erythrocytosis pattern is characterized by increased hemoglobin along with an increased RBC count. It is normal, however, for the hemoglobin level, the red blood cell mass, and the MCV to be high in the first month of life.

Erythrocytosis can be caused by an autonomous proliferation of erythroid precursors (i.e. primary erythrocytosis) or can be secondary to either tissue hypoxia (e.g. high altitude, pulmonary diseases, smoking, congenital cyanotic heart disease, and high oxygen-affinity hemoglobins) or inappropriate erythropoietin production. Inappropriate erythropoietin production can occur in the following neoplasms: renal tumors, cerebellar hemangioblastoma, hepatoma, extremely large uterine leiomyomas, and adrenal tumors. Clinical information and laboratory data are necessary to separate primary from secondary polycythemia.

Primary congenital polycythemia, also known as idiopathic erythrocytosis or familial polycythemia is a rare disorder that is diagnosed by exclusion. Most cases are asymptomatic and the erythrocytosis is discovered incidentally. Features of an MPD (splenomegaly, thrombocytosis, basophilia, marrow panhyperplasia) and clinical complications are absent. This heterogeneous group of disorders is not associated with hemoglobin mutations or enzyme abnormalities. Some cases demonstrate increased crythropoietin production and others have normal or decreased erythropoietin levels. Family studies may be helpful.

In the erythrocytosis pattern, the presence of basophilia, a moderate thrombocytosis (in the range of $500–800 \times 10^9$/l) (Figure 6.1) or hypochromic, microcytic RBCs suggests the diagnosis of PRV, a myeloproliferative disorder. Basophilia is a feature common to most MPDs. It is present in about 65% of cases of PRV. If basophilia is not present, and the patient has been venesected, the blood picture in PRV can simulate that of thalassemia minor/trait. The hypochromia and microcytosis reflect iron deficiency due to the marked erythroid expansion. Rare NRBCs may be present. Repeated venesections, often used as part of the therapy for PRV, accentuate the iron deficiency.

**Professor Petrushka
Case 47**

In PRV, there is usually an associated leukocytosis and neutrophilia with a mild left shift. However, these features may also be seen in secondary polycythemias, such as those induced by pulmonary disorders or chronic heavy smoking.

Splenomegaly, due to large splenic red cell pools, is a key clinical feature that separates PRV from secondary polycythemias. Extramedullary hematopoiesis is minimal.

Symptoms related to hyperviscosity are also prominent clinical findings in PRV. Hyperviscosity can cause phlebitis (with resulting gangrene of the lower extremities), transient ischemic attacks, and pruritus. The most serious consequences are cerebrovascular accidents.

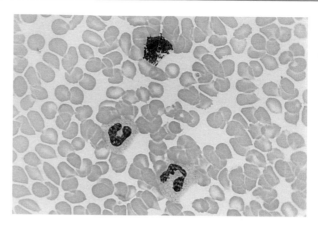

Figure 6.1 Sample from a patient with polycythemia vera exhibiting a markedly increased Hgb level (19 g/dl) and RBC count, which account for crowding of the red cells even in the zone of morphology. The patient also had mild basophilia and mild neutrophilia

According to the Polycythemia Vera Study Group, there are three major and three minor criteria to be used in the diagnosis of PRV. The major criteria are increased RBC mass, normal oxygen saturation and splenomegaly. Total RBC mass can be measured by isotopic dilution studies. This test can be omitted if the hemoglobin is greater than 20 g/dl. The minor criteria are a platelet count greater than $400 \times 10^9/l$, a WBC count greater than $12 \times 10^9/l$, and either a leukocyte alkaline phosphatase score greater than 100 (in the absence of inflammation) or a serum B_{12} level of greater than 900 pg/ml. A presumed diagnosis of PRV is made if all three major criteria are met or if the first two major criteria are met along with any two minor criteria. The diagnosis should be confirmed with a bone marrow aspirate and biopsy. In PRV, the bone marrow will demonstrate panhyperplasia (a feature shared with other MPDs) and an absence of stainable iron. Cytogenetic abnormalities may be present.

Table 6.1 lists six sequential steps that can be applied to differentiate PRV from other causes of erythrocytosis.

Table 6.1 Sequential steps to differentiate PRV from other causes of erythrocytosis

1. Measurement of total RBC mass. A normal RBC mass indicates a relative polycythemia.
2. If the RBC mass is increased, measure arterial oxygen saturation.
3. If oxygen saturation is greater than 92%, proceed to a measurement of carboxyhemoglobin. An arterial oxygen saturation below 92% indicates a secondary polycythemia due to a cardiopulmonary disorder.
4. If carboxyhemoglobin is normal, look at the Hgb–oxygen dissociation curve. Increased carboxyhemoglobin indicates smoker's polycythemia.
5. If the Hgb–oxygen dissociation curve results are normal, then measurement of erythropoietin (EPO) in serum and/or urine is indicated. If the oxygen pressure at which hemoglobin is half saturated is low, it indicates a secondary polycythemia due to a high oxygen affinity hemoglobin.
6. If EPO is decreased, perform erythroid colony growth to confirm PRV. Increased EPO production indicates a secondary polycythemia possibly due to autonomous EPO production by an underlying neoplasm. Decreased or absent EPO is strongly suggestive of PRV. Erythroid colony growth is an *in vitro* assessment of EPO requirements. In PRV, the erythroid precursors require little or no EPO to grow. In primary congenital polycythemia, erythroid colony formation only occurs when EPO is added.

Thrombocytosis pattern

Thrombocytosis can occur as the sole peripheral blood feature or in association with other pathology. In the latter instance, other peripheral blood findings predominate over the raised platelet count, which is usually moderate rather than marked.

Similar to erythrocytosis, thrombocytosis can be classified as either primary or secondary. Primary thrombocytosis results from an autonomous proliferation of megakaryocytes, as seen in ET and other MPDs. Secondary thrombocytoses are 'reactive' thrombocytoses occurring in several conditions including occult malignancies, infections, status post-splenectomy and rebound from prior thrombocytopenia. The relationship between the degree of thrombocytosis and the other CBC parameters helps to make this distinction. For example, in occult malignancy the mild to moderate thrombocytosis ($< 1000 \times 10^9/l$) is overshadowed by the coexisting anemia. With a more severe thrombocytosis, however, the distinction between a primary and secondary thrombocytosis is more difficult. Other clinical and laboratory findings aid in the differential diagnosis.

The degree of thrombocytosis required for consideration of a diagnosis of ET varies between institutions. Although the Polycythemia Vera Study Group recommends $600 \times 10^9/l$ as the cut-off, the studies were conducted on patients with at least $1000 \times 10^9/l$. This higher threshold is more useful since more than 90% of patients with ET present with platelet counts above that level. A lower threshold results in a higher overlap with reactive conditions.

It should be noted that even among patients with platelet counts above $1000 \times 10^9/l$, a substantial number do not have ET. Prior to diagnosing ET, the two most important differential diagnoses to consider are malignancy and infection/inflammation. Both conditions may be occult, and both can produce peripheral blood findings indistinguishable from those of ET, including platelet counts of $1000–1500 \times 10^9/l$ along with a mild to moderate leukocytosis. It is extremely rare for the platelet count to exceed $2000 \times 10^9/l$ in a reactive thrombocytosis. At that level, the diagnosis is either ET or another MPD.

Furthermore, the peripheral blood findings in ET (Figure 7.1) can overlap with those in other MPDs. For instance, in CML under therapy, fluctuations in the peripheral counts may result in a blood picture indistinguishable from ET. Variation in platelet size and abundant giant platelets are common in straightforward cases of ET (Figure 7.2a). However, this feature is not always present, particularly in those cases that need to be differentiated from secondary thrombocytosis. Furthermore, variation in platelet size, platelet aggregates, and abnormal platelets (e.g. giant and/or hypogranulated platelets) also feature in other MPDs (Figure 7.2b) and in reactive thrombocytoses.

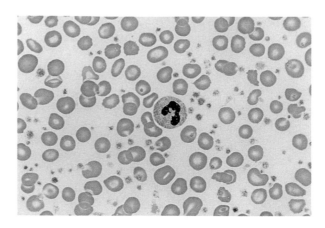

Figure 7.1 Severe thrombocytosis (platelet count 1300 $\times$ 10^9/l) in a case of essential thrombocythemia. There is minimal variation in the size of the platelets

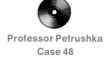

Professor Petrushka
Case 48

Conversely, a small number of patients with ET have normal or slightly elevated platelet counts. The diagnosis rests on the clinical manifestations (thromboembolism, bleeding). These features can also be found in PRV, however. Additional helpful studies include *in vitro* culture of bone marrow precursors and testing for platelet stickiness.

The current diagnostic criteria for ET are listed in Table 7.1. These criteria indicate the importance of ruling out other MPDs (such as PRV, AMM and

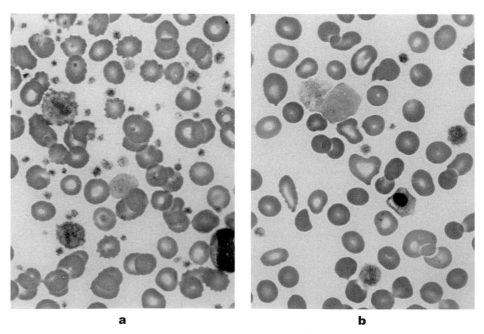

a   b

Figure 7.2 Giant platelets in ET (a) and AMM (b)

Table 7.1 Criteria for the diagnosis of ET

- A persistent elevated platelet count, preferably on three different blood counts separated from each other by 3-month intervals.
- Hemoglobin less than 13 g/dl or a normal RBC mass (males <30 ml/kg, females <32 ml/kg).
- A bone marrow with stainable iron on the aspirate (or normal MCV and ferritin levels). The presence of stainable iron is more reliable than either a normal MCV or serum ferritin.
- No collagen fibrosis in the bone marrow biopsy. Recently, it has been accepted that if collagen fibrosis is present then it should occupy less than one-third of the biopsy area and neither splenomegaly nor a leukoerythroblastic reaction should be present.
- No evidence of the Philadelphia chromosome and no *bcr-abl* rearrangement.
- No evidence (especially cytogenetically) of an MDS.
- No known cause for a reactive thrombocytosis.

CML) and myelodysplastic syndromes with thrombocytosis (e.g. RARS or an MDS associated with abnormalities of chromosome 3). The diagnosis of ET is predominantly a diagnosis of exclusion.

CHAPTER 8

Absolute lymphocytosis pattern

Absolute lymphocytosis is defined as a lymphocyte count greater than $4 \times 10^9/l$ in adults. Since lymphocyte counts are normally higher in children than adults, higher thresholds are used to define absolute lymphocytosis in infants ($> 10 \times 10^9/l$ at less than 2 years of age) and children ($> 7 \times 10^9/l$ between 2 and 10 years of age).

An absolute lymphocytosis, as reported by the automated analyzers, can be composed of either normal-appearing lymphocytes (e.g. small lymphocytes, plasmacytoid lymphocytes, large granular lymphocytes) and/or lymphoid cells with 'abnormal' morphology, which may trigger suspect flags for blasts or variant lymphocytes. The 'abnormal mononuclear cell' pattern (see Chapter 5) is applicable if cells with 'abnormal' morphology are seen on the blood film (e.g. cerebriform cells, circulating lymphoma cells or Downey cells) irrespective of any lymphocytosis. The 'absolute lymphocytosis' pattern applies when the lymphocytosis is composed of cells with normal-appearing morphology.

The differential diagnosis between a neoplastic lymphocytosis (i.e. a lymphoproliferative disorder) and a benign lymphocytosis is straightforward if the lymphocyte count is marked (at least $15 \times 10^9/l$ in an adult). The distinction can be more problematic with a lesser degree of absolute lymphocytosis, unless FCM immunophenotyping and/or other pertinent clinical and laboratory data are available. The lymphocytosis is benign if the proliferation is mature and there is no evidence of either monoclonality or an aberrant T-cell phenotype.

8.1 Benign (reactive) lymphocytoses

Reactive lymphocytoses can be secondary to stress, infections or splenectomy. Transient (stress) lymphocytosis is occasionally observed in patients with emergency medical conditions including trauma (e.g. sickle cell crisis, acute myocardial infarcts and motor vehicle accidents). The lymphocytosis is usually mild to moderate (i.e. $5–10 \times 10^9/l$) and of short duration. The lymphocyte count returns to normal within 48 hours. The cause of stress lymphocytosis is thought to be endogenous release of epinephrine. In these conditions, the lymphoid population is composed predominantly of small, mature-appearing lymphocytes with occasional reactive-appearing cells.

Infectious lymphocytosis occurs in young children secondary to various viral illnesses. A marked lymphocytosis ($> 10 \times 10^9/l$) is also a significant part of the laboratory picture in *Bordetella pertussis* infection ('whooping cough') (Figure 8.1). A small number of lymphocytes with nuclear indentations (similar to

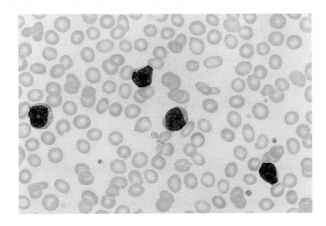

Figure 8.1   Lymphocytosis in an 8-year-old child with whooping cough and iron deficiency. Note the hypochromic and microcytic RBCs

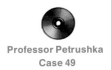

Professor Petrushka
Case 49

those seen in circulating small lymphoma cells) is common in normal children (Figure 8.2).

It is very important to know the age of the patient when reviewing the peripheral blood film in order to avoid a misdiagnosis of a malignant lymphoproliferative disorder. In viral-related lymphocytosis, the reactive population is usually a mixture of small lymphocytes, plasmacytoid lymphocytes and frequently a few Downey cells (see Section 5.11).

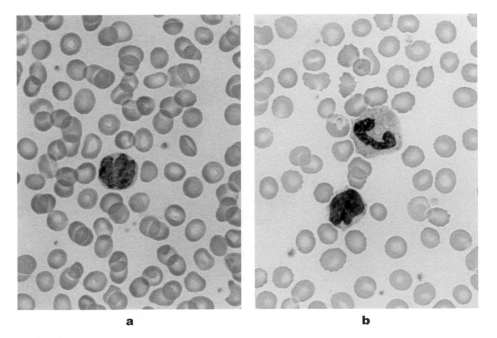

a   b

Figure 8.2   (a), (b) Blood films from two different children, showing nuclear indentations in normal lymphocytes

Mild absolute lymphocytosis (usually 4–$6 \times 10^9/l$) is normal after splenectomy. The lymphocytes are morphologically unremarkable and are accompanied by the telltale presence of Howell-Jolly bodies. In older subjects, the distinction between benign lymphocytosis secondary to splenectomy and early CLL may be difficult. The age of the patient and immunophenotyping to rule out monoclonality are the keys to establishing the correct diagnosis.

8.2 Lymphoproliferative disorders (LPDs)

In neoplastic lymphocytosis, the cell population can be composed predominantly of small round lymphocytes, plasmacytoid lymphocytes or large granular lymphocytes (LGLs). Disorders with a mixture of small round lymphocytes, plasmacytoid lymphocytes and some prolymphocytes belong to the general category of CLL and related disorders, including LPC lymphoma-leukemia, Waldenstrom's macroglobulinemia (WM) and CLL/PL.

Plasmacytoid lymphocytes (Figure 8.3) can be recognized by the following features which are presumptive evidence of protein synthesis, activation and/or progression towards plasma cell differentiation:

- A larger, eccentrically placed nucleus, with a small distinct nucleolus, condensed chromatin and moderate to ample pale blue cytoplasm. The larger

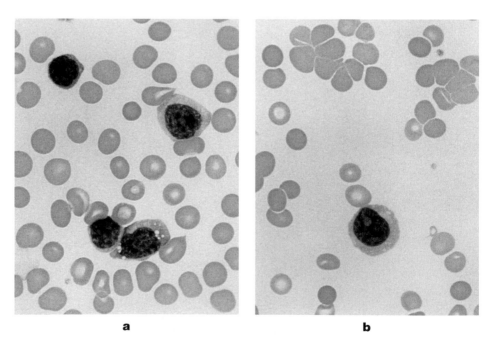

a   b

Figure 8.3 (a) Two plasmacytoid lymphocytes and two small round lymphocytes from a case of LPC lymphoma-leukemia. One of the plasmacytoid lymphocytes has a more basophilic cytoplasm (with vacuoles) and a less distinct nucleolus. (b) A plasmacytoid lymphocyte and rouleaux formation in Waldenstrom's macroglobulinemia

nucleus is still within the range of a small cell, i.e. about twice the diameter of an RBC.

- With increasing differentiation towards the plasma cell stage, the cytoplasm becomes more basophilic, the chromatin more cartwheel, and the nucleolus is no longer visible (these cells may referred to as plasmacytic lymphocytes). Occasional cytoplasmic vacuoles may be present. Small lymphoid cells with a bit of eccentric cytoplasm should not be enumerated as plasmacytoid lymphocytes (Figure 8.4).

Large granular lymphocytes also have eccentrically placed nuclei. However, they can be identified by the presence of small azurophilic granules. In rare instances, neoplastic LGLs are agranular and therefore can be easily mistaken for plasmacytoid lymphocytes (Figure 8.5b).

8.2.1 Chronic lymphocytic leukemia (CLL)

Chronic lymphocytic leukemia, an indolent B-cell disorder, is the most common of the chronic leukemias, accounting for approximately 70% of LPDs. The disease is seen more frequently in men (male/female ratio of 2.5:1) and occurs very rarely before age 40. The degree of lymphocytosis is variable, depending on the stage of the disease at presentation. A significant number of patients are asymptomatic, with the lymphocytosis discovered incidentally during a routine blood examination.

8.2.1.1 Peripheral blood findings in CLL

In most cases, the leukemic population is homogeneous and composed of quasi-normal-appearing small lymphocytes with scant cytoplasm, round nuclei, and

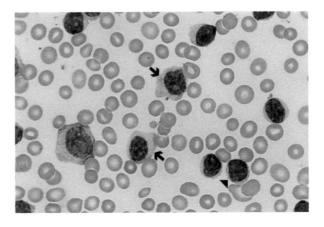

Figure 8.4 Lymphoplasmacytoid lymphoma-leukemia (with strong expression of B-cell antigens, monoclonal surface light chain, and no expression of CD5, CD10 or CD23), composed of a mixture of plasmacytoid lymphocytes (arrow), small round lymphocytes (arrowhead) and occasional prolymphocytes. In this patient, plasmacytoid lymphocytes (arrow) constituted the majority of the neoplastic cells

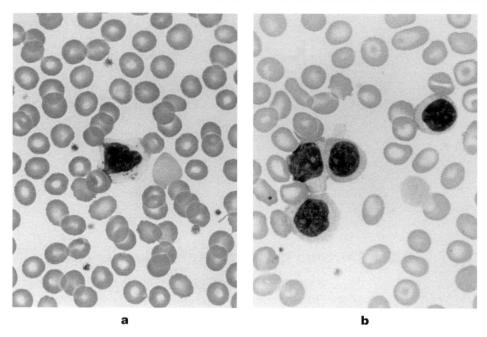

a   b

Figure 8.5 (a) A large granular lymphocyte in normal blood. (b) Neoplastic 'agranular' LGLs

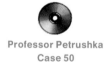

Professor Petrushka
Case 50

clumped chromatin (Figure 8.6). The fragility of CLL cells accounts for the frequently observed 'smudge cells'. Smudge cells are not pathognomonic for CLL, however, and can occur in other leukemias and in normal blood following prolonged storage. When cells are smudged, their identity is uncertain (e.g. lymphocyte vs. prolymphocyte). Therefore, they should not be included in the manual differential.

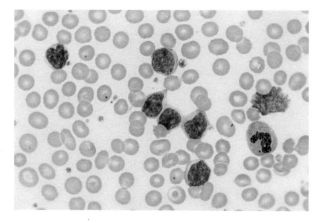

Figure 8.6 Chronic lymphocytic leukemia in a 60-year-old male. One of the lymphocytes (top left) exhibits nuclear irregularities. The patient had long-standing disease and was given different chemotherapy regimens over the years. Note the nuclear fragment in the neutrophil, indicative of chemotherapy effects. The patient also had his spleen removed (Howell-Jolly bodies)

The neoplastic population may also include:

1. A variable proportion of plasmacytoid lymphocytes (Figure 8.7). In general, the number of plasmacytoid cells in CLL should be much less than the number of small lymphocytes, whereas the reverse is true in LPC leukemia-lymphoma/Waldenstrom's macroglobulinemia.
2. A few cells with clefted nuclei ($\leqslant 5\%$), similar to circulating lymphoma cells. This feature is common in long-standing CLL. Ensure that the nuclear irregularity is not an artifact secondary to delayed processing.
3. Prolymphocytes ($\leqslant 10\%$). Disorders with more than 10% prolymphocytes, i.e. CLL/PL and PLL, are discussed in Chapter 5.

8.2.1.2 Other features in CLL

Anemia and/or thrombocytopenia ultimately develop in CLL, primarily due to decreased hematopoietic reserve as a consequence of the progressively increased bone marrow tumor burden. Immune thrombocytopenia occurs in only 1–2% of patients in CLL.

The anemia in CLL is normocytic or mildly macrocytic. A macrocytic anemia may reflect disturbed erythropoiesis associated with malignancy/chemotherapy or unsuspected B_{12}/folate deficiency, common in elderly patients with CLL. A sudden severe drop in Hgb may indicate superimposed red cell aplasia caused by parvovirus B19 infection.

Approximately 10–20% of patients with CLL are Coombs-positive, but less than half of these develop overt autoimmune hemolytic anemia (AIHA) with frequent spherocytes (Figure 8.8). The severity of the AIHA bears no relationship to the stage of the CLL. Polychromasia may be absent/minimal because of decreased bone marrow hematopoietic reserve.

Other clinical features of CLL include lymphadenopathy and hepatosplenomegaly. Lymphadenopathy is present in up to 70–90% of patients with CLL.

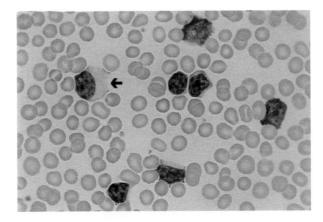

Figure 8.7 Chronic lymphocytic leukemia. The neoplastic population is composed predominantly of small lymphocytes. An occasional plasmacytoid lymphocyte (arrow) is present

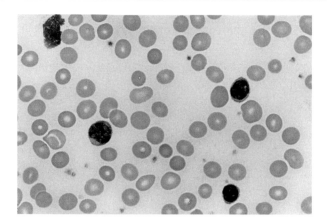

Figure 8.8 Occasional spherocytes in a case of CLL with mild autoimmune hemolytic anemia

The lymph node counterpart of CLL is small lymphocytic lymphoma (SLL). This is just a semantic distinction. Chronic lymphocytic leukemia and SLL are two different initial presentations of the same disease. Patients with peripheral blood disease, i.e. CLL, invariably develop lymphadenopathy. Conversely, those with initial nodal-based disease (SLL) ultimately demonstrate leukemic manifestations.

8.2.1.3 Differential diagnosis of CLL

Morphologically, the differential diagnosis of CLL includes reactive lymphocytosis, NHL in leukemic phase, Waldenstrom's macroglobulinemia and LPC lymphoma-leukemia. A reactive lymphocytosis cannot be excluded if the lymphocytosis is less than $15 \times 10^9/l$ and the patient is less than 40 years of age. An abundance of cells with indented nuclei suggests circulating lymphoma cells. The degree of lymphocytosis, the morphology of the lymphoid cells, the age of the patient, the lymph node findings and FCM immunophenotyping are all useful in establishing the correct diagnosis. In CLL, the lymph node histology is that of an SLL, with proliferation centers present in the great majority of cases.

8.2.1.4 Recommended work-up for CLL

The most important steps in the diagnostic work-up for CLL are FCM immunophenotyping, a bone marrow aspirate/biopsy and assessment of serum immunoglobulins. A lymph node biopsy, if lymphadenopathy exists, and molecular genetics may be useful. The characteristic immunophenotype in CLL (CD19$^+$, CD5$^+$, CD23$^+$, weak CD20 and weak monoclonal sIg) is distinctive enough to rule out reactive lymphocytoses and separate CLL from an NHL in leukemic phase.

Often, bone marrow studies are omitted at diagnosis in CLL and are only performed because of anemia or thrombocytopenia. An Hgb of less than 10 g/dl and a low platelet count (i.e. $< 100 \times 10^9/l$) are poor prognostic factors in CLL if they are secondary to bone marrow infiltration. In clinical trials, a bone marrow is often done at presentation to establish the baseline tumor burden and hematopoietic reserve.

Serial serum protein immunoelectrophoresis over the disease course is useful to separate CLL from Waldenstrom's macroglobulinemia/LPC lymphoma-leukemia. Patients with CLL invariably develop hypogammaglobulinemia during the course of their disease and an IgM or IgA monoclonal band is not present.

Although not usually included in the routine work-up, a lymph node biopsy with FCM immunophenotyping can be essential to identify NHL in leukemic phase (which may be overlooked as CLL morphologically) or transformation of CLL into high-grade lymphoma (Richter's syndrome). This infrequent complication can be suspected when the clinical course deteriorates with development of fever, night sweats, and/or weight loss.

8.2.2 Waldenstrom's macroglobulinemia and lymphoplasmacytoid lymphoma-leukemia

Waldenstrom's macroglobulinemia is an indolent disease, similar to CLL, but with morbidity caused by the monoclonal (M) protein and increased plasma viscosity. The clinical manifestations may be preceded by several years of so-called 'monoclonal gammopathy of undetermined significance' (MGUS). With disease progression, splenomegaly, lymphadenopathy, and the consequences of hyperviscosity replace the initial vague constitutional symptoms.

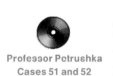

**Professor Petrushka
Cases 51 and 52**

Waldenstrom's macroglobulinemia can present with either a relative lymphocytosis or an absolute lymphocytosis. Closely related to and overlapping with Waldenstrom's macroglobulinemia is the category of LPC lymphoma-leukemia. Lymphadenopathy is more common in the latter group, whereas the M-spike is at least 20 g/l in the former. The relationship between the two disorders is discussed in Section 39.2.1.

In either disorder, the neoplastic population consists mostly of plasmacytoid lymphocytes (see Section 8.2), with a lesser number of small lymphocytes (Figure 8.9). Note that neoplastic plasmacytoid lymphocytes may be mistaken for reactive lymphocytes (Figure 5.43). Occasional prolymphocytes or immunoblasts are usually present. The degree of rouleaux depends on the level of M protein (Figure 8.10). Excessive M protein results in plasma hyperviscosity, leading to visual impairment, headaches and polyneuropathies. The M protein also interacts with coagulation factors and/or causes abnormal platelet function resulting in increased bleeding.

The diagnostic work-up mentioned in Section 8.2.1 applies to Waldenstrom's macroglobulinemia. The diagnosis of Waldenstrom's macroglobulinemia rests on the identification and quantitation of the M protein by immunoelectrophoresis (or immunofixation) and bone marrow studies. The M protein, usually an IgM or less commonly an IgA, can be quantitated by nephelometry. In some patients, the M protein is present in the urine. The differential diagnosis includes multiple myeloma and MGUS.

The features necessary for a diagnosis of MGUS are shown in Table 8.1. Since a substantial number of patients initially diagnosed as MGUS subsequently exhi-

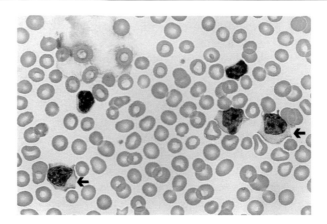

Figure 8.9 Lymphoplasmacytoid lymphoma-leukemia in a 58-year-old male with a small monoclonal IgM band. The neoplastic population is composed predominantly of plasmacytoid lymphocytes (arrow)

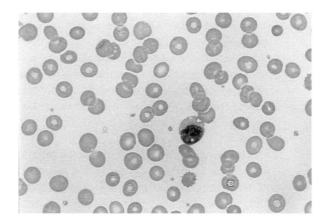

Figure 8.10 Waldenstrom's macroglobulinemia: rouleaux and plasmacytoid lymphocytes with cytoplasmic vacuoles

Table 8.1 Diagnostic features of MGUS

- No lymphadenopathy.
- No Bence-Jones proteinuria.
- Normal liver and spleen.
- No evidence of lytic bone lesions.
- A stable low level of serum M protein (<2.5 g/dl) over a long period.

bit the full clinical and pathologic picture of multiple myeloma or Waldenstrom's macroglobulinemia, MGUS requires careful follow-up.

The distinction of Waldenstrom's macroglobulinemia from multiple myeloma is based on bone marrow morphology, the immunologic profile and the clinical and laboratory features including the results of serum immunoelectrophoresis. In Waldenstrom's macroglobulinemia, there is a mixture of small lymphocytes and plasmacytoid lymphocytes. In multiple myeloma, the predominant cells are plasma cells and plasmablasts.

Unlike CLL, Waldenstrom's macroglobulinemia does not have a 'fingerprint' immunologic profile. In Waldenstrom's macroglobulinemia, the malignant lymphoid cells are B cells with a variable expression of CD5, CD38, and CD23 (see Section 27.5.5). The sIg staining intensity is usually strong. The lack of a well-defined immunologic profile partly reflects the lack of uniform criteria to define lymphoplasmacytic neoplasms. Most cases are negative for CD5 and CD23.

8.2.3 Large granular lymphocytosis/leukemia

Large granular lymphocytosis has been the subject of much confusion. Prior to the era of DNA gene rearrangement studies, it was not possible to firmly establish the neoplastic nature of the disease. Proliferations of LGLs are a heterogeneous group of disorders, including reactive conditions, indolent clonal disease and aggressive malignancies. There is a marked overlap in the clinical features, hematological findings and immunologic profile between the reactive conditions and the indolent clonal proliferations. Diagnosis is often problematic.

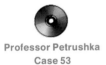

Professor Petrushka
Case 53

It is easier to appreciate LGLs on peripheral blood films than on bone marrow smears. Large granular lymphocytes constitute about 10–20% of peripheral blood lymphocytes in normal subjects (Figure 8.5a). Various conditions (e.g. AIDS, chemotherapy and malignant lymphomas) may be associated with a mild relative or absolute increase in LGLs overlapping with the LGL levels seen in indolent LGL leukemia. Occasionally, the neoplastic LGLs appear agranular by light microscopy and therefore may be mistaken for plasmacytoid lymphocytes (Figure 8.11).

Several terminologies (T-CLL, T-γ lymphocytosis) have been used to designate indolent LGL leukemia. With the widespread use of the FAB classification of chronic lymphoproliferative disorders, T-CLL has become a 'nonentity'. Indolent LGL leukemia is frequently associated with autoimmune disease (rheumatoid arthritis in 20–30% of patients), isolated unexplained neutropenia or, less commonly, red cell aplasia. Although the disease can occur in any age group, including young adults, it is rare in children. The majority of patients are asymptomatic unless the accompanying neutropenia is severe enough to result in recurrent infections. Lymphocytosis is mild to moderate (5–15 $\times$ 10^9/l) with LGLs comprising 60–90% of the lymphocytes.

The proposed diagnostic criteria for LGL leukemia include: (1) an unexplained increase in the absolute LGL count of at least 2 $\times$ 10^9 LGLs/l; or (2) LGLs should constitute greater than 50% of lymphocytes and the increase should persist for at least 6 months. There should be no evidence of viral infection, underlying

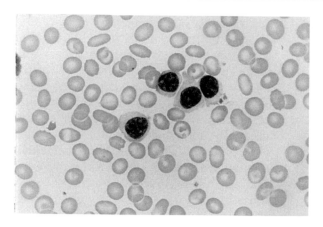

Figure 8.11 A CD3^{+} LGL leukemia in which the neoplastic cells are agranular by light microscopy. The enlarged spleen (secondary to tumor involvement) had been previously removed

malignancy or chemotherapy. The diagnosis can be made with less than 2×10^9LGLs/l if other features supportive of malignancy (visceral involvement, karyotypic abnormalities) are present. These manifestations are unusual in indolent LGL leukemia, however.

The aggressive forms of LGL leukemia manifest with rapidly progressive lymphocytosis and widespread systemic involvement (see Section 40.5.2.4). In aggressive disease, the neoplastic lymphocytes are often larger with fewer granules and less condensed nuclear chromatin (Figure 8.12).

The diagnosis and immunologic classification of LGL disorders requires peripheral blood FCM immunophenotyping and *TCR* gene rearrangement studies to determine clonality (see Section 28.4).

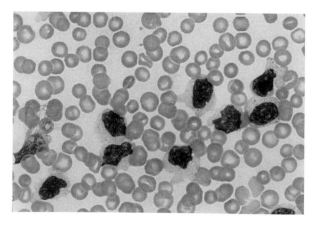

Figure 8.12 Aggressive LGL leukemia composed of large neoplastic cells. The patient presented with massive hepatosplenomegaly, extensive bone marrow involvement and rising leukocytosis, and expired 6 months after diagnosis

8.2.4 Acute lymphoblastic leukemia (ALL)

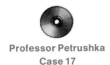

**Professor Petrushka
Case 17**

Most cases of ALL trigger flagging for 'blasts', 'variant lymphocytes' or 'large unstained cells' on the automated analyzer. No flag may be triggered if the blasts are small, close to the size of normal lymphocytes, however. The resulting hemogram may only indicate a lymphocytosis, accompanied by an inappropriately severe anemia and thrombocytopenia. The 'missed' blasts are usually picked up on examination of the blood film. Not infrequently, however, small blasts with homogeneous nuclear chromatin may be overlooked as normal lymphocytes.

To avoid misidentification of small blasts as lymphocytes, one should keep in mind that the nuclear diameter of small lymphocytes with scant cytoplasm is approximately that of an erythrocyte. Benign/reactive lymphocytes with a larger nuclear diameter have an accompanying increase in the amount of cytoplasm. Therefore, any 'lymphocyte' with a nuclear size equal to or greater than 2–2.5 times the size of an erythrocyte, but with a thin rim of cytoplasm, should be thought of as abnormal, and a small blast must be considered (Figure 5.7).

Thrombocytopenia pattern

The thrombocytopenia pattern is defined by platelet counts below the lower limit of normal (usually $150 \times 10^9/l$). Thrombocytopenia can result from impaired production of platelets (either congenital or acquired) or peripheral destruction of platelets.

In primary platelet disorders, thrombocytopenia usually occurs as an isolated abnormality. When accompanied by either leukopenia or anemia, the thrombocytopenia is usually secondary to another disease process (e.g. acute leukemia, MDS or severe B_{12}/folate deficiency). In these instances, other peripheral blood findings predominate over the decreased platelet count.

9.1 Morphologic findings

Peripheral blood film examination is important to confirm that the low platelet count reported by the automated analyzer is not an artifact, i.e. there should be no evidence of platelet clumping, phagocytosis of platelets, or platelet satellites around neutrophils (Figure 9.1). Platelet morphology, mean platelet volume, and platelet distribution width are of limited diagnostic significance in most cases. Although the presence of giant platelets suggests peripheral destruction, this finding can also be seen in MPDs and hereditary platelet abnormalities.

**Professor Petrushka
Case 54**

In some diseases, the constellation of findings associated with the thrombocytopenia can suggest the final diagnosis. The combination of thrombocytopenia with giant platelets and distinct, large Döhle-like bodies in granulocytes and monocytes is pathognomonic for May-Hegglin anomaly (Figure 3.6). In addition, when thrombocytopenia is associated with anemia and abundant schistocytes, then thrombotic thrombocytopenic purpura (TTP), hemolytic uremic syndrome (HUS), or disseminated intravascular coagulation (DIC) should be considered.

The work-up of isolated thrombocytopenia requires thorough clinical information. Special platelet function studies (e.g. aggregation tests) may be useful in some instances. In the older age group, thrombocytopenia may be the sole manifestation of underlying malignancy (e.g. light chain multiple myeloma). A bone marrow study may be worthwhile before rendering a diagnosis of chronic idiopathic thrombocytopenic purpura (ITP) in such instances.

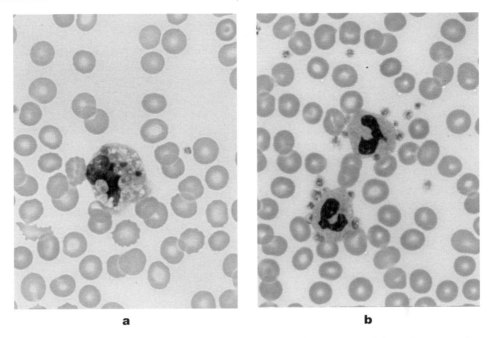

a   b

Figure 9.1   (a) Phagocytosis of platelets, an infrequent cause of thrombocytopenia.
(b) Platelet satellites

9.2 Classification of thrombocytopenia

Thrombocytopenias are usually divided into the hereditary and acquired types. The acquired thrombocytopenias are further subdivided on the basis of the pathophysiologic mechanism involved, peripheral destruction or impaired production.

9.2.1 Acquired thrombocytopenias

Acquired thrombocytopenias secondary to impaired production of platelets include both drug-induced and viral-induced bone marrow suppression. Drug-induced bone marrow suppression can be caused by antibiotics, thiazide, chemotherapy or heavy alcohol consumption. Viruses known to be associated with bone marrow suppression include varicella, rubella, Coxsackie, CMV and herpes simplex.

Thrombocytopenias secondary to peripheral destruction of platelets include ITP, drug-induced immune thrombocytopenia (e.g. quinine/quinidine, gold salts, sulfonamides and heparin) and neonatal immune thrombocytopenias. In drug-induced thrombocytopenia, if a patient is on multiple medications, the offending drug may be difficult to identify. Heparin is a common offender in hospitalized patients. Paradoxically, patients with heparin-induced thrombocytopenia are at higher risk of developing thrombotic complications.

9.2.1.1 Idiopathic thrombocytopenic purpura (ITP)

Acute ITP occurs mainly in children, usually associated with a recent viral infection. The clinical course is self-limited. The diagnosis is based on the peripheral blood examination and clinical features unless: (1) the presenting clinical features suggest a different disorder; (2) the thrombocytopenia persists for more than 6–12 months; or (3) the low platelet counts are unresponsive to intravenous immunoglobulin therapy. Additional laboratory investigations (e.g. anti-platelet antibodies) and a bone marrow study are often unnecessary. When suspected, HIV testing should be performed, however. A bone marrow aspirate/biopsy may be also necessary if the peripheral blood demonstrates other abnormalities (e.g. neutropenia or unexplained anemia) to rule out bone marrow infiltrative disorders including ALL. In the majority of children with ITP, the platelet count recovers to normal within 2 months. Progression to chronic ITP, defined as a platelet count less than $150 \times 10^9/l$ for more than 6 months, is uncommon. The following features appear to be associated with an increased risk of such progression: female sex, patients older than 10 years of age, and the presence of purpura for 2–4 weeks prior to diagnosis.

Chronic ITP occurs mainly in adults (predominantly women). The disorder can have potentially severe clinical manifestations, especially if left untreated. Spontaneous remission is infrequent. In comparison to children, there is a higher risk of bleeding, including fatal intracranial hemorrhage. Currently, most patients are treated with glucocorticoids. Splenectomy is best reserved for patients who do not respond to steroids.

Because of the high association between chronic ITP and autoimmune diseases, the work-up should focus on the search for underlying disorders such as rheumatoid arthritis or SLE. In addition, HIV infection and other causes of isolated thrombocytopenia such as splenomegaly secondary to liver disease, unsuspected LPD/NHL and drug-induced thrombocytopenia should be excluded.

9.2.1.2 Immune thrombocytopenia in infants and neonates

In neonates and infants, other causes of immune thrombocytopenia (e.g. maternal alloantibodies, or autoantibodies from a mother with chronic ITP) are more prevalent than ITP associated with viral infection. Neonatal alloimmune thrombocytopenia is analogous to Rh hemolytic disease of the newborn. Congenital disorders with thrombocytopenia (e.g. congenital megakaryocytic hypoplasia) also need to be excluded in this age group, especially if the thrombocytopenia becomes persistent.

9.2.2 Hereditary thrombocytopenias

The hereditary thrombocytopenias are a diverse group of relatively rare diseases. The most notable are congenital megakaryocytic hypoplasia/aplasia, May-Hegglin anomaly, Wiskott-Aldrich syndrome, and the giant gray platelet syndromes. Congenital megakaryocytic hypoplasia refers to a heterogeneous group of rare and fatal disorders including thrombocytopenia with absent radii syndrome.

Wiskott-Aldrich syndrome is an X-linked immune disorder defined by the clinical triad of recurrent infection, thrombocytopenia and eczema. The patients develop cervical lymphadenopathy and progressive lymphocytopenia (with a decrease in T cells) during the course of the disease. The keys to the diagnosis are the unique immunoglobulin profile (decreased IgM, increased IgA and IgE, normal IgG) and a poor antibody response to polysaccharide antigen. Platelet aggregation (with epinephrine, ADP and collagen) is deficient.

Several qualitative platelet disorders manifest morphologically as giant gray platelets on blood films. One of these is Bernard-Soulier syndrome, a rare autosomal recessive disease characterized by deficient glycoprotein Ib on the platelet surface. Glycoprotein Ib is necessary for the interaction between von Willebrand Factor (vWF) and platelets, to induce aggregation in the initial phase of clot formation. In Bernard-Soulier syndrome, platelet aggregation is normal with ADP or collagen, but deficient with thrombin, vWF and ristocetin.

Eosinophilia pattern

The eosinophilia pattern is defined by an absolute increase in the number of eosinophils (i.e. $> 0.8 \times 10^9$/l). Peripheral blood eosinophilia generally reflects an increased tissue demand for eosinophils, which can be mediated by chemotactic agents or cytokines (e.g. interleukin-3 and interleukin-5) secreted by mast cells, basophils, and T lymphocytes. In contrast, the absolute eosinophilia in CML is not the predominant finding, since it is part of the uncontrolled hematopoiesis releasing blasts and immature myeloid precursors into the blood.

The most common causes of eosinophilia are allergic diseases (e.g. asthma, hay fever, drug allergies), parasitic infections, and cutaneous disorders (e.g. pemphigus). Other, less common, causes include collagen-vascular diseases (e.g. Churg-Strauss syndrome), malignancies (Sezary syndrome, other non-Hodgkin's lymphomas and Hodgkin's disease), hereditary/congenital immunodeficiencies (e.g. Wiskott-Aldrich syndrome), and idiopathic hypereosinophilic syndrome (HES).

Idiopathic hypereosinophilic syndrome is a diagnosis of exclusion. The criteria include persistent eosinophilia, greater than 1.5×10^9/l for at least 6 months, without an obvious etiology, and signs/symptoms of tissue damage due to organ infiltration by eosinophils (especially heart, lung, kidney, liver, spleen and skin).

The hypereosinophilic syndrome is actually a heterogeneous group of disorders, either reactive (to unknown allergens) or neoplastic (as confirmed by cytogenetic abnormalities, e.g. trisomy 8, trisomy 15). Because of this heterogeneity, the clinical course and survival reported in HES is highly variable. Neoplastic HES exhibits features of an MPD similar to CML but with a marked increased in eosinophilic precursors. Cases of neoplastic HES can progress to a blast crisis.

10.1 Peripheral blood morphology in eosinophilia

In most cases of eosinophilia, the eosinophils are morphologically normal. Knowledge of the clinical setting is extremely helpful during blood film examination. For instance, the severe degree of eosinophilia in some patients with MF may obscure the lower number of circulating Sezary cells. The presence of significant numbers of abnormal eosinophils with monolobed or hypersegmented nuclei, cytoplasmic vacuolation or hypogranulation (Figure 10.1) is associated with idiopathic HES. The hypogranulation is related to a decrease in both the size and number of eosinophilic granules. These qualitative abnormalities can also occur in MPD, MDS and immunocompromised patients, how-

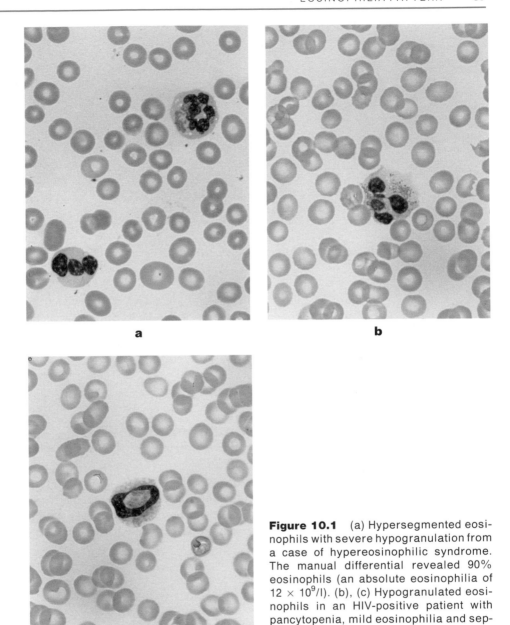

Figure 10.1 (a) Hypersegmented eosinophils with severe hypogranulation from a case of hypereosinophilic syndrome. The manual differential revealed 90% eosinophils (an absolute eosinophilia of 12×10^9/l). (b), (c) Hypogranulated eosinophils in an HIV-positive patient with pancytopenia, mild eosinophilia and sepsis. One eosinophil is hypersegmented (b) and one has a ring-shaped nucleus (c)

ever. Marked hypogranulation may result in eosinophils being counted as neutrophils by the analyzer, giving rise to an erroneous automated differential (see Section 1.5).

Parasitic infection, especially with parasites that invade tissue (e.g. trichinosis), is a common cause of eosinophilia in developing countries. Nematode infestation (discussed here for completeness) does not result in eosinophilia. In the maturation cycle of certain nematodes, such as the filariae species *Wuchereria bancrofti*

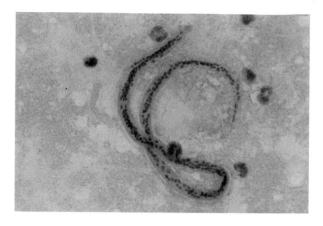

Figure 10.2   Microfilariasis (Wuchereria bancrofti)

(Figure 10.2) and *Loa loa*, there are stages during which the parasites circulate through the blood. Microfilaria should be carefully searched for if the patient has been traveling or residing in an endemic area. The exact identification of the species, based on the morphology of the tail of the parasite, is best referred to the microbiology department.

10.2 Diagnostic work-up for eosinophilia

The appropriate work-up relies heavily on the clinical history (e.g. allergies, medications, underlying malignancies) and nonhematological tests such as a search for parasites. A bone marrow aspirate/biopsy with cytogenetics (including molecular genetics) should be performed in protracted unexplained eosinophilia.

Monocytosis pattern

Absolute monocytosis is defined as a monocyte count greater than $1 \times 10^9/l$. Since automated analyzers count other large mononuclear cells as monocytes (see Section 1.5), it is important to confirm an absolute monocytosis microscopically.

Monocytosis can represent a reactive phenomenon or a neoplastic disorder involving monocytes and their precursors. The threshold of $1 \times 10^9/l$ set by the FAB group to define chronic myelomonocytic leukemia (CMMoL) is rather low and does not aid in the distinction between reactive and neoplastic monocytosis. In reactive conditions with leukocytosis, the high WBC count is sufficient to bring the monocyte level beyond $1 \times 10^9/l$, as illustrated in the following example from a child with bacterial infection: WBC count $20 \times 10^9/l$, neutrophils and bands 73%, lymphocytes 16%, eosinophils 2%, and monocytes 9%. The resulting absolute monocytosis is $1.8 \times 10^9/l$. A mild monocytosis is therefore a common accompanying feature in reactive neutrophilia. The diagnosis of reactive monocytosis necessitates correlation with other clinical and laboratory findings.

A variety of conditions can raise the monocyte count, including autoimmune disorders (e.g. rheumatoid arthritis, SLE and inflammatory bowel disease), chronic infections (e.g. mycobacteria or listeria infections), underlying solid tumors, hemolytic anemias, cyclic neutropenia, and chronic neutropenia. The monocytes in these conditions are mature-appearing. In neutropenic patients, the monocytosis represents a compensatory phenomenon. If the patient is receiving G-CSF therapy, hypergranulated intermediate myeloid precursors will also be present.

11.1 Neoplastic monocytosis

The presence of promonocytes (see Section 5.3) suggests a neoplastic monocytosis, namely CMMoL (Figure 11.1) or AML with monocytic differentiation (FAB subtypes M4 and M5). Rarely, promonocytes may be seen in CML. If a neoplastic monocytosis is suspected, the work-up should include a bone marrow aspirate and biopsy with cytogenetics and cytochemistries. Complementary tests, such as serum and/or urine lysozyme levels, may be helpful.

In AML with monocytic differentiation, the circulating cells of monocytic lineage may appear more 'mature' in the peripheral blood than in the bone marrow. Nevertheless, the leukemic population is composed predominantly of blasts and promonocytes, leading to the abnormal mononuclear cell pattern in the peripheral

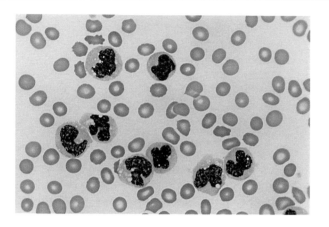

Figure 11.1   Severe monocytosis in a case of CMMoL

blood (see Sections 5.2 and 5.3). The subclassification of these leukemias is based on the bone marrow findings.

In CML, the marked leukocytosis raises the monocyte count above the $1 \times 10^9/l$ threshold. The relative proportion of monocytes is not increased, however. The increase in promyelocytes, myelocytes, and metamyelocytes, usually with circulating NRBCs and/or blasts, overshadows the monocytosis in CML.

11.1.1 Chronic myelomonocytic leukemia (CMMoL)

The main neoplastic disorder to be considered under the monocytosis pattern is CMMoL. The criteria set by the FAB, which classifies CMMoL as an MDS, are ill-defined apart from the peripheral absolute monocyte count of $1 \times 10^9/l$. Cases with leukocytosis and cases with a decreased WBC count can both be classified as CMMoL according to the FAB definition.

Patients with CMMoL who present with a high WBC count exhibit similar features to those with an MPD, including splenomegaly, frequent hepatomegaly, skin lesions and lymph node involvement. Increased serum and urine lysozyme levels and polyclonal hypergammaglobulinemia may also be present. These patients respond to cytoreductive therapy (hydroxyurea) as expected. In the very early stage, the WBC count is usually near the upper limit of the normal range, but with an overt preponderance of monocytes. The peripheral blood picture is more informative than the bone marrow appearance, which may be indistinguishable from that of CML unless an NSE stain is performed to identify monocytes and promonocytes with certainty. In this proliferative form of CMMoL, the circulating cells are composed of a spectrum of promonocytes and monocytes, with monocytes predominating. There should be fewer than 5% circulating blasts, a feature that distinguishes CMMoL from AML with monocytic differentiation. Qualitative abnormalities in other cell types (e.g. hypogranulated, hyposegmented neutrophils and macrocytic RBCs) can be present. These cytologic abnormalities do not necessarily imply that the underlying condition is myelodysplasia.

The main differential diagnosis of CMMoL includes CML and a CML-like MPD. A helpful diagnostic clue is the relationship between the monocytic elements and the circulating intermediate myeloid precursors. In CMMoL, the proportion of monocytes and promonocytes exceeds the number of intermediate myeloid precursors, whereas the reverse is true in CML and CML-like MPD. Most cases of CML demonstrate at least 15% circulating intermediate myeloid precursors. Cytogenetics or molecular genetics may further help to resolve the differential diagnosis.

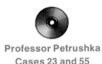

Professor Petrushka
Cases 23 and 55

The form of 'CMMoL' which presents with a relatively low WBC count, absolute monocytosis and qualitative abnormalities is virtually indistinguishable from an MDS with peripheral monocytosis. The common presentation is either pancytopenia, or bicytopenia (low WBC, along with a decreased Hgb or platelet count) with a mild stable monocytosis (usually in the $1.5–2.5 \times 10^9/l$ range). The therapeutic approach in these patients is similar to that used for an MDS. Therefore, it is best to designate this group of 'CMMoL' as MDS with peripheral monocytosis (either refractory anemia or RAEB, depending on the percentage of blasts in the peripheral blood and bone marrow) and avoid confusion with true CMMoL.

CHAPTER 12
Bicytopenia/pancytopenia pattern

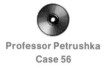

Professor Petrushka
Case 56

Pancytopenia refers to the peripheral blood pattern in which the hemoglobin, platelet count, and WBC count are all decreased. In bicytopenia, any two of the three are decreased (however, if anemia is present, it must not be hypochromic or microcytic). In general, bicytopenia/pancytopenia implies impaired hematopoiesis.

Bicytopenia/pancytopenia can be caused by bone marrow infiltration, usually secondary to neoplastic disorders (Table 12.1), and can occur in non-neoplastic conditions associated with diminished hematopoiesis (Table 12.2). In bicytopenia, the combination of anemia and thrombocytopenia can be the result of peripheral destruction of platelets and RBCs, as seen in TTP, HUS or DIC. Clonal disorders resulting in bone marrow hypoplasia such as aplastic anemia, paroxysmal nocturnal hemoglobinuria (PNH) and various congenital disorders (e.g. Chediak-Higashi syndrome) can also result in pancytopenia.

Table 12.1 Neoplastic diseases causing bone marrow infiltration

- Acute and chronic leukemias.
- Myeloproliferative disorders (especially AMM)
- Myelodysplastic syndromes
- Malignant lymphomas
- Multiple myeloma
- Metastatic carcinomas

Table 12.2 Non-neoplastic causes of impaired hematopoiesis

- Recent chemotherapy and/or radiation therapy.
- Drugs other than chemotherapeutic agents (e.g. sulfonamides).
- Severe B_{12} or folate deficiency.
- Advanced HIV infection.

12.1 Morphologic features in bicytopenia/pancytopenia

Macrocytes, including oval macrocytes (Figure 12.1), elliptocytes, stomatocytes and basophilic stippling (Figure 12.2) are common RBC abnormalities in pancytopenia. These dyserythropoietic features are nonspecific and do not necessarily imply an underlying stem cell disorder. Polychromasia is minimal and the absolute reticulocyte count is inappropriately low for the degree of anemia.

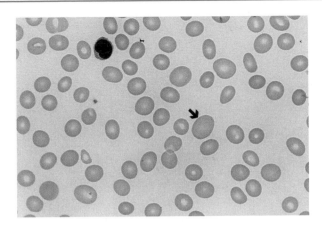

Figure 12.1 Pancytopenia and macrocytosis in a case of PNH. The mixture of macrocytes, oval macrocytes (arrow) and normocytic RBCs results in a dimorphic blood picture

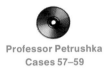

**Professor Petrushka
Cases 57–59**

Relatively more specific RBC abnormalities, if present, may be a helpful clue to the underlying process. The presence of rouleaux, abundant teardrop cells, or many schistocytes would suggest a possible underlying multiple myeloma, bone marrow infiltration with myelofibrosis, or TTP/HUS/DIC, respectively (Figure 12.3). In these diseases, the pattern is usually bicytopenia (Hgb/PLT). Oxidative injury in patients on a multidrug regimen (e.g. HIV-positive patients) can present with abundant bite cells and/or irregularly contracted cells. An absolute reticulocyte count is helpful to determine whether the decreased hemoglobin is due to peripheral destruction or bone marrow impairment.

Qualitative abnormalities in granulocytes (e.g. hyposegmentation, hypogranulation) can be seen in stem cell disorders (e.g. MDS, acute leukemias) as well as

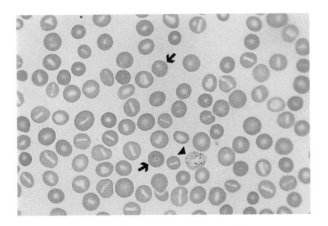

Figure 12.2 Peripheral blood film from a patient on chemotherapy for a myeloproliferative disorder, showing macrocytes and numerous stomatocytes. Basophilic stippling can be seen in two RBCs (arrow) and Pappenheimer bodies in another RBC (arrowhead)

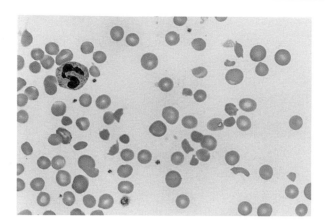

Figure 12.3 Hemolytic uremic syndrome in a 5-year-old child. The hemoglobin level and platelet count were decreased, accompanied by numerous schistocytes

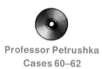

Professor Petrushka
Cases 60–62

HIV infection (Figure 12.4). The abnormal granulopoiesis secondary to chemotherapy can manifest as nuclear fragments (round or rhomboid) in leukocytes (Figure 12.5). Hypersegmentation in the context of pancytopenia is suggestive of B_{12}/folate deficiency. In addition, the blood films should be examined carefully for the presence of small numbers of abnormal mononuclear cells (e.g. blasts, hairy cells) especially along the edges and tail of the film. The presence of rare blasts suggests an acute leukemia, MDS or recent chemotherapy.

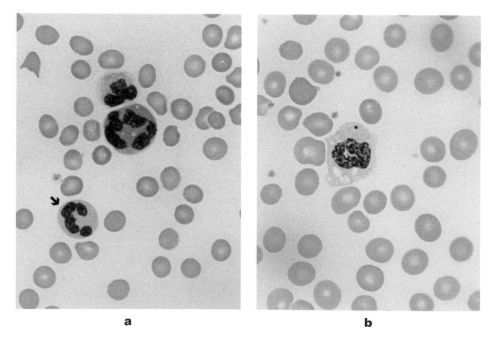

a   b

Figure 12.4 Blood films from two patients with pancytopenia. (a) One hypogranulated neutrophil (arrow) and one giant neutrophil from a myelodysplastic syndrome. (b) A hypogranulated neutrophil with a nuclear fragment in an HIV-positive patient

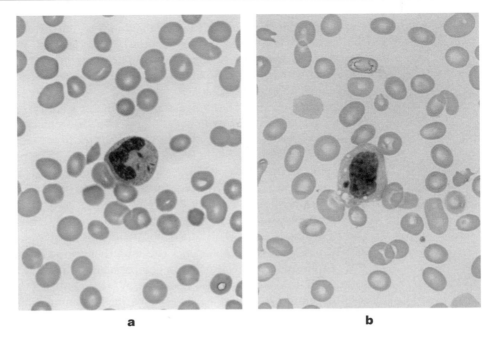

a   b

Figure 12.5 Blood films from two different pediatric oncology patients. (a) Several rhomboid nuclear fragments in a neutrophil. (b) A nuclear fragment in a monocyte. The morphology here can simulate Chediak-Higashi anomaly

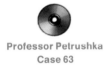

Professor Petrushka
Case 63

Unless the clinical history can account for the bicytopenia/pancytopenia, a bone marrow aspirate/biopsy may be necessary to determine the underlying etiology. When performing a bone marrow for bicytopenia/pancytopenia, appropriate material should be saved for potential ancillary studies such as cytogenetics and immunophenotyping. Table 12.3 lists additional tests that may be indicated.

Table 12.3 Additional tests which may be indicated in the work-up of bicytopenia/pancytopenia

- B_{12}/folate levels.
- An absolute reticulocyte count.
- A sucrose hemolysis test and FCM studies if PNH or aplastic anemia is suspected.
- Coagulation studies, i.e. prothrombin time, PTT (activated partial thromboplastin time), bleeding time, fibrinogen levels and fibrin split products, if TTP, HUS or DIC is suspected.
- HIV testing.

12.2 Paroxysmal nocturnal hemoglobinuria

Paroxysmal nocturnal hemoglobinuria is a clonal stem cell disorder of insidious onset, prolonged course and diverse peripheral blood manifestations. Because of the varied clinical and peripheral blood presentations, PNH should be suspected in any patient with unexplained chronic intravascular hemolysis (with acute exacerbations and hemoglobinuria), pancytopenia, intractable iron deficiency or recurrent venous thrombosis. The acute hemolytic episodes are often associated with abdominal pain, which most likely represent transient occlusion of the large abdominal veins.

Depending on the severity and stage of the disease, PNH can present with an NCNC anemia (with or without mild anisocytosis), a macrocytic anemia, a persistent hypochromic, microcytic anemia (Figure 12.6) caused by excessive loss of iron in the urine, bicytopenia (WBC/Hgb or Hgb/PLT) or pancytopenia. Paroxysmal nocturnal hemoglobinuria can masquerade as iron deficiency. In many cases, the disease can only be recognized after iron therapy.

The peripheral blood cells in PNH have been recently identified to be deficient in glycosylphosphatidylinositol (GPI)-linked surface antigens, secondary to altered synthesis of the GPI anchor protein. This results in increased sensitivity of RBCs to lysis by complement. The underlying molecular defects involve the *PIG-A* (phosphatidylinositol glycan complementation group A) gene on chromosome Xp22.1 in hematopoietic stem cells. A large number of mutations spreading over the entire *PIG-A* gene have been identified and more than one mutated clone can exist in the same patient. The resulting abnormalities in the PIG-A enzyme involved in GPI anchor protein synthesis influence the PNH phenotype and severity of the disease.

12.2.1 Laboratory studies for PNH and congenital dyserythropoietic anemia type II

The traditional tests for PNH are based on the susceptibility of PNH red cells to lysis by small amounts of complement. A simple screening test is the

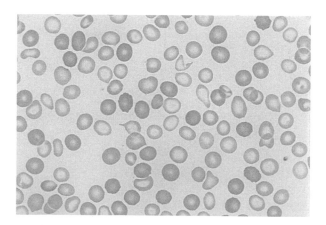

Figure 12.6 Blood film from a 33-year-old female with PNH following blood transfusion. The patient had protracted loss of iron in the urine and severe iron deficiency anemia (Hgb 5g/dl) which necessitated transfusion. The mixture of the patient's RBCs (hypochromic and microcytic) and the transfused RBCs (normochromic and normocytic) results in anisochromasia and dimorphism

sucrose-water test that induces RBCs to adsorb complement at low ionic concentration.

Until recently, the acidified serum test (Ham test) was the diagnostic test for PNH. In the acidified serum test, the patient's RBCs are incubated in compatible acidified serum at 37°C. If hemolysis occurs (i.e. positive result), it indicates PNH or congenital dyserythropoietic anemia type II (CDA II). Adding magnesium chloride increases the sensitivity. To exclude possible false-positive results, the patient's RBCs are incubated in fresh (i.e. nonacidified) normal serum and in heat-inactivated normal serum. Hemolysis in fresh serum suggests a technical error, i.e. incompatible serum. Hemolysis in heat-inactivated serum is seen in congenital and acquired spherocytosis. With PNH cells, there should be no lysis under either of the control conditions.

> Congenital dyserythropoietic anemia type II is also known as hereditary erythroid multinuclearity with positive acidified-serum lysis test (HEMPAS). It can be distinguished from PNH by the fact that, in CDA II, the sucrose hemolysis test is negative, hemolysis does not occur in the patient's own acidified serum, and the Ham test is positive in only about 30% of normal sera. The Ham test is positive in those sera that contain an IgM antibody reacting to the unique antigen present on HEMPAS cells.

A recent and more sensitive diagnostic test for PNH is FCM analysis of GPI-linked surface antigens, e.g. CD59, a membrane glycoprotein that protects cells from lysis by the complement membrane attack complex. This test is also useful for following the patient's response to therapy. With this technique, the proportion of PNH III cells (those with complete absence of GPI-anchored proteins) and PNH II cells (which have residual GPI-anchored protein expression) can be determined accurately. By testing for antigens that are not only present on RBCs but also on granulocytes (e.g. CD59, CD66), the sensitivity of the FCM analysis is further increased. The lifespan of PNH granulocytes is normal and their number is unaffected by RBC transfusion. Therefore, decreased to absent expression of CD59 or CD66 on granulocytes identifies patients with a small unsuspected PNH clone. With the routine use of FCM methods, GPI-deficient cells are found in one-third to one-half of patients with aplastic anemia. This finding suggests a close relationship between aplastic anemia and PNH. Furthermore, the manifestations of bone marrow failure in PNH can be as severe as those in aplastic anemia; and a substantial number of patients with aplastic anemia develop overt PNH over the course of their disease.

12.3 Non-neoplastic disorders with bicytopenia or pancytopenia

In infants and neonates, overwhelming sepsis may cause neutropenia and anemia. The WBC count may be normal if there is a compensatory monocytosis.

In children under 10 years old, bicytopenia (Hgb/WBC), or, less commonly, pancytopenia, can be a manifestation of the 'accelerated' phase of Chediak-Higashi disease (congenital gigantism of peroxidase granules). This rare, presumably

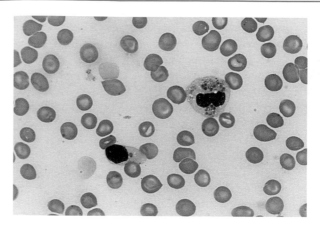

Figure 12.7 Chediak-Higashi syndrome in a 5-year-old male. Large gray inclusions in a granulocyte and a large azurophilic inclusion in a lymphocyte are apparent

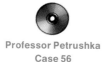

Professor Petrushka
Case 56

autosomal recessive disorder, is characterized by partial ocular and cutaneous albinism, recurrent pyogenic infections, an increased bleeding tendency, and the presence of Chediak-Higashi inclusions (Figure 12.7). The granules, which presumably result from progressive aggregation of azurophilic and specific granules, are most easily detected in neutrophils. There are multiple defects in neutrophil function contributing to the increased susceptibility to infections. Lymphadenopathy, splenomegaly and hepatomegaly, due to a widespread lymphohistiocytic infiltrate in tissues (easily mistaken for NHL), are also present during the 'accelerated' phase.

CHAPTER **13**	Neutropenia/leukopenia pattern

The definition of the neutropenia/leukopenia pattern is either a decreased WBC count ($<4 \times 10^9/l$ in adults) or a decreased number of granulocytes ($<1.5 \times 10^9/l$ in adults). In most situations, neutropenia and leukopenia occur together. The WBC count in normal black individuals is usually lower than in other ethnic groups (the absolute neutrophil count can be as low as $1.0 \times 10^9/l$).

Impaired production, peripheral destruction and an abnormal distribution of neutrophils can cause low numbers of circulating granulocytes. Neutropenia due to impaired production is caused by a stem cell defect as seen in cyclic neutropenia and familial agranulocytosis. Immune-mediated neutropenia, severe infection and hypersplenism can cause peripheral destruction of neutrophils. Neutrophils are abnormally distributed when there is an increase in the marginated pool (on the walls of blood vessels) and in the so-called lazy leukocyte syndrome where there is defective bone marrow release of granulocytes. In practice, more than one of these mechanisms may work in concert. For example, drug therapy with phenothiazines, antidepressants or trimethoprim-sulfamethoxazole can cause neutropenia by inhibiting myelopoiesis, immune destruction of neutrophils, and other poorly understood complex mechanisms.

13.1 Acquired neutropenias

The common causes of non-neoplastic acquired neutropenia include drugs, certain infections and autoimmune neutropenia. Drug-induced neutropenia predominates in adults and can result from a variety of medications, e.g. analgesics, antibiotics and anticonvulsants.

Overwhelming infection is the leading cause of neutropenia in neonates and infants. Several mechanisms can be involved, including bone marrow suppression by the infectious organisms and neutrophil utilization which exceeds bone marrow production. Widespread infection is also the leading cause of neutropenia among chronic alcoholics and malnourished elderly patients. Typhoid and paratyphoid fever, brucellosis, tularemia, most rickettsial infections, and some viral infections (hepatitis, AIDS) are the main diseases in which neutropenia is observed instead of neutrophilia.

13.1.1 Drug-induced immune neutropenia

There are two underlying mechanisms in drug-induced immune neutropenia:

1. High dose penicillin (or derivatives) can induce IgG antibodies directed against the antibiotic that can become bound to neutrophils. This results in a gradual onset of neutropenia that promptly subsides when the antibiotic is discontinued.
2. Drug–antibody complexes can adsorb onto neutrophils with complement activation, resulting in an abrupt onset of severe neutropenia.

13.1.2 Autoimmune neutropenia

Autoimmune neutropenia can occur at any age but is most common in adults. In adults, it is often associated with an underlying disorder such as SLE or rheumatoid arthritis. There may be an increased number of LGLs in the blood and/or bone marrow. The neutropenia is usually self-limited with spontaneous recovery after 2–3 years. The site of granulocyte destruction can be either the peripheral blood or bone marrow. In the latter instance, the bone marrow exhibits an apparent maturation arrest at the myelocyte stage. In some patients, the LGL proliferation is neoplastic (see Sections 28.1 and 28.4). The constellation of neutropenia, splenomegaly and severe rheumatoid arthritis is recognized clinically as Felty's syndrome.

In contrast, autoimmune neutropenia in infants is not associated with an underlying autoimmune disorder. The disease usually occurs within the first 2 years of life and resolves within 1–2 years. Autoimmune neutropenia in this age group needs to be differentiated from other causes of neutropenia in infancy including alloimmune neutropenia (which can last up to 6 months) and the less common constitutional neutropenias. The diagnosis of autoimmune neutropenia rests on the finding of granulocyte-specific antibodies using immunofluorescence and/or agglutination tests. Because of the low antibody titers, the tests should be repeated two or three times at 2–4 week intervals.

13.2 Constitutional neutropenias

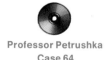

**Professor Petrushka
Case 64**

Uncommon causes of neutropenia include the hereditary neutropenias and cyclic neutropenia. Because the peripheral blood and bone marrow manifestations of the various hereditary neutropenias are similar to each other, the diagnosis rests primarily on the clinical picture and family studies. The peripheral blood demonstrates either a leukopenia or a compensatory monocytosis.

The main neutropenias in infants and children include Kostmann's disease (infantile genetic agranulocytosis) and cyclic neutropenia. Kostmann's disease is a rare autosomal recessive disorder in which the onset of symptoms occurs shortly after birth. Prior to the use of G-CSF, the disease was invariably fatal within the first year of life.

The main differential diagnosis of Kostmann's disease is chronic benign granulocytopenia of infancy and childhood. Evidence suggests that this condition is an autoimmune process. Parvovirus infection may be implicated in the pathogenesis. Despite the chronic clinical course, the disease spontaneously resolves around the age of 4 years in most patients.

Cyclic neutropenia is a rare disorder characterized by the periodic production failure of granulocytes, presumably at the stem cell level. The disease usually begins in infancy or childhood and gradually subsides as the patient gets older. The symptomatic episodes of fever and mild infections, usually with cervical lymphadenopathy, recur approximately every 3–4 weeks. The neutropenic periods, lasting 3–6 days, are associated with infections of mucosal sites (e.g. oropharynx, upper respiratory tract or rectal mucosa). Because RBCs and platelets also fluctuate (not necessarily in synchrony with the neutropenia), the disease is more appropriately termed cyclic hematopoiesis.

13.3 Peripheral blood findings in neutropenia/leukopenia

In infection-associated neutropenia, toxic granulation, Döhle bodies, and vacuoles may be seen in the neutrophils. The finding of intracellular bacterial or fungal organisms (Figure 13.1) within leukocytes indicates overwhelming septicemia and a poor prognosis. In neutropenic patients, a compensatory monocytosis may be present, elevating the WBC count into the normal range. In many cases, this reactive monocytosis helps to prevent recurrent infections.

In the recovery phase after neutropenia, rebound neutrophilia is the rule. Frequently, one finds circulating intermediate myeloid precursors (mainly metamye-

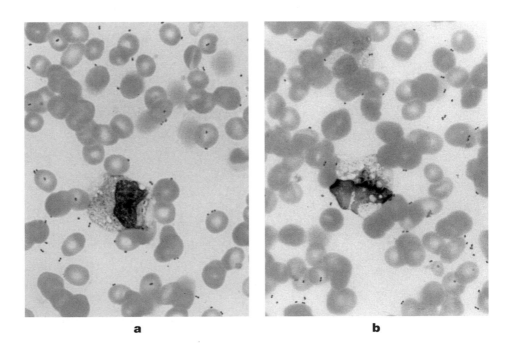

a   b

Figure 13.1 Terminal sepsis in a severely leukopenic patient. (a) Numerous extracellular and intracellular diplococci. (b) Intracellular Candida organisms are also present

locytes and myelocytes). The blood picture may be indistinguishable from a neutrophilia secondary to infection. Hypergranulation is present if G-CSF has been given.

In adults, large granular lymphocytosis/leukemia should be suspected if neutropenia is persistent, associated with a normal (or increased) WBC count, and more than half of the lymphocytes are LGLs (see Section 8.2.3).

13.4 Diagnostic work-up of neutropenia/leukopenia

Review of the clinical history is important to rule out drug exposure and underlying illnesses such as autoimmune diseases and to determine the frequency and duration of infections (i.e. a cyclic pattern). Bone marrow examination may be necessary, especially in adults, if the clinical history is noncontributory. Various techniques are available to assay for antibodies to neutrophils.

Hypochromia/microcytosis pattern

The hypochromia/microcytosis pattern is seen in hemoglobin synthesis disorders. Hypochromia (indicated by a decreased MCH) usually precedes overt microcytosis (decreased MCV) and is therefore a more sensitive indicator of the impaired synthesis which affects either the globin chains or the heme component. Hypochromia and/or microcytosis can occur in the absence of anemia.

Iron deficiency and thalassemias are the two leading candidates in the differential diagnosis of the hypochromia/microcytosis pattern. Less common causes of hypochromia and/or microcytosis are congenital sideroblastic anemia and sideroblastic anemia secondary to lead (or other heavy metals) poisoning.

The effect of lead poisoning on erythropoiesis results from complex mechanisms, including inhibition of enzymes involved in heme synthesis and reduction of the intracellular iron supply to the site of heme synthesis. The basophilic stippling seen in lead poisoning represents acquired pyrimidine $5'$ nucleotidase deficiency.

A normal serum ferritin level in renal patients does not exclude iron deficiency unless the lower limit of normal is raised appropriately for this clinical setting. Microcytic anemia in renal patients on hemodialysis can be the result of either aluminum toxicity or iron deficiency secondary to blood loss in the dialysis apparatus.

Other conditions can give rise to isolated hypochromia or microcytosis. Severe anemia of chronic disease can result in hypochromia. Microcytosis alone can be observed in various hemoglobinopathies (e.g. Hgb C, Hgb E and hereditary persistence of Hgb F). When numerous fragmented cells and microspherocytes are present, as seen in some hemolytic anemias (e.g. hereditary pyropoikilocytosis), the MCV can be low, resulting in an apparent microcytic anemia.

14.1 Peripheral blood findings in hypochromia/microcytosis

The extent of RBC abnormalities depends on the severity of the underlying disorder. The following morphologic features can be observed:

1. **Hypochromic RBCs**, which have an increase in the central pallor to more than one-third of the red cell diameter (Figure 12.6).
2. **Microcytes**, i.e. RBCs with a decreased volume and a decreased diameter (Figure 12.6). Microcytes are invariably hypochromic. The nucleus of a resting lymphocyte can be used as a guide to the diameter of a normal RBC.
3. **Dimorphism and/or anisochromasia** (Figure 12.6). When hypochromic and/or microcytic cells constitute only a portion of the RBC population, the

result is a mixture of cells with dimorphism and/or anisochromasia. Dimorphism is two populations of RBCs that differ in cell volume (e.g. microcytes plus normocytes). Anisochromasia is a mixture of cells with different staining characteristics (i.e. hypochromic cells plus normochromic cells). In the context of a hypochromic, microcytic pattern, dimorphism and/or anisochromasia are seen in sideroblastic anemias, early iron deficiency, and iron deficiency following therapy or transfusion.

4. **Poikilocytosis** (e.g. elliptocytes/ovalocytes, target cells and/or teardrop cells). The terms 'elliptocytes' and 'ovalocytes' can be used interchangeably since there are no accepted rules (with respect to the ratio of the short diameter of the RBC to the long diameter) to define these cell types. In addition, they tend to occur together. An ovalocyte is a 'fat' elliptocyte and an elliptocyte (Figure 14.1) is a 'long' ovalocyte. In normal blood, these cells constitute less than 2% of RBCs. A moderate number of elliptocytes can be seen in anemias of various etiologies, e.g. iron deficiency, thalassemia, B_{12}/folate deficiency, and the anemia associated with myelofibrosis.

Target cells (Figure 14.2) have an increased cell surface to cell volume ratio. This may be the result of either decreased hemoglobin content and/or an increased surface membrane. Decreased hemoglobin content in red cells is observed in hemoglobin synthesis disorders and certain hemoglobinopathies (e.g. Hgb C, Hgb E, Hgb D or Hgb S). An increased surface membrane results from deranged lipid metabolism as seen in obstructive jaundice or severe liver disease. The combination of hypochromia/microcytosis and 3+ target cells can be seen in hereditary persistence of fetal hemoglobin (HPFH), thalassemia, Hgb C and Hgb E. Target cells are commonly present (nonspecifically) in other conditions (e.g. after splenectomy).

Teardrop cells (Figure 14.3) are an acquired deformity of erythrocytes. When present in small numbers, the changes are relatively nonspecific. Significant numbers of teardrop cells occur in two situations. Erythrocyte inclusions (such as precipitated excess α chains in thalassemia) can render

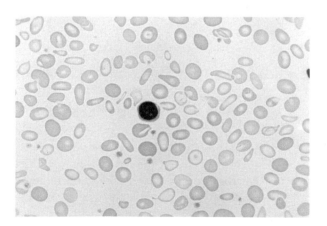

Figure 14.1 Blood film from a young male with congenital sideroblastic anemia, showing dimorphism, anisochromasia, abundant elliptocytes/ovalocytes and hypochromic, microcytic RBCs

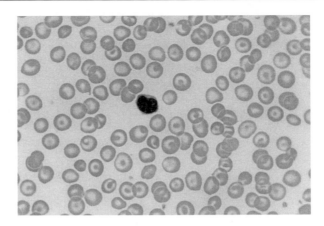

Figure 14.2 Numerous target cells in a black individual without anemia. The subsequent work-up established the diagnosis of HPFH

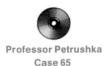

Professor Petrushka
Case 65

the RBC less deformable and less able to withstand splenic filtration. In addition, transit of RBCs through deformed marrow sinuses or diseased splenic cords can cause teardrop cells. This is a common finding in bone marrow infiltrative disorders, especially those with fibrosis.

5. **Basophilic stippling** (Figure 14.4a) represents aggregates of ribosomes and degenerating mitochondria. In the context of hypochromia/microcytosis, basophilic stippling occurs in thalassemias, congenital sideroblastic anemia and heavy metal poisoning (e.g. lead, mercury). Other dyserythropoietic states such as unstable hemoglobins, pyrimidine $5'$ nucleotidase deficiency, CDA and stem cell disorders (e.g. acute leukemia, MDS) can also manifest with basophilic stippling. The MCV in these diseases is not low, however.

6. **Siderotic granules**, known as **Pappenheimer bodies** (Figure 14.4b), are mainly seen in congenital sideroblastic anemia and the severe forms of thalassemia. The presence of Pappenheimer bodies indicates iron overload. In

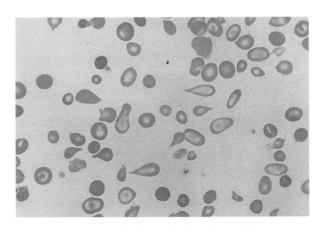

Figure 14.3 Frequent teardrop cells along with target cells, hypochromic and microcytic RBCs from a case of Hgb E β-thalassemia

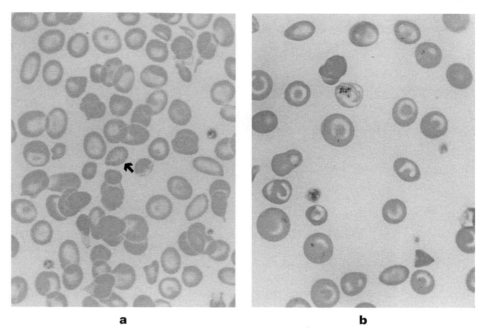

a   b

Figure 14.4 (a) Basophilic stippling (arrow) surrounded by numerous target cells from a case of Hgb H disease. A few elliptocytes and teardrop cells are present. (b) Pappenheimer bodies in a case of transfusion-dependent Hgb S β-thalassemia

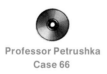

Professor Petrushka
Case 66

thalassemia, this is the result of repeated transfusion and increased gastrointestinal absorption of iron.

7. **Irregularly contracted cells** (IRCs). The affected RBCs contain molecules of abnormal hemoglobin, such as abnormal or excess globin chains, a defective heme component or oxidized hemoglobin. The abnormal molecules are presumably removed by the phagocytic system, resulting in an irregularly shrunken red cell. Small numbers of IRCs can be found in the thalassemias and some hemoglobinopathies. A large number of IRCs along with numerous target cells and a low MCH/MCV is strongly suggestive of a combined Hgb C/thalassemia disorder (Figure 14.5). The anemia is much less severe than that seen in most sickle-β thalassemia disorders. A leukoerythroblastic blood picture is unusual in Hgb C-thalassemia.

Thrombocytosis can be seen as an associated finding in cases of hypochromic, microcytic anemia. If hypersegmented neutrophils are seen, B_{12}/folate values should be checked to rule out a combined deficiency of iron and other nutritional factors. Circulating NRBCs may be found when the anemia is severe.

As noted above, certain features (e.g. basophilic stippling, Pappenheimer bodies, frequent teardrop cells, large numbers of circulating NRBCs and 3+ target cells), when present in the context of a hypochromic, microcytic pattern, suggest a process other than iron deficiency. In addition, a marked microcytosis with minimal or no anemia (i.e. the low MCV is out of proportion to the Hgb

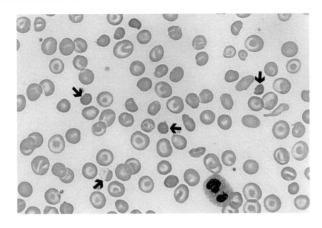

Figure 14.5 Frequent irregularly contracted RBCs (arrow) and numerous target cells in a case of Hgb C β-thalassemia. The densely stained, irregularly contracted RBCs may be misinterpreted as spherocytes

level) favors thalassemia minor or thalassemia trait. These findings can also be seen in treated PRV with iron deficiency.

Various formulae based on RBC indices (MCV, MCH, RDW, RBC count) have been tested in an attempt to separate iron deficiency from thalassemia trait. In general, these formulae only work well in straightforward cases. They are often least helpful when they are most needed, for example in thalassemia trait with iron deficiency in a pregnant woman. Note that in a substantial number of cases, the peripheral blood film morphology and hemogram data offer no clues to discriminate thalassemia trait from iron deficiency.

14.2 Diagnostic work-up of hypochromia/microcytosis

Proper assessment of a case with hypochromia and/or microcytosis often requires access to both clinical information and other laboratory studies. The patient's ethnic background, family history, dietary habits and a search for any medical disorders that can cause chronic hemolysis or blood loss can be important. There is a high prevalence of thalassemia among people of Mediterranean extraction (Italy, Greece, Cyprus, and Turkey), South-East Asians (Thailand and China) and those of African descent. A family history of hemoglobinopathy, thalassemia, or congenital sideroblastic anemia can also be a clue to the cause of hypochromia and/or microcytosis. A history of gastrointestinal bleeding (from ulcers, inflammatory bowel disease or hookworm infestation), heavy and prolonged menstruation in women of childbearing age, or episodic paroxysmal intravascular hemolysis with loss of iron in the urine (e.g. PNH; see Section 12.1) indicate iron deficiency.

Since iron deficiency is so common, the determination of the patient's iron status is the first step in the diagnostic work-up of hypochromia/microcytosis.

If the iron status is normal or indicates iron overload, then proceed to hemoglobin electrophoresis for the detection of thalassemias or hemoglobinopathies. Cellulose acetate electrophoresis at pH 8.6 (alkaline) and citrate agar electrophoresis at pH 6.2 (acid) are sufficient for diagnosing most hemoglobinopathies. When the hemoglobin electrophoresis is noncontributory, bone marrow studies may be indicated, especially if there is a strong suspicion of congenital sideroblastic anemia. Family studies and genetic counseling are recommended for the above-mentioned hereditary disorders.

A number of laboratory tests of variable sensitivity and specificity have been used for testing a patient's iron status including: (1) serum iron, total iron binding capacity (TIBC) and per cent saturation; (2) serum ferritin; and (3) RBC ferritin. The information obtained from the combined results of serum iron, TIBC and per cent saturation are the least helpful in the diagnosis of iron deficiency. The wide diurnal variation in iron levels, plus the high turnover rate of the iron pool limit the usefulness of the serum iron determination. The methodologies for TIBC are empirical and none is quite satisfactory. The two preferred tests are serum and RBC ferritin.

Serum ferritin is an iron storage compound that correlates with total body iron stores. Determination of serum ferritin is done by enzyme immunoassay using antibodies against liver or spleen ferritin. With the exception of certain conditions which increase the ferritin level and can therefore mask iron deficiency (infection/inflammation, liver damage, prolonged fasting, chronic renal failure, hematopoietic malignancy), serum ferritin is a reliable and sensitive indicator of iron deficiency. Decreased ferritin levels precede changes in the serum iron, TIBC, RBC indices and RBC morphology.

RBC ferritin is an even better indicator of iron status because it is only minimally affected by the conditions that can give rise to a 'falsely' elevated serum ferritin. The assay method is stringent, however, requiring a hemolysate free of RBC stroma obtained from a pure RBC suspension without any WBC contamination. RBC ferritin is especially useful in detecting early iron deficiency, iron deficiency in anemia of chronic disease, and iron deficiency in heterozygous β-thalassemia.

A promising tool for the diagnosis of iron deficiency, especially in the presence of concomitant inflammatory disorders, is the determination of soluble transferrin receptor (TfR). The level of soluble TfR is not affected by the acute phase response. Elevated levels are seen not only in iron deficiency, but also in conditions that induce increased erythropoiesis, such as hemolysis or B_{12} deficiency. Studies are still needed to establish the utility of this test in separating iron deficiency from thalassemia. It is not clear whether the test is as sensitive as RBC ferritin determination.

14.3 Iron deficiency

There are three stages in iron deficiency:

Stage I   Iron depletion
Stage II Iron deficient erythropoiesis

Stage III Iron deficiency anemia

Professor Petrushka
Case 67

Stage I can only be diagnosed by serum and/or RBC ferritin. RBC abnormalities occur late in iron deficiency. Table 14.1 lists the abnormalities at each stage.

Table 14.1 Laboratory abnormalities at each stage of iron deficiency

	Stage I	Stage II	Stage III
RBC ferritin	D	D	D
Serum ferritin	D	D	D
Serum iron	N	D	D
TIBC	N	I	I
Hgb	N	N	D
MCH	N	N/D	D
MCV	N	N	D

D – decreased; N – normal; I – increased.

14.4 Congenital sideroblastic anemia

Congenital sideroblastic anemia (Figure 14.1) is a rare disease that can be confused with iron deficiency anemia since the dominant features are hypochromia and microcytosis. The anemia is of variable severity. In the majority of cases, the inheritance is X-linked. Female carriers demonstrate hypochromia and dimorphism but are not anemic. The diagnosis can be established with a bone marrow aspirate/biopsy (to look for increased numbers of ring sideroblasts) and family studies.

The biochemical abnormality in X-linked sideroblastic anemia is deficient aminolevulinic acid synthetase activity. Approximately 50% of patients respond to high doses of pyridoxine with an improvement in the hemoglobin to normal despite persistence of the hypochromia and microcytosis. Late in the clinical course, patients develop hypersplenism (with or without hepatomegaly) due to iron overload. Table 14.2 compares the results of iron studies in congenital sideroblastic anemia with those in iron deficiency.

Table 14.2 Iron studies in sideroblastic anemia and iron deficiency

	Sideroblastic anemia	Iron deficiency anemia
Serum ferritin	High	Low
RBC ferritin	High	Low
Serum iron	Normal/high	Low
TIBC	Normal/low	High
Transferrin saturation	Normal/high	Low

Professor Petrushka
Case 68

14.5 Thalassemias

The thalassemias are a group of hereditary hemolytic anemias characterized by decreased or absent synthesis of one of the globin subunits in the hemoglobin molecule. In normal subjects, the synthesis of α and β globin chains is balanced, and the genotype is $\alpha\alpha/\alpha\alpha$, β/β. Hgb A_2 (composed of α chains and δ chains) normally constitutes about 2.5–3.2% of the total hemoglobin. In thalassemia, the clinical and hematological picture is caused by an imbalance in the production of α and β chains. The reduction or absence of one of these chains results in altered globin synthesis, and therefore a decrease in hemoglobin production.

Based on the severity of the clinical manifestations, the thalassemias are divided into three groups:

1. Thalassemia major
2. Thalassemia minor (trait)
3. Thalassemia intermedia

**Professor Petrushka
Case 4**

In thalassemia major, the patient is transfusion-dependent due to a severe anemia (Hgb usually <5 g/dl). Skeletal abnormalities (due to marked hematopoiesis), growth retardation, and cardiopulmonary complications of iron overload (i.e. hemosiderosis) are also present.

Patients with thalassemia minor have little or no anemia and no clinical symptoms from the disease. Thalassemia intermedia exhibits a moderate to severe anemia (Hgb in the 7–9 g/dl range). Such patients are less transfusion-dependent than patients with thalassemia major. There are no growth abnormalities, but these patients ultimately suffer the complications of hemosiderosis.

14.5.1 α-Thalassemias

Normal individuals have four α genes ($\alpha\alpha/\alpha\alpha$). There are four clinical phenotypes of α-thalassemia: (1) silent carrier state; (2) α-thalassemia minor; (3) Hgb H disease (Figure 14.6); and (4) Hgb Bart's, i.e. hydrops fetalis (Figure 14.7).

In most cases, the silent carrier state corresponds to the deletion of one α gene ($-\alpha/\alpha\alpha$). Since this condition has no effect on the hemoglobin level or RBC morphology, silent carriers are picked up when family studies of a symptomatic α-thalassemia patient are carried out. Definitive identification requires gene mapping. Individuals who are heterozygous for Hgb Constant Spring also exhibit a silent carrier state with no overt hematological problems.

The α-thalassemia minor phenotype can result from various genotypes. The heterozygous phenotype with both deletions inherited from one parent ($- - /\alpha\alpha$) is common among Asians, and the homozygous phenotype with a deletion inherited from each parent ($-\alpha/ - \alpha$) is common among blacks. A less common genotype can result from inheritance of a single α gene deletion from one parent, plus a nondeletional mutation in an α gene from the other parent. Clinically, patients with α-thalassemia minor have normal or slightly reduced hemoglobin levels with obvious microcytosis and/or hypochromia. Hemoglobin electrophoresis is normal with normal levels of Hgb A_2 and Hgb F. This distin-

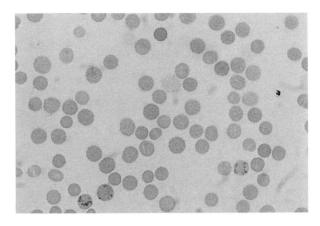

Figure 14.6   Supravital stain: the 'golf ball' appearance of the precipitated Hgb H is pathognomonic for the disorder

guishes the condition from β-thalassemia minor. Definitive diagnosis can be established by either globin chain synthesis studies or gene mapping analysis.

Hgb H disease can be the result of various genotypes which effectively cause the loss of three of the four α genes. The two most common genotypes (encountered primarily in Asia) are $- - / - \alpha$ and $- - / \alpha\alpha^{cs}$, where cs is the Constant Spring variant of the α chain. Hemoglobin Constant Spring, which results in decreased α chain synthesis and an abnormal hemoglobin containing the structurally abnormal α^{cs} chain, accounts for about 50% of the Hgb H disease in South-East Asia. Clinically, patients with Hgb H present with moderate anemia and splenomegaly. The peripheral blood picture includes hypochromia, microcytosis and anisopoikilocytosis. Excess β chains form precipitated tetramers (i.e. Hgb H) which are seen as fine inclusions (with the RBCs having a 'golf ball' appearance) on supravital staining (Figure 14.6). The presence of Hgb H can be confirmed by cellulose acetate electrophoresis. If the patient has the $- - / \alpha\alpha^{cs}$ genotype, the band corresponding to hemoglobin Constant Spring will be seen.

Hydrops fetalis results from the deletion of all four α genes (Figure 14.7). The resulting hemoglobin (Hgb Bart's) has a high oxygen affinity and is therefore useless in supplying oxygen to the tissues. The result is a fatal anemia *in utero* by the third trimester.

14.5.2 β-Thalassemias

The subclassification of β-thalassemias can be based on genotype or clinical manifestations.

14.5.2.1 Genetic classification of β-thalassemia

Many, but not all, α-thalassemias are caused by gene deletions. In contrast, most mutations in β-thalassemias are nondeletional, resulting in alterations in mRNA transcription or mRNA processing. There are at least 100 different

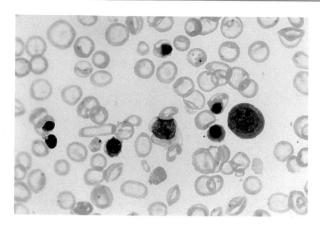

Figure 14.7 Severe hypochromia and numerous circulating NRBCs in a case of Hgb Bart's

known mutations causing β-thalassemia. Two main subgroups are recognized: (1) mutations which completely suppress β chain synthesis in the homozygous state are designated as β^0 genes; and (2) mutations which, in the homozygous state, only result in a decreased production of β chains are called β^+ genes.

Hgb Lepore syndromes (encountered in all ethnic groups) are produced by a combination of mutations resulting in a hybrid gene plus a defect in mRNA production. The hybrid gene, δβ *Lepore*, is composed of sequences from the δ gene (at the $5'$ end) and sequences from the β gene (at the $3'$ end). Hgb Lepore moves electrophoretically in the same position as Hgb S.

Also grouped together with the β-thalassemias are the δβ-thalassemias, in which the deletional mutations result in a decrease or absence of both δ and β chains in the homozygous state. In these conditions, a partial compensatory production of γ chains alleviates globin chain imbalance and decreases disease severity. In HPFH, there is full compensation from γ chain synthesis. Homozygous patients with HPFH are therefore asymptomatic. There are two main categories of HPFH based on whether Hgb F is uniformly distributed in RBCs (the pancellular type) or not (the heterocellular type). Homozygosity for the pancellular type of HPFH has been seen in blacks only. It is characterized by normal to increased hemoglobin levels (100% Hgb F), a low to normal MCV and abundant target cells on the blood film (Figure 14.2). Individuals affected with the heterozygous form of pancellular HPFH have no anemia, slight hypochromia and/or microcytosis, and abundant target cells. Hemoglobin A_2 levels are decreased and there is a moderate increase in Hgb F (10–36%). Individuals with the heterocellular form of HPFH, whether homozygous or heterozygous, are clinically and hematologically normal. They have decreased Hgb A_2 levels and increased Hgb F (19–21% for homozygous and 1–13% for heterozygous).

14.5.2.2 Clinical classification of β-thalassemia

The β-thalassemias manifest clinically as three major groups: (1) β-thalassemia major; (2) β-thalassemia intermedia; and (3) β-thalassemia minor (trait). Identification of the exact underlying genotype in overtly symptomatic patients is usually not necessary.

The most common genotypes causing β-thalassemia major are β^0/β^0, β^0/β^+ and homozygous Hgb Lepore. In these conditions, hemoglobin electrophoresis shows Hgb F as the predominant component with absent to trace Hgb A and an increased ratio of Hgb A_2 to Hgb A. If the patient has Hgb Lepore, it makes up about 10–20% of the total hemoglobin. The severity of β-thalassemia major (Figure 14.8) is due to the excess of free α chains, which aggregate within erythroid precursors. This causes marked dyserythropoiesis and excessive intramedullary destruction. It is in this group of patients that the most dramatic RBC changes are found (i.e. NRBCs, basophilic stippling, Pappenheimer bodies, teardrop cells and severe hypochromia).

A large number of genotypes can manifest as β-thalassemia intermedia, including patients with Hgb Lepore in combination with other defects, and patients with δβ-thalassemia. When the δ gene is affected, Hgb A_2 is decreased to absent. Hgb F is the predominant hemoglobin in all of these patients.

Heterozygosity for β^0 or β^+ are the most common genotypes causing β-thalassemia minor. These two genotypes can only be distinguished by determining the globin chain synthesis ratio in peripheral blood reticulocytes. The key diagnostic feature of β-thalassemia minor is an increase in Hgb A_2 (3.5–8%). This can be masked by iron deficiency, which causes the Hgb A_2 levels to be normal or low. In that case, the β-thalassemia trait can only be uncovered once the iron deficiency is treated. In Hgb Lepore trait (i.e. heterozygous Hgb Lepore), Hgb A_2 is less than normal and Hgb Lepore is present along with Hgb A.

The differential diagnosis between thalassemia minor and iron deficiency may not be straightforward, since the two conditions can coexist. In endemic areas, it is also important to screen potential mothers for thalassemia and other structural hemoglobinopathies (e.g. Hgb S, Hgb E). If the woman is positive, it is prudent to screen the woman's partner in order to council the prospective parents, and hopefully avoid any severe thalassemic syndrome in the offspring. With the currently

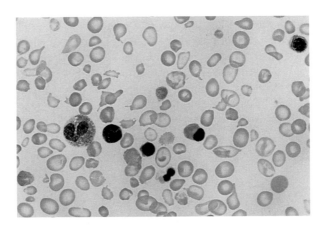

Figure 14.8 β-Thalassemia major in an untreated 9-month-old infant, showing NRBCs and severely hypochromic RBCs which can easily become fragmented. The polychromatophilic cells are also poorly hemoglobinized

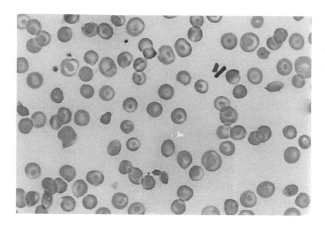

Figure 14.9 Two Hgb C crystals in a case of Hgb C disease

available restriction endonucleases, it is possible to perform prenatal diagnosis on fetal DNA obtained from amniocentesis to detect gene deletions/mutations.

14.6 Hemoglobinopathies presenting with a hypochromia/ microcytosis pattern

Hemoglobin C disease (C-C) and Hgb E disease (E-E) can present as hypochromic, microcytic anemias.

Hemoglobin C disease is found among blacks, but is rare. The MCV may be microcytic or in the normal range. The diagnosis rests on hemoglobin electrophoresis. The peripheral blood contains abundant target cells. On rare occasions, the pathognomonic Hgb C crystals (Figure 14.9) are found.

Hemoglobin E disease, most common among South-East Asians, is characterized by a decreased MCV with little or no anemia. Again, the predominant finding on the peripheral blood film is abundant target cells. Individuals with Hgb E trait also have a decreased MCV but without anemia. In South-East Asia, double inheritance for Hgb E and β^0-thalassemia is common, manifesting clinically as thalassemia major (Figure 14.3).

Macrocytosis pattern

Although reference ranges for MCV differ between laboratories, it is generally accepted that an MCV greater than 100 is indicative of macrocytosis. Several conditions can give rise to a falsely elevated MCV.

15.1 Factitious macrocytosis

Factitious macrocytosis can result from:

1. **RBC agglutination** (Figure 15.1). This is caused by cold agglutinins, resulting in doublets and triplets of RBCs which are counted as single cells. Clumps of cells greater than the upper threshold of the analyzer are excluded from the enumeration. These factors result in a falsely low RBC count and a falsely high MCV, which in turn leads to a falsely high MCHC. This condition can be suspected when the hemogram demonstrates a lack of concordance between the RBC count, Hgb, and Hct, along with a high MCV and a marked elevation of the MCIIC. An RBC agglutination suspect flag should also be present. Warming the blood to 37°C will reverse the effect.

2. **Hyperosmolar conditions**, e.g. severe hyperglycemia (blood glucose of 800–2000 mg/dl) as seen in uncontrolled diabetes mellitus. With severe hyperglycemia, the RBCs become hyperosmolar (glucose-loaded). When these cells are mixed with the isotonic diluent, water moves more rapidly than electrolytes and glucose across the cell membrane, causing the cells to swell. The MCV is falsely elevated. In turn, the Hct is falsely elevated and the MCHC falsely decreased. On the blood film, the RBC size does not reflect the 'increased' MCV. Indeed, the process may have masked a microcytosis. The problem can be corrected by pre-diluting the specimen with isotonic diluent to allow osmotic equilibrium to be achieved. A more accurate Hct can be determined from a spun microhematocrit, if necessary.

3. A **marked leukocytosis** (especially $> 100 \times 10^9$/l). This can lead to a falsely elevated Hgb and a falsely high MCV. The Hgb and Hct may need to be determined manually. Since the primary problem is a white cell disorder, the factitious macrocytosis is of little consequence to the overall interpretation of the hemogram.

4. Prolonged specimen storage.

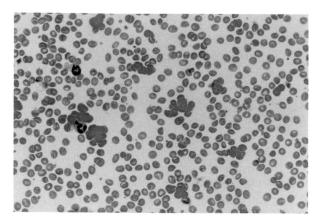

Figure 15.1   RBC agglutination

15.2 Macrocytosis secondary to increased reticulocytes

Increased release of reticulocytes from the bone marrow can raise the MCV. Reticulocytes are about 20% larger than mature erythrocytes. In stressful conditions with accelerated bone marrow production of RBC precursors, cell division may be skipped during the maturation process, resulting in the release of 'macroreticulocytes' which can be twice the size of normal RBCs. This mechanism accounts for the macrocytosis seen in severe hemolytic anemias, including thalassemia, where the marked reticulocytosis may result in a normal or even high MCV.

15.3 True macrocytosis

Macrocytosis can result from abnormalities in DNA synthesis or alterations in the lipid content of the RBC membrane:

1. Macrocytosis occurs when DNA synthesis and cell division are delayed and out of synchronization with the synthesis of cytoplasmic components such as hemoglobin. This mechanism accounts for the increased MCV seen in B_{12}/folate deficiency, chemotherapy, myelodysplastic syndromes and hematopoietic malignancies. The result of asynchronous nuclear/cytoplasmic maturation in erythroid precursors is an RBC with increased volume, diameter and thickness. The hemoglobin concentration is increased in proportion to the cell size (i.e. the cell is normochromic). On blood films, the increased thickness is seen as a loss of central pallor.
2. In liver disease, or status post-splenectomy, increased cholesterol in RBC membranes results in increased surface area without an increase in cell volume. On the peripheral blood film, RBCs may appear either as macrocytes with an increased diameter and enlarged central pallor (i.e. a thin

macrocyte), or as target cells. In alcoholic liver disease, macrocytosis can be due to a combination of mechanisms including impaired DNA synthesis and reticulocytosis, in addition to the RBC membrane abnormalities.

15.4 Conditions with macrocytosis

Macrocytosis can manifest with or without anemia. Mild macrocytosis (MCV 100–110) without anemia can represent a 'physiologic' state or be due to several underlying causes (e.g. ethanol consumption, early B_{12}/folate deficiency, or hydroxyurea therapy in PRV).

'Physiologic' macrocytosis occurs in both neonates and elderly patients. A moderate to marked macrocytosis (MCV 110–130) is normal at birth. Thereafter, the MCV decreases steadily until normal 'adult' levels (i.e. MCV < 100) are reached. During this time there is also a steady decrease in hemoglobin levels ('physiologic anemia' of the newborn) caused by the postnatal fall in erythropoietin production. The blood film of normal newborns is characterized by macrocytic RBCs, mild polychromasia and a few NRBCs that usually disappear after the first week. A few fragmented cells and target cells can be present. This physiologic neonatal macrocytosis in healthy newborns does not require any diagnostic work-up. According to several studies, mild macrocytosis is a frequent occurrence in apparently healthy elderly individuals, especially in association with smoking. The hemoglobin level in the elderly is lower than that in younger adults, and can fall into the 'anemic' range when compared to laboratory reference ranges that have been established using young healthy adults. In the geriatric age group, there is an increased incidence of malignancies, however. Therefore, caution must be observed before concluding that macrocytosis in an older person, with or without anemia, is due to age and not some underlying illness.

A large number of disorders can present with macrocytic anemia, including B_{12}/folate deficiency, MDS, bone marrow infiltration, chemotherapy and hemolytic anemias. The peripheral blood morphology may give clues to the underlying process, such as the presence of hypersegmented or hyposegmented neutrophils, or an overwhelming number of target cells or stomatocytes.

In addition to blood film examination, an absolute reticulocyte count is a helpful first step in the diagnostic work-up of a macrocytic anemia. An automated reticulocyte count is the method of choice, since it is more accurate and less labor intensive than the manual method. An increased absolute reticulocyte count indicates active erythropoiesis. The conditions that can manifest as a macrocytic anemia with an increased absolute reticulocyte count include hemolytic anemias (see Chapter 17), hemorrhage (see Chapter 16) and treated B_{12}/folate deficiency. In macrocytic anemia secondary to decreased production, the absolute reticulocyte count is either normal or decreased.

Additional laboratory tests, B_{12}/folate levels, liver function tests including γ-glutamic transferase, and clinical information (e.g. a history of malignancy or chemotherapy) can help narrow the differential diagnosis. Bone marrow studies may be necessary to establish the definitive diagnosis.

15.5 B₁₂/folate deficiency

Macrocytic anemia caused by B_{12}/folate deficiency has been traditionally called 'megaloblastic' anemia. Since the term 'megaloblast' refers to giant erythroblasts observed in the bone marrow and only rarely present in peripheral blood, it is more correct to limit the designation 'megaloblastic' to bone marrow diagnoses. Depending on the severity of the B_{12} and/or folate deficiency, the peripheral blood manifestation of the disorder can be NCNC anemia, a mild macrocytosis (MCV 100–110) without anemia, macrocytic anemia alone, or macrocytic anemia with leukopenia and/or thrombocytopenia.

15.5.1 Peripheral blood findings in B₁₂/folate deficiency

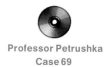

Professor Petrushka
Case 69

Morphologic abnormalities in overt cases of B_{12} and folate deficiency, such as hypersegmented neutrophils (Figure 15.2a) and oval macrocytes (Figure 15.3a), are easily identified. These features are not specific for B_{12}/folate deficiency, however. They can occur in macrocytosis secondary to folate antagonists and hydroxyurea (Figure 15.2b). Oval macrocytes can also be found in MDS (Figure 15.3b) and in the rare disorder, South-East Asian ovalocytosis. With severe anemia (Hgb < 7–8 g/dl), other nonspecific RBC abnormalities may be present including teardrop cells, fragmented cells, basophilic stippling, Howell-Jolly

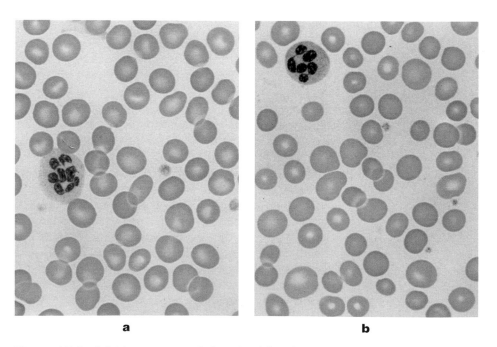

a   b

Figure 15.2   (a) A hypersegmented neutrophil and macrocytosis in folate deficiency. (b) Similar features in a patient with CML on hydroxyurea therapy (normal WBC count)

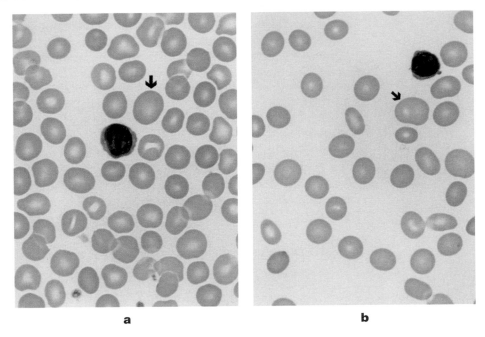

a   **b**

Figure 15.3 An occasional oval macrocyte (arrow) in folate deficiency (a) and a mye-lodysplastic syndrome (b)

bodies and NRBCs exhibiting nuclear/cytoplasmic asynchrony. Knowledge of the clinical background is often a helpful clue. An increased propensity for B_{12}/folate deficiency exists among certain groups of individuals, namely pregnant females, HIV-positive patients, patients with multiple myeloma and the elderly.

The peripheral blood manifestations of B_{12}/folate deficiency can be masked by coexisting iron deficiency, thalassemia trait or pre-existing hematological conditions that are accompanied by marked RBC morphologic abnormalities. Patients with chronically stressed hematopoiesis (e.g. with hemoglobinopathies or thalassemia major) have increased requirements for folate. Under these circumstances, folate stores can be quickly depleted but the MCV may not rise above the normal range and macrocytes may be difficult to detect on the peripheral blood film. Since hypersegmented neutrophils can occasionally occur in iron deficiency alone, their presence does not necessarily indicate coexisting B_{12}/folate deficiency.

15.5.2 Determination of B_{12}/folate levels

Assays of B_{12}/folate levels are necessary to determine the exact deficiency. The tests should be performed as a panel since individual test values may overlap in folate deficiency and B_{12} deficiency. If the levels are determined by microbiologic assay (rather than isotope techniques), it is necessary to ensure that the patient is not on any medications which can interfere with the assay (e.g. antibiotics, folate antagonists or chlorpromazine). Although microbiologic assays for B_{12} and folate are more time-consuming than isotope methods, they yield the most consistently reliable results.

Serum folate levels fluctuate with short-term variations in vitamin intake. Low serum folate, therefore, does not necessarily indicate folate deficiency. RBC folate levels are a better index of tissue folate stores. In folate deficiency, both serum and RBC folate levels are decreased. In B_{12} deficiency, serum folate may be increased and RBC folate may be decreased, since tissue and RBC uptake of serum folate requires the presence of vitamin B_{12}.

Most of the B_{12} in the serum is bound to transcobalamin I, a carrier protein, and is in equilibrium with tissue stores. Therefore, serum B_{12} levels are a reliable index of body stores when known causes of spurious B_{12} results are not present. The circumstances that can give rise to spuriously low levels of B_{12} are shown in Table 15.1.

Table 15.1 Circumstances giving rise to spuriously low levels of vitamin B_{12}

- Drugs interfering with the microbiologic assay of vitamin B_{12}.
- Megadose vitamin C.
- Pregnancy or birth control pills.
- Folate deficiency.
- Transcobalamin I deficiency (a rare congenital disorder).

15.5.3 Underlying causes of B_{12}/folate deficiency

The most common cause for folate deficiency is insufficient dietary intake of folate secondary to either malnutrition or excessive cooking of vegetables. Deficiency can also result from elevated folate requirements (i.e. increased cell turnover or proliferation) as seen in pregnancy, severe hemolytic anemia, bone marrow malignancies and exfoliative skin disorders. Less frequent causes of folate deficiency include intestinal malabsorption due to extensive small bowel resection, gluten-sensitive enteropathy, long-term anticonvulsant therapy and oral contraceptives. Folate deficiency in chronic alcoholism results from several factors including poor nutrition, inhibition of folate absorption by ethanol, and a direct toxic effect of ethanol on the bone marrow.

In contrast to folate, dietary B_{12} deficiency is rare, even in strict vegetarians. The two major causes of B_{12} deficiency are food-bound B_{12} malabsorption and gastric/small bowel disorders causing intrinsic factor (IF) deficiency.

Food-bound B_{12} malabsorption is the inability to release B_{12} from its binders in food. This mechanism accounts for 30–40% of B_{12} deficiency among the elderly. In these patients, IF-mediated absorption of free B_{12} is normal. Therefore, the condition cannot be detected by the Schilling test. Possible underlying causes of food-bound B_{12} malabsorption include decreased gastric secretion (either from gastric atrophy or secondary to acid suppressive therapy) and micro-organisms (such as *Helicobacter pylori*). Since the absorption of free B_{12} is unaltered, B_{12} depletion secondary to this mechanism progresses at a much slower rate than in pernicious anemia (PA). Most affected patients demonstrate little or no clinical symptoms. However, overt symptoms can develop promptly if the patients are exposed to factors that further interfere with B_{12} metabolism (e.g. nitrous oxide exposure during surgery).

Pernicious anemia is caused by a deficiency of IF, the glycoprotein carrier involved in the transport of vitamin B_{12} to the specific mucosal receptors in the distal ileum where B_{12} passes into the bloodstream. The fundamental abnormality in PA is gastric atrophy. It is presumed to be an autoimmune disorder because autoantibodies to parietal cells and/or IF can be detected in the serum, saliva, or gastric fluid of many patients. Antibodies to IF are of two forms: (1) blocking antibodies, which occlude the binding site on IF, thereby preventing the formation of an IF-B_{12} complex; and (2) binding antibodies, which prevent the attachment of IF or the IF-B_{12} complex to ileal receptors. Useful diagnostic tests to confirm the diagnosis of PA include direct estimation of IF in gastric fluid, detection of IF antibodies in the serum by sensitive techniques (e.g. radioimmunoassay) and the Schilling urinary excretion test. Some patients with PA may present with a pronounced neuropathy without overt anemia.

In the Schilling test, the fasting patient is injected with a large 'flushing' dose of nonradioactive B_{12} intramuscularly, and, at the same time, is given an oral physiologic dose of radiolabeled B_{12}. The radioactivity of the urine collected over 24 hours is measured to assess the absorption of vitamin B_{12}. A low urinary excretion of radioactivity indicates malabsorption. To confirm that malabsorption is due to IF deficiency, a second Schilling test is performed 5 or more days after the first test. In the second test, purified IF is given orally along with the radiolabeled B_{12}. Increased urinary excretion of radioactivity indicates IF deficiency. No change between the results of the first and second tests indicates that malabsorption is due to small bowel disease. The major sources of error in the Schilling test are incomplete urine collection and renal dysfunction. If direct measurement of IF, or detection of IF antibodies yields a positive result for PA, a Schilling test becomes unnecessary.

Other less frequent causes of B_{12} deficiency include gastric surgery, hemodialysis, extensive disease or surgery of the ileum, and fish tapeworm (*Diphyllobothrium latum*) infestation.

15.6 Drug-induced macrocytic anemia

Most cases of drug-induced macrocytosis/macrocytic anemia are caused by chemotherapeutic agents that interfere with DNA synthesis. There are two broad categories: folate antagonists and antimetabolites. Folate antagonists, such as methotrexate and aminopterin, are powerful inhibitors of dihydrofolate reductase. Administering a prophylactic high dose of folinic acid can prevent the toxic effect. Antimetabolites can be purine analogs (e.g. azathioprine, 6-mercaptopurine, 6-thioguanine, and high dose acyclovir) or pyrimidine analogs (e.g. 5-fluorouracil, 6-azauridine, and AZT). Other antimetabolites interfere with ribonucleotide reductase (e.g. hydroxyurea) or DNA polymerase (e.g. cytosine arabinoside).

Rapid onset of macrocytic anemia ('acute megaloblastic anemia') can result from nitrous oxide anesthesia. The active (reduced) form of B_{12} is oxidized into an inactive form, resulting in impairment of folate metabolism and other B_{12}-dependent metabolic pathways. Megaloblastic effects in the bone marrow occur within 6–24 hours after nitrous oxide exposure. The effects of nitrous oxide reverse after 1–2 days. Giving a prophylactic high dose of folinic acid can prevent the problem.

15.7 Other causes of macrocytic anemia

The other major causes of macrocytic anemia include alcoholic liver disease, MDS and congenital disorders. A macrocytic anemia can occur in alcoholic liver disease in the absence of folate or B_{12} deficiency because ethanol has a direct toxic effect on hematopoiesis. The peripheral blood manifestations can simulate those of B_{12} or folate deficiency and the blood counts reflect the severity of the disorder. With increasing severity, the patient develops bicytopenia or pancytopenia.

In the context of a high MCV, the finding of abundant target cells and/or stomatocytes without accompanying hypersegmented neutrophils is suggestive of alcoholic liver disease. Stomatocytes are cup-shaped (i.e. uniconcave) RBCs which appear as cells with a slit-like mouth on peripheral blood films. Hemorrhage and hemolysis (common in ethanol abuse) will cause reticulocytosis that further increases the MCV. Useful laboratory studies include liver function tests (with determinations of γ-glutamic transferase), and B_{12}/folate levels to exclude concomitant deficiency.

The differential diagnosis of macrocytosis with little or no anemia accompanied by abundant stomatocytes also includes hereditary stomatocytosis (Figure 15.4), a heterogeneous group of disorders characterized by RBC swelling due to increased intracellular sodium and water. The underlying pathogenesis includes various

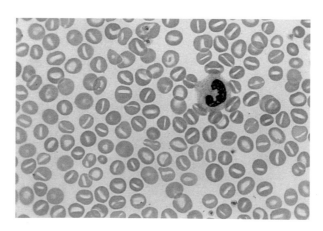

Figure 15.4 Hereditary stomatocytosis

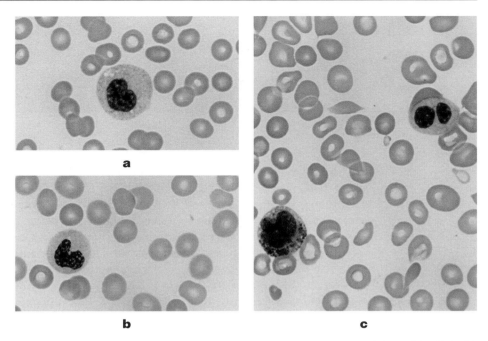

Figure 15.5 Hyposegmented neutrophils in three different conditions: (a) MDS; (b) HIV infection; and (c) treated CML

membrane defects. Hereditary stomatocytosis usually presents with a normal MCV. An increased MCV may be observed after splenectomy.

The peripheral blood manifestations of MDS can be similar to those of $B_{12}/$ folate deficiency. Hypogranulation and hyposegmentation in neutrophils (i.e. pseudo-Pelger-Huët anomaly) suggest MDS but can also occur in other disorders (Figure 15.5). Red cell changes in MDS may include teardrop cells, stomatocytes, a mixture of hypochromic and normochromic cells, basophilic stippling and occasional NRBCs. The RBC morphologic changes are not specific to MDS, however. The definitive diagnosis and classification is based on bone marrow findings.

Congenital/hereditary disorders are rare causes of macrocytic anemia. These include:

- Metabolic abnormalities, such as inborn errors of folate (e.g. dihydrofolate reductase deficiency), pyrimidine (e.g. hereditary orotic aciduria), or purine metabolism (e.g. Lesch-Nyhan syndrome).
- Deficiency of the protein carrier transcobalamin II, which is responsible for transport of B_{12} to the appropriate receptor sites in tissue cells.
- Congenital dyserythropoietic anemia type I (autosomal recessive) and CDA type III (autosomal dominant). These disorders may present as a mild to moderate macrocytic anemia. Bone marrow evaluation and family studies are necessary to establish the diagnosis.

Normochromic, normocytic anemia pattern

Normochromic, normocytic anemias occur in a large number of settings in which RBC survival is shortened and/or bone marrow erythropoiesis is affected. Depending on the etiology and severity of the anemia, variations in RBC size (anisocytosis) and RBC shape (poikilocytosis) can range from imperceptible/minimal to extremely marked. Currently, automated analyzers are not capable of identifying specific types of poikilocytes. The assessment of anisocytosis, on the other hand, has already been automated and is expressed by the RDW. Most instruments calculate the RDW as the standard deviation of the distribution of RBC volumes divided by the MCV. The upper limit of normal for RDW is usually set to a value between 14 and 15. In addition to the large category of anemia of chronic disease, NCNC anemia with a normal RDW can also occur in liver, renal and endocrine disorders. Normochromic, normocytic anemias with a high RDW are covered in Chapter 17.

16.1 Absolute reticulocyte count

Normochromic, normocytic anemia may be the sole manifestation or the first incidental evidence of a potentially serious systemic disease. Since the RBC morphology is often relatively unremarkable, the list of diagnostic possibilities is long. Therefore, identifying the underlying cause requires correlation with other clinical and laboratory data. A useful test is the absolute reticulocyte count to determine if the bone marrow response is appropriate for the degree of anemia. The traditional manual microscopic method for reticulocytes, using the supravital stain new methylene blue, is tedious and poorly reproducible. Automated reticulocyte counting achieves a higher degree of precision and efficiency since it utilizes a much larger (thereby more representative) sample and eliminates interobserver variation. In addition, since the amount of RNA remaining in a reticulocyte is inversely proportional to the age of the cell, the degree of reticulocyte maturation can be determined by automated methods. The younger the reticulocytes, the higher the fluorescence intensity. A relatively high proportion of brightly fluorescent reticulocytes is an early indicator of bone marrow recovery following bone marrow transplantation.

The absolute reticulocyte count, obtained by multiplying the percentage of reticulocytes by the RBC count, is the appropriate way to report reticulocytes. Expressing the reticulocyte count as a percentage alone can be misleading since the percentage can be increased either from a higher number of circulating reticulocytes or a decreased number of mature RBCs. An increased absolute reticulocyte count in the presence of anemia indicates an appropriate bone marrow response in an effort to compensate for the anemia. If the absolute reticulocyte count is decreased despite the anemia, it indicates a problem with bone marrow erythropoiesis. The reticulocyte data are least helpful when the absolute value falls within the 'normal' range (40,000–100,000/μl).

Acute blood loss (hemorrhage) and hemolytic anemias account for most of the NCNC anemias with an increased absolute reticulocyte count. With intact bone marrow function, and in the absence of complicating factors, the reticulocyte response is seen within 3–5 days and disappears after 10–14 days following an acute episode of hemorrhage/hemolysis. In most cases, the reticulocytosis does not result in frank anisocytosis. The hemoglobin level is restored after 6–8 weeks. In hospitalized patients, the physiologic response is altered and therefore less evident if the patient is transfused.

Reticulocytosis also occurs in hemolytic anemias. Hemolytic anemias are usually accompanied by an increased RDW and are discussed in Chapter 17. If the anemia is very mild or the disease is in the quiescent phase (e.g. G6PD or pyruvate kinase deficiency in the absence of oxidative stress), the hemolytic anemia may present as an NCNC anemia with only minimal RBC abnormalities and no increase in RDW.

A variety of disorders (mostly systemic diseases) can manifest as NCNC anemia without an apparent reticulocytosis. These include anemia associated with infections/inflammatory conditions, malignancies (in which the bone marrow remains uninvolved), renal insufficiency, liver disease, endocrine disease, early iron or B_{12}/folate deficiency (including B_{12}/folate deficiency masked by coexisting iron deficiency), bone marrow infiltration and chemotherapy. Similar anemias can be the result of erythroid hypoplasia, either congenital (i.e. Blackfan-Diamond syndrome) or acquired (as the result of viral infections such as parvovirus B19, or in association with neoplasms such as a thymoma).

To narrow this list of differential diagnoses, correlation with clinical history and other laboratory data is necessary (Table 16.1).

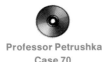

Professor Petrushka
Case 70

Table 16.1 Laboratory tests which may be helpful in the work-up of NCNC anemia

- Iron studies (serum ferritin, RBC ferritin).
- Serologies (e.g. rheumatoid factor, antinuclear antibodies, antibodies to double-stranded DNA) if autoimmune disease is suspected.
- Serum B_{12}/folate and RBC folate levels.
- BUN/creatinine.
- Liver function tests (including γ-glutamic transferase).
- Serum protein electrophoresis and immunoelectrophoresis.
- Hormone assays (e.g. thyroid hormones, growth hormone, cortisol) if an endocrine disease is being considered.
- Bone marrow aspirate/biopsy if the clinical and laboratory data yield no answer in the face of a persistent or worsening anemia.

16.2 Peripheral blood film findings

**Professor Petrushka
Case 71**

In most NCNC anemias with a normal RDW, RBC abnormalities are minimal (1 +). In some instances, the blood film demonstrates a particular preponderant (2 + /3 +) RBC abnormality, namely target cells, echinocytes, or rouleaux, which may suggest the underlying cause of the anemia. Morphologic changes in the WBCs may also provide a clue to the etiology. For example, hypersegmented neutrophils suggest early B_{12}/folate deficiency and hypogranulation together with hyposegmentation suggests an underlying bone marrow disorder.

Target cells have less value as a clue to the diagnosis in NCNC anemia than in the setting of an increased MCV, or a decreased MCV/MCH. The formation of target cells can be due to either excess RBC membrane (liver disease, status post-splenectomy) or decreased Hgb content (hemoglobinopathy, thalassemia). The combination of NCNC anemia and a preponderant population of target cells (but no Howell-Jolly bodies) suggests either liver disease or a mild/stable hemoglobinopathy. Howell-Jolly bodies are present along with a significant number of target cells in hyposplenic states.

Echinocytes (burr cells, crenated cells) are erythrocytes with 10–30 short, blunt evenly spaced spicules (Figure 16.1). This RBC change is often unhelpful since the most common cause of the abnormality is a delay in making the peripheral blood film (old blood). Echinocyte formation is presumed to be secondary to decreased ATP or accumulation of fatty acid/lysolecithin on the cell surface. In addition to prolonged blood storage, this finding can occur in pyruvate kinase deficiency, splenectomized patients and conditions with RBC/plasma metabolic alterations (uremia or heparinized patients on cardiopulmonary bypass).

Rouleaux formation (Figure 1.12) occurs with high levels of high molecular weight proteins (immunoglobulins, α2-macroglobulin, fibrinogen). Therefore, the presence of rouleaux suggests a plasma cell dyscrasia (multiple myeloma or Wal-

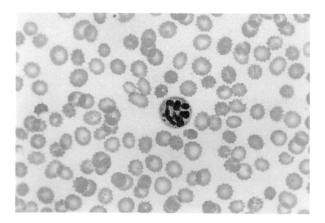

Figure 16.1 Numerous echinocytes in a case of chronic renal failure. Note the hypersegmented neutrophil with a nuclear fragment. The patient was treated for an underlying solid tumor. Serum and RBC folate levels were normal

denstrom's macroglobulinemia), inflammatory conditions (all of the high molecular weight proteins are increased) or pregnancy (increased fibrinogen).

16.3 Anemia of chronic disease

Anemia of chronic disease is one of the most frequently diagnosed NCNC anemias. The main causes are malignancies and chronic inflammatory disorders. Typically, the anemia is mild to moderate and is characterized by a decreased serum iron, decreased TIBC, increased transferrin saturation, and normal or increased iron stores.

Since ferritin is one of several acute phase reactants, otherwise known as C-reactive proteins, serum ferritin values are often increased in inflammatory disorders, thereby masking any coexisting iron deficiency. It has been suggested that a level of 60 mg/l be used as the lower limit of normal for serum ferritin in inflammatory conditions such as rheumatoid arthritis. C-reactive protein levels are a more sensitive and specific measure of active inflammation than the erythrocyte sedimentation rate. Red blood cell ferritin levels should be used to assess iron reserves in a patient with increased C-reactive protein and serum ferritin values in the normal/high range.

In anemia of chronic disease, the reticulocyte count is not appropriately increased for the degree of anemia, despite increased erythropoietin release. The underlying mechanism is not fully understood. Current evidence points to cytokines (e.g. γ-interferon, IL-1, and tumor necrosis factor) playing a role in inhibiting erythropoiesis. Cytokines may also be responsible for the altered iron metabolism.

16.4 Anemia in renal disease

In renal failure, the two mechanisms responsible for anemia are: (1) impaired erythropoietin secretion, and (2) retention of toxic substances which results in decreased erythroid production in the bone marrow and shortened survival of both the patient's own RBCs and transfused RBCs. The proposed toxic substances have not yet been identified but presumably they are not dialyzed. In renal disease, RBC morphology is essentially normal, although variable numbers of echinocytes may be present. When patients with renal failure undergo dialysis, the most common superimposed complication is iron deficiency resulting from blood lost in the hemodialysis apparatus. Iron deficiency can also develop as the patient responds to recombinant human erythropoietin treatment. Another possible cause for microcytic anemia in patients undergoing dialysis is aluminum toxicity, since aluminum interferes with incorporation of iron into erythroid precursors.

16.5 Anemia in liver disease

The anemia in liver disease may be an NCNC anemia with or without anisocytosis or may be a macrocytic anemia. Thrombocytopenia can also be present. Target cells and macrocytes (including oval macrocytes) are common. In a small number of patients with liver failure, a stable/nonprogressive anemia suddenly changes into a progressive/fatal hemolytic anemia characterized by numerous acanthocytes (see Section 17.2.6).

The underlying mechanisms of anemia in liver disease can include any of the following: (1) acute hemorrhage; (2) B_{12}/folate deficiency; (3) hypersplenism (which can cause trapping of both RBCs and platelets); and (4) direct toxic effect on bone marrow RBC production, especially in liver disease related to alcohol.

16.6 Anemia in endocrine disease

The anemia associated with endocrine deficiencies is presumed to be an 'adaptive' anemia. The hormone deficiency causes decreased metabolic activity (i.e. decreased tissue consumption of oxygen). Therefore, the body responds by decreasing erythropoietin, which results in less bone marrow production of RBC precursors. Red blood cell abnormalities are usually absent unless there is superimposed iron or folate deficiency (a frequent occurrence in patients with hypothyroidism). In hyperthyroidism, the mechanism of anemia is unknown.

Anemia with anisocytosis pattern

The definition of the anemia with anisocytosis pattern is decreased hemoglobin, a normal MCV and an increased RDW (i.e. an NCNC anemia with a high RDW). Alterations in RBC shape (poikilocytosis) often result in changes in RBC size, and therefore affect the RDW. In most laboratories, the upper limit of normal for RDW is set between 14 and 15. Values greater than this cut-off signify anisocytosis. There is little advantage in arbitrarily setting this cut-off too low. Setting the limit for anisocytosis at 14 results in a high number of cases with a slightly increased RDW (flagged by the analyzer as 'abnormal'), most if not all of which would reveal virtually no RBC changes on examination of a peripheral blood film. The authors' preference is to set the upper limit of normal for RDW at 15.

The peripheral blood picture in an anemic patient depends on several factors, including: (1) when in the course of the disease the patient is examined; (2) the severity of the disease; and (3) the presence or absence of complications or therapeutic intervention. For this reason, several types of NCNC anemia can present with or without anisocytosis.

17.1 Differential diagnosis of an anemia with anisocytosis

The differential diagnosis of NCNC anemia with anisocytosis includes: (1) early iron or B_{12}/folate deficiency; (2) anemia secondary to systemic diseases; (3) bone marrow infiltration; and (4) hemolytic anemias. Since so many diseases can result in anemia with anisocytosis, it is important to examine the blood film with knowledge of the patient's clinical history.

In early iron or B_{12}/folate deficiency, if the MCV is in the normal range, the patient may present with an anemia with anisocytosis pattern. The recovery phase of iron or B_{12}/folate deficiency may result in a similar set of RBC parameters after appropriate replacement therapy. In anemia secondary to systemic disease (e.g. chemotherapy, renal failure) anisocytosis becomes noticeable as the anemia worsens.

Bone marrow infiltration occurs in metastatic carcinomas (most commonly breast, lung or prostate), hematological malignancies (especially bone marrow involvement by NHL, Hodgkin's disease or early MDS), granulomata, and metabolic disorders (e.g. Gaucher's disease). Bone marrow involvement by NHL usually causes little structural damage in the marrow, and the resulting mild anemia is accompanied by only mild anisocytosis. In contrast, metastatic carcinomas and AMM result in an anemia with a high degree of anisocytosis and poikilocytosis that may progress to a leukoerythroblastic picture.

17.1.1 Hemolytic anemias

Most hemolytic disorders (excluding thalassemias and severe hemoglobinopathies) manifest as mild to moderate anemia with anisocytosis. Worsening of the anemia often results in a leukoerythroblastic picture. The underlying category of hemolytic anemia can be suspected when the blood film reveals a predominant and/or specific RBC abnormality. In pyruvate kinase (PK) deficiency and hemolytic disorders with intravascular hemolysis, however, the RBC abnormalities are minimal apart from polychromasia.

Pyruvate kinase is the main enzyme deficiency in which the resulting hemolytic anemia usually shows no distinctive RBC abnormalities. In some cases, especially after splenectomy, abundant echinocytes are present. Since echinocytes commonly occur as an artifact, they have little diagnostic value. Several different mutants of the PK enzyme exist with variable clinical manifestations. Pyruvate kinase deficiency blocks the glycolytic pathway by which ATP is generated in mature RBCs, thereby altering membrane permeability and shortening RBC survival. The resulting anemia ranges from mild to severe, usually with bland RBC morphology and reticulocytosis. Similar to G6PD, PK activity is higher in reticulocytes. Marked reticulocytosis may give a false normal result on a PK assay. Therefore, the PK assay should be performed on reticulocyte-depleted samples.

Disorders with intravascular hemolysis include:

Professor Petrushka
Case 72

- PNH (see Section 12.2).
- Intermittent hemolysis associated with IgG hemolysins.
- Hemolysis secondary to severe excercise or physical trauma.
- Hemolysis secondary to infection or parasitic infestation. This occurs in infection by *Clostridium welchii*, certain gram-negative bacilli, *Babesia*, malarial parasites (Figure 17.1) and extracellular micro-organisms (Figure 17.2).

Although thick films can be used for the quick detection of parasites, identification of *Plasmodium* species is done on a thin film. Because the parasite count may be very low, it has been recommended to scan 100–200 fields with 1000 × magnification before signing out a slide as negative. For clinical purposes, the identification of *P. falciparum* (Figure 17.1a) is most important since infection with this organism can be fatal if left untreated. The identification is facilitated by the characteristic banana shape of the gametocytes of *P. falciparum* and the frequent multiple infection of red cells (i.e. two or more ring forms within the same RBC).

The *Babesia* parasite (Figure 17.3) occurs as ring forms within RBCs and can be easily confused with *Plasmodium*. The formation of a Maltese cross by four organisms in contact with each other is a diagnostic clue. The diagnosis can be confirmed by an indirect immunofluorescence antibody test on the serum. Hyposplenic individuals are particularly susceptible to babesiosis.

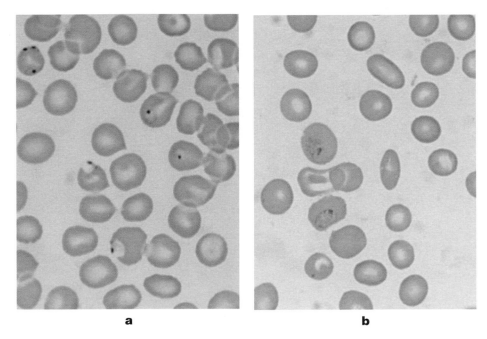

Figure 17.1 Malarial parasites: (a) Plasmodium falciparum trophozoites – some RBCs are infected by more than one organism; (b) Plasmodium vivax trophozoites

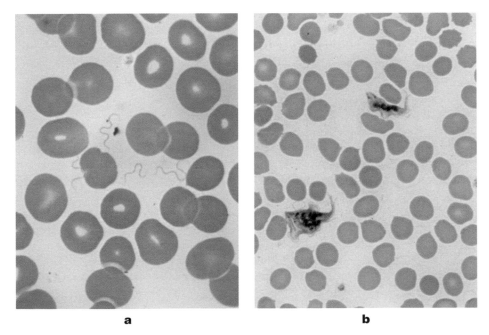

Figure 17.2 Extracellular micro-organisms in the blood: (a) Borrelia; (b) Trypanosoma gambiense

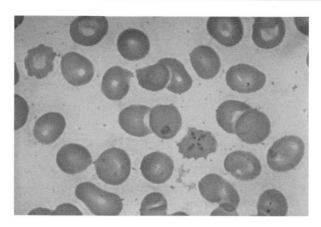

Figure 17.3 Diagnostic 'Maltese cross' formation in babesiosis. The patient is hyposplenic (Howell-Jolly bodies)

Bartonella bacilliformis is a gram-negative bacillus visible on Romanovsky-stained films. It causes a severe and sometimes fatal hemolytic anemia in certain areas of Central and South America.

17.2 Red cell abnormalities

As mentioned in Section 1.4, certain RBC abnormalities are more specific than others and several RBC abnormalities can be mistaken for each other (Table 17.1). In anemia with anisocytosis, the choice of confirmatory test(s) to narrow the differential diagnosis is made easier when a predominant and/or specific RBC abnormality is seen on the peripheral blood film.

17.2.1 Polychromasia

Significant polychromasia is a reflection of an increased percentage of reticulocytes, but not necessarily an increased absolute reticulocyte count. The polychromatophilic erythrocytes visible on a blood film correspond to young reticulocytes with high amounts of residual RNA. Polychromasia can be seen in: (1) neonates; (2) as a response to hemorrhage or hemolysis; (3) in response to iron or B_{12}/folate therapy in a previously deficient patient; (4) during recovery from bone marrow failure (especially after engraftment of a bone marrow

Table 17.1 RBC abnormalities that can be confused with each other

- Irregularly contracted cells: invariably misinterpreted as spherocytes.
- Bite cells: often identified as schistocytes.
- Echinocytes and acanthocytes: can be confused with each other.
- Distorted sickle cells (in S-C disorder): overlooked as schistocytes.
- Spherocytes: mislabeled as microcytes.

transplant); and (5) bone marrow infiltration. A large group of disorders are represented by the term bone marrow infiltration, including AMM. In this group of diseases, the absolute reticulocyte count is either decreased or within the noncontributory 'normal' range and the degree of polychromasia bears no relationship to the reticulocyte count.

In chronic hemolytic anemia, the absolute reticulocyte count is inversely proportional to the level of hemoglobin, unless there is a superimposed aplastic or megaloblastic crisis. An aplastic crisis can be caused by parvovirus B19 infection. A megaloblastic crisis can be the result of folate stores being depleted by chronic erythroid hyperplasia. The more severe the hemolytic anemia, the greater the chance of an aplastic or megaloblastic crisis.

With marked reticulocytosis, the MCV may be increased to greater than 100. Accelerated erythropoiesis can also demonstrate circulating NRBCs and basophilic stippling. Young reticulocytes have a tendency to stick to each other when present in high numbers (Figure 17.4). This phenomenon is different from the agglutination of mature RBCs and bears no relationship to the cold agglutinin syndrome. Therefore, warming the blood to 37°C has no effect on reticulocyte agglutinates.

17.2.2 Sickle cells

Sickle cells are pathognomonic for sickling disorders with clinical manifestations. The severity of the disease depends on the extent of the sickling process. The amount of sickling is determined by: (1) the concentration of deoxygenated Hgb S; (2) the presence of other hemoglobins in the RBCs (e.g. Hgb F); (3) low oxygen tension; and (4) other factors such as acidosis, vascular stasis or infection. The sickle cells are RBCs in which the sickling process has become irreversible.

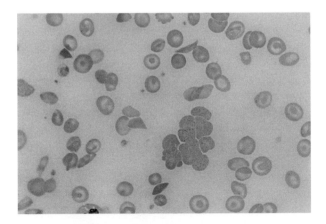

Figure 17.4 Agglutination of young polychromatophilic RBCs (reticulocytes) in Hgb S β-thalassemia with severe anemia. Basophilic stippling is visible in many of the reticulocytes. Note the presence of hypochromic and microcytic RBCs, abundant target cells and some sickle cells

The substitution of valine for glutamic acid in the sixth position of the β chain leads to polymerization of deoxygenated Hgb S molecules. With repeated polymerization and depolymerization while the erythrocytes circulate from peripheral tissues back to the lungs, the RBC membrane becomes altered, resulting in permanently sickled cells that do not revert to a normal shape even with vigorous reoxygenation. The most important determinant in this process is low oxygen tension.

Hemoglobin F interferes with the polymerization of Hgb S and thereby helps to prevent sickling. The amount of Hgb F varies from cell to cell in patients with S-S disease. Only those cells that are endowed with a high content of Hgb F are protected from sickling. In patients who are double heterozygous for Hgb S and HPFH, each RBC contains increased levels of Hgb F resulting in no sickling and no clinical disease. The protective effect of high levels of Hgb F is also evident in neonates with S-S disease who remain asymptomatic for the first 8–10 weeks of life. Variability in Hgb F production appears to be an important factor in the clinical severity of the disease. For example, Arabs with S-S disease have a mild anemia because of high Hgb F levels, in contrast to the severe anemia found among black patients. Hydroxyurea increases Hgb F production in most patients with S-S disease and has therefore been introduced as a treatment modality. Other hemoglobins do cause sickling when they interact with Hgb S, but the interaction is not as strong as the S-S interaction and there is some interference with the polymerization resulting in a somewhat milder disease. These hemoglobins include Hgb C, Hgb D, and Hgb O_{Arab}.

In general, sickle cells are easily found in S-S anemia, S $β^0$-thalassemia, and S-O_{Arab}. Anemia is less severe, with few to rare sickle cells in S-C, S $β^+$-thalassemia, S α-thalassemia and S-D. The sickle cells may be overlooked if they are 'plump' (Figure 17.5) or deformed (Figure 17.6a), as seen in S-C disease. On rare occasions, both sickle cells and Hgb C crystals (Figure 17.6b) can be found. An overwhelming number of sickle cells against a leukoerythroblastic background is typical of sickle cell crisis.

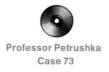

Professor Petrushka
Case 73

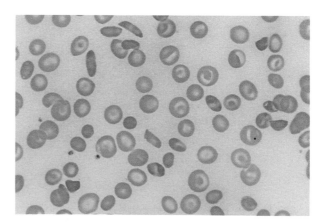

Figure 17.5 'Plump' sickle cells, numerous target cells and a Howell-Jolly body in sickle cell anemia

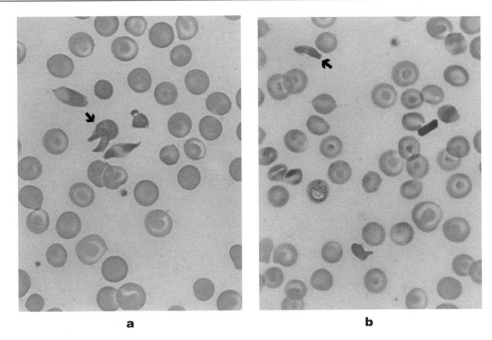

a   b

Figure 17.6 S-C disease: (a) a deformed sickle cell (arrow) and abundant target cells; (b) a sickle cell (arrow) and a rare Hgb C crystal in the same field

Additional RBC changes which may accompany sickle cells include abundant target cells (Figure 17.7), Howell-Jolly bodies (Figure 17.7a), Pappenheimer bodies (Figure 17.7b), IRCs and NRBCs. Howell-Jolly bodies (remnants of nuclear material) indicate the 'asplenic' state that usually results from repeated splenic infarction in adults with severe sickle cell disorders. The absence of Howell-Jolly bodies does not rule out S-S anemia, however, since young children with the disease have splenomegaly. Splenomegaly may persist into adulthood if the patient is infected with malarial organisms.

When easily detected basophilic stippling is present, along with a decreased MCH, decreased MCV and sickle cells, the findings are strongly suggestive of double heterozygosity for Hgb S and thalassemia (Figure 17.4). The MCH and MCV may also be decreased in S-S anemia if there is superimposed iron deficiency secondary to therapeutic venesection (Figure 17.7b).

The diagnosis of sickle cell disorders (whether symptomatic or not) relies on laboratory tests ranging from simple screening tests to sophisticated DNA analysis. The sickle solubility test (e.g. the commercially available Sickledex) is based on the insolubility of deoxy-Hgb S in a concentrated phosphate buffer. False-negative results are not uncommon when the level of Hgb S is low, such as in neonates or recently transfused patients. Another screening test for sickling uses sodium metabisulfite added to a drop of blood to induce the formation of deoxy-Hgb S. Under these conditions, RBCs containing Hgb S will become sickle cells, detectable by microscopic examination of a wet mount.

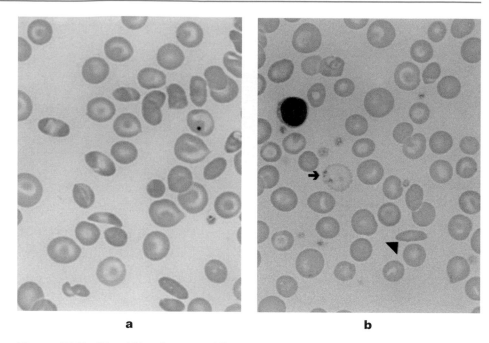

a   b

Figure 17.7 Blood films from two different patients with sickle cell anemia. (a) Sickle cells, target cells, a rare spherocyte and a Howell-Jolly body. (b) A rare Pappenheimer body (arrow) and a sickle cell (arrowhead). Note the hypochromic and microcytic RBCs. This patient also had iron deficiency induced by repeated therapeutic venesection

17.2.3 Target cells

In NCNC anemia, abundant target cells are commonly found in hemoglobino-pathies, liver disease and after splenectomy. The common hemoglobinopathies with numerous target cells include Hgb C trait, S-C, C-C, S-D, and homozy-gous Hgb O_{Arab}. If there is no evidence of liver disease or splenectomy, a care-ful search should be made for sickle cells and Hgb C crystals (Figure 17.6). The crystals are uncommon, but when present are pathognomonic for Hgb C. They can be found in C-C disease, S-C, and C β-thalassemia. In C-C disease, a low MCV is common. The classification of the hemoglobinopathies is made by Hgb electrophoresis.

17.2.4 Spherocytes

A spherocyte is an RBC with the same volume as a normal RBC but with a smaller diameter. Since one views cells as two-dimensional elements on a peri-pheral blood film, spherocytes appear smaller than normal RBCs (they are not microcytes), more deeply stained, and without the central pallor (Figure 17.8). Spherocytes may result from: (1) an inherited membrane defect, as in hereditary spherocytosis (HS); (2) acquired damage to the RBC membrane (e.g. heat damage from extensive burns (Figure 17.9); or (3) removal of part of the RBC

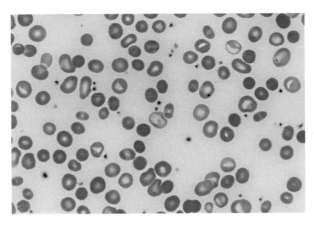

Figure 17.8 Hereditary spherocytosis: spherocytes, polychromasia and a Howell-Jolly body (status post-splenectomy) are visible

membrane by macrophages (as in immune hemolytic anemia). Rarely, the phagocytosis of spherocytes by leukocytes may be seen on the blood film.

Spherocytes may occur in small numbers in: (1) immune hemolytic anemia secondary to LPDs, IM or mycoplasma pneumonia; (2) acute attacks of paroxysmal cold hemoglobinuria; and (3) hereditary pyropoikilocytosis. In these conditions other, more specific, RBC/WBC abnormalities and the clinical presentation are more important in establishing the diagnosis.

The main differential diagnosis of large numbers of spherocytes includes HS and the immune hemolytic anemias. The term 'immune hemolytic anemias' encompasses warm AIHA, drug-induced immune hemolytic anemia, hemolytic disease of the newborn, and alloimmune hemolytic anemia (i.e. delayed transfusion reactions involving alloantibodies to minor blood group antigens). The majority of immune hemolytic anemias are positive for the direct antiglobulin (Coombs) test. Immunohematologic tests performed by the blood bank are

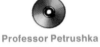

Professor Petrushka
Case 2

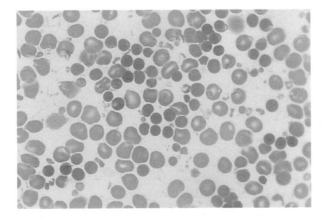

Figure 17.9 Numerous spherocytes, 'microspherocytes' and RBC stroma in a case of extensive third degree burns

required to determine the specific subtype. Careful attention to clinical information (e.g. recent transfusions and medications) is helpful in choosing the appropriate tests.

Microspherocytes are RBCs with a decreased cell surface/volume ratio (like spherocytes) but also a decreased cell volume. They are found mainly in extensive second or third degree burns and the severe forms of hereditary elliptocytosis (HE), i.e. HE with infantile poikilocytosis, hereditary pyropoikilocytosis and homozygous HE.

17.2.4.1 Hereditary spherocytosis (HS)

Hereditary spherocytosis is not a single disease entity, but a heterogeneous group of inherited disorders leading to RBC membrane defects. Table 17.2 lists the various defects that can be present. These defects lead to the weakening of the vertical connections between the cell skeleton and the lipid bilayer in the membrane. The areas of the membrane not supported by the skeleton are prone to form microvesicles and later detach from the cell, resulting in a decreased cell surface area.

The membrane defects cause a decreased cell surface area (along with a decreased surface/volume ratio) and the formation of spherocytes. The spherocytes have decreased deformability and altered membrane permeability. The altered membrane permeability causes mild cellular dehydration that is reflected as an increased MCHC in about 50% of patients with HS.

The different membrane defects and modes of inheritance are reflected in the heterogeneity of the clinical manifestations of HS. The hemoglobin level can range from normal to severely decreased. Patients with normal hemoglobin levels are diagnosed as part of the family studies of a symptomatic relative or during a work-up for hemolysis from other causes. In most instances, the typical HS patient has mild anemia, jaundice, splenomegaly, and a peripheral blood film characterized by abundant sphcrocytes and polychromasia (Figure 17.8). Howell-Jolly bodies and an increased platelet count may be present in HS patients who have undergone splenectomy.

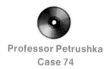

Professor Petrushka
Case 74

The direct antiglobulin test (DAT) and the measurement of osmotic fragility in hypotonic saline are adequate to diagnose HS and differentiate it from AIHA. Osmotic fragility evaluates the ratio of surface area to volume in RBCs. As this ratio decreases, the RBC becomes more sensitive to osmotic lysis. The test does not measure the mechanical 'strength' of the RBC membrane. The osmotic fragility test can be performed on freshly drawn blood or on blood incubated at 37°C for 24 hours. Incubating the blood at 37°C accentuates the degree of spherocytosis.

Table 17.2 Membrane defects in hereditary spherocytosis

- Isolated partial deficiency of spectrin.
- Combined partial deficiency of spectrin and ankyrin (the most common type).
- Partial deficiency of band 3 protein.
- Deficiency of protein 4.2.

Increased osmotic fragility and a negative DAT characterize HS. The osmotic fragility is improved but not normalized after splenectomy. Although AIHA may also have increased osmotic fragility, the DAT is positive.

17.2.4.2 Immune hemolytic anemia in the neonatal period

It is not unusual to find a few spherocytes in normal newborns. When a significant number of spherocytes are present in the neonatal period, one should consider hemolytic disease of the newborn (HDN). The cause of HDN can be antibodies against the D antigen of the Rhesus blood group system (Rh-HDN), anti-A and/or anti-B (ABO-HDN) or antibodies to minor blood group antigens (Kell, Duffy, Kidd or MNS).

The number of spherocytes in HDN does not necessarily reflect the severity of the disease. Abundant spherocytes are seen in ABO-HDN even though the anemia is mild (Figure 17.10a). The reverse is often true in Rh-HDN (Figure 17.10b). The initial cord blood hemoglobin and bilirubin levels better reflect the severity of the disease. Sequential bilirubin measurements determine whether exchange blood transfusion is necessary. Although the DAT on cord blood is usually positive, a negative DAT does not exclude HDN (especially ABO-HDN), due to the relative paucity of A and B antigen sites on the RBCs of the newborn. The best test for ABO-HDN is the indirect antiglobulin test (indirect Coombs) in which adult RBCs from blood groups A_1, B and O are incubated with a concentrated eluate from the newborn's RBCs.

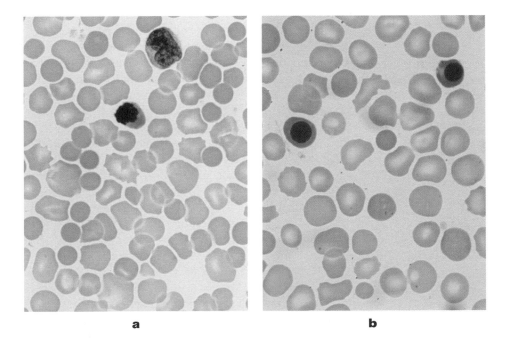

a   b

Figure 17.10 Blood films from two different neonates. (a) Frequent spherocytes in ABO-HDN. Note also the nuclear indentations in the normal lymphocyte. (b) An occasional spherocyte in Rh-HDN

Hereditary spherocytosis, hereditary pyropoikilocytosis, and hereditary ellipto-cytosis can also cause a congenital hemolytic anemia with a significant number of spherocytes in neonates.

17.2.4.3 Autoimmune hemolytic anemia (AIHA)

The hemolysis in AIHA is either extravascular or intravascular depending on the subtype of the autoantibodies. Autoimmune hemolytic anemia can be idio-pathic or secondary to disorders such as SLE, infection, or an LPD.

Eighty to ninety per cent of AIHAs are caused by warm autoantibodies that result in extravascular removal of the altered RBCs by macrophages in the spleen. The antibodies are usually IgG and most have anti-Rh specificity. Spherocytes are formed when the RBCs coated with the autoantibodies get trapped in the spleen and are partially phagocytized by macrophages. The degree of spherocytosis parallels the severity of the anemia. In AIHA, the DAT is positive and can show three patterns of reaction: (1) reaction with anti-IgG only; (2) reaction with anti-complement antisera only; and (3) reaction with both IgG and comple-ment. In the first step of the DAT, a broad-spectrum reagent containing antibo-dies to both IgG and complement is used. If this is positive, the test is repeated with anti-IgG and anti-C3 antisera.

A small percentage of AIHAs are due to cold autoantibodies that mainly result in intravascular hemolysis. Cold autoantibodies are of two types:

1. **Cold agglutinins.** These are IgM antibodies, with either anti-I or anti-i (reacting with cord blood) specificity. They are mostly found in adults either as an idiopathic disorder or associated with IM, mycoplasma pneu-monia or lymphoma (mainly LPC lymphoma-leukemia). The cold aggluti-nins bind to RBCs at 28–31°C in the blood vessels of the skin. This is followed by adsorption and partial activation of complement on the cell surface. At the higher temperature in the body core, the antibodies disas-sociate from the cells. RBCs coated with complement are lysed intravascu-larly or phagocytized in the spleen.

2. **IgG hemolysins** (Donath-Landsteiner antibodies). These are associated with viral infections occurring in children. Most IgG hemolysins have spe-cificity against P blood group antigens. Antibody binding to RBCs at low temperatures is followed by activation of the complement cascade, result-ing in intravascular lysis at 37°C in the central circulation. The term 'par-oxysmal cold hemoglobinuria' refers to such episodic and massive hemolytic anemia brought on by exposure to cold. In many instances, the attacks are not related to cold exposure but to viral infections. The typi-cal clinical picture is that of a sudden sharp drop in Hgb of 2–3g/dl, with red plasma and dark brown to black urine. The blood film may not reveal any red cell changes although a few spherocytes or RBC aggluti-nates may be present. The DAT reaction with anti-complement antisera is positive.

The main differential diagnosis of paroxysmal cold hemoglobinuria includes PNH (also characterized by episodic intravascular hemolysis) and cold agglutinin disease. Cold agglutinins with high thermal amplitude can result in intravascular hemolysis of the same intensity as paroxysmal cold hemoglobinuria.

17.2.4.4 Drug-induced immune hemolytic anemia

In drug-induced hemolytic anemia, the number of spherocytes can range from few to many depending on the offending drug and its mechanism of action. The immune hemolytic anemia may be the result of:

- Production of autoantibodies against RBCs. The prime example is α-methyldopa. The mechanism is unknown. Although approximately one-third of patients on this drug demonstrate a positive DAT, less than 1% actually develop hemolytic anemia. The autoantibodies react against epitopes on the Rh complex.
- IgG antibodies against the drug which have a high affinity for RBCs. The typical example is prolonged therapy with high dose penicillin in patients with anti-penicillin antibodies. A high number of spherocytes is common. In this situation, the RBCs are innocent bystanders.
- Ternary complex formation. The prototype for this mechanism is quinidine. The antibody only recognizes the drug when it is bound to a particular structure on the RBC membrane. RBC lysis is mediated via complement activation. In this scenario, a small dose of the offending drug is sufficient to precipitate severe intravascular hemolysis.

17.2.5 Elliptocytes and ovalocytes

In normal individuals, elliptocytes are usually less than 5% of RBCs. Mild to moderate numbers of elliptocytes are frequent in various disorders such as iron deficiency, B_{12}/folate deficiency and bone marrow infiltration (including MPD, MDS, and metastatic disease).

In HE, the number of elliptocytes can range from 15 to 100%, and the blood film may exhibit additional RBC poikilocytosis in the form of teardrop cells and

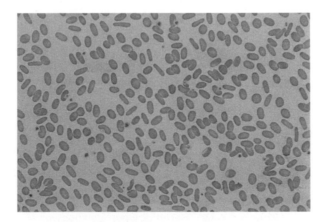

Figure 17.11   Hereditary elliptocytosis

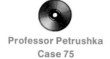

Professor Petrushka
Case 75

schistocytes. Therefore, unless the peripheral blood film contains an overwhelming number of elliptocytes (Figure 17.11), it is not always possible to distinguish HE from other disorders.

Hereditary elliptocytosis is a heterogeneous group of disorders that include common HE (the most prevalent form), spherocytic HE and stomatocytic HE. The spherocytic and stomatocytic forms are rare.

Common HE is itself heterogeneous with regards to molecular defects and clinical manifestations. Most of the defects involve mutations in the α or β chain of spectrin in the vicinity of the contact site that forms a functional spectrin tetramer. Failure to form tetramers results in RBC membrane instability. The spectrin content in the cells and the percentage of abnormal spectrin molecules are the two main factors affecting the severity of the disease.

Most patients with common HE have a very mild anemia and the disorder is incidentally diagnosed during a routine CBC when abundant elliptocytes are found on the peripheral blood film. In the presence of superimposed stress (e.g. infection), the hemolytic anemia can become more severe and additional poikilocytosis (e.g. schistocytes) may develop.

In neonates and infants (especially those of African descent), the finding of severe hemolytic anemia with other RBC poikilocytosis in addition to elliptocytosis raises the differential diagnosis of HE with infantile poikilocytosis versus hereditary pyropoikilocytosis (Figure 17.12). In HE with infantile poikilocytosis, the blood picture improves by 6 months to 1 year of age and converts to mild common HE. Presumably, the high level of Hgb F in neonates indirectly alters the interaction of RBC membrane skeletal proteins, thus worsening the already existing membrane instability. Hereditary pyropoikilocytosis is now recognized as a subset of HE rather than a separate disease, since relatives often have mild common HE. In these two disorders (as well as homozygous HE), the peripheral blood contains a mixture of elliptocytes, microspherocytes and schistocytes. The large numbers of microspherocytes and schistocytes often result in a low MCV ('apparent' microcytic anemia).

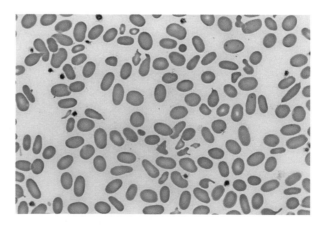

Figure 17.12 Hereditary pyropoikilocytosis in an infant, showing abundant elliptocytes/ovalocytes, frequent schistocytes and occasional spherocytes

17.2.6 Acanthocytes

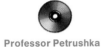

Acanthocytes, also known as spur cells (Figure 17.13), are densely stained RBCs without central pallor, but with multiple irregular projections that vary in width, length and surface distribution. They need to be differentiated from echinocytes (Figure 16.1) and schistocytes. The confusion between these three RBC abnormalities is more frequent than expected. Since moderate numbers of acanthocytes (often accompanied by target cells) may be present in hyposplenism/splenectomy, the blood film should be carefully examined for the telltale presence of Howell-Jolly bodies. The differential diagnosis of anemia with moderate to abundant acanthocytes includes spur cell hemolytic anemia (Figure 17.14), abetalipoproteinemia and the McLeod phenotype.

Spur cell hemolytic anemia is a severe and usually fatal anemia caused by severe liver disease such as alcoholic cirrhosis or neonatal hepatitis. An alteration of plasma lipoproteins leads to accumulation of cholesterol (out of proportion to phospholipid) in the RBC membrane. This leads to altered membrane deform-

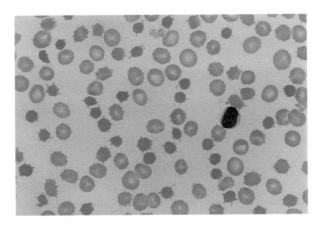

Figure 17.13 Abetalipoproteinemia: numerous acanthocytes are visible

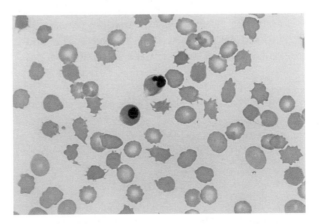

Figure 17.14 End-stage liver failure manifesting as spur cell hemolytic anemia

ability. When normal erythrocytes are transfused into these patients, they become acanthocytes.

Abetalipoproteinemia is a rare autosomal recessive disorder with defective liver cell synthesis of apoprotein B. The resulting absence of chylomicrons, low-density lipoproteins and very low-density lipoproteins causes impairment of triglyceride transport from the intestine. Serum triglycerides are virtually absent and cholesterol is markedly decreased. Cholesterol content in the RBC membrane is normal, however. The anemia is usually mild with a large number of acanthocytes. Retinal damage and neuromuscular manifestations are progressive and fatal.

McLeod phenotype is a rare disorder characterized by the absence of an antigen of the Kell blood group system on RBCs. The anemia is mild. Some patients also have X-linked chronic granulomatous disease.

17.2.7 Schistocytes

Schistocytes are fragmented red cells. Red blood cell fragmentation can be caused by mechanical damage secondary to turbulent blood flow around a prosthetic heart valve or from contact with fibrin strands, tumor cells, or an abnormal vessel wall. Schistocytes take a variety of appearances such as crescents, helmets or triangles.

In most instances, the presence of appreciable numbers of schistocytes signifies a microangiopathic hemolytic anemia (MAHA) (Figure 17.15). Since the peripheral blood picture does not provide any clue to the underlying disease, the etiology needs to be determined on the basis of other laboratory tests and clinical information. There may be coexisting thrombocytopenia or granulocytosis with or without a left shift. The main diseases to consider in the differential diagnosis of MAHA are shown in Table 17.3.

Hemolytic uremic syndrome typically occurs in children, usually following enteric infection by verotoxin-producing strains of *Escherichia coli*, or *Shigella dysenteriae*. It can also occur in adults in the context of pregnancy, chemotherapy (high dose mitomycin C), AIDS and organ transplant (including bone marrow transplant). Depending on the degree of platelet consumption, there may be thrombocytopenia in addition to MAHA. Thrombotic thrombocytopenic purpura is a syndrome with multiple causes. Because of the overlap in clinical and laboratory manifestations between TTP and HUS, those two entities are often considered to represent the same disease.

Table 17.3 Differential diagnosis of microangiopathic hemolytic anemia

- Hemolytic uremic syndrome
- Thrombotic thrombocytopenic purpura
- Pregnancy or postpartum complications
- Malignant hypertension
- Disseminated carcinoma
- Disseminated intravascular coagulation
- Infection/sepsis
- Generalized vasculitis in an autoimmune disorder
- Hemangiomas

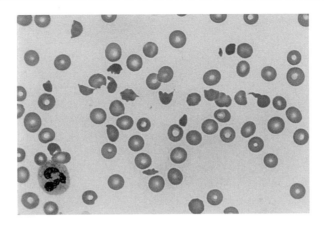

Figure 17.15 Microangiopathic hemolytic anemia, exhibiting numerous schisto-cytes. The patient had DIC secondary to sepsis

Microangiopathic hemolytic anemia is an infrequent occurrence in patients with disseminated carcinoma. Most cases are the result of mucin-producing tumors (gastric carcinoma accounts for more than 50% of the cases), followed by breast, lung and prostate cancer. In many patients, there may be laboratory evidence of DIC and/or bone marrow metastases. The peripheral blood manifestations of metastatic disease are highly variable, including marked neutrophilia, a leukoerythroblastic reaction, pancytopenia, or just anemia with anisocytosis. Microangiopathic hemolytic anemia can also occur in certain bacterial or viral infections (including HIV) without DIC being present.

With chronic intravascular hemolysis secondary to RBC fragmentation, hemoglobin released from RBCs binds to haptoglobin. Once haptoglobin becomes saturated, free hemoglobin is lost in the urine. This may ultimately result in iron deficiency, further worsening the anemia.

17.2.8 Bite cells/Heinz bodies

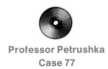

Professor Petrushka
Case 77

Heinz bodies represent hemoglobin denatured because of oxidative injury. Bite cells (Figure 17.16) are presumably formed when splenic macrophages remove a Heinz body from an erythrocyte. Therefore, the presence of appreciable numbers of bite cells suggests Heinz body hemolytic anemia, e.g. glucose-6-phosphate dehydrogenase (G6PD) deficiency. The diagnostic value of this finding is limited, however, since it is present only during the hemolytic attacks and the morphology of bite cells is easily confused with that of schistocytes with few horns. It is preferable to perform supravital staining with either brilliant cresyl blue or crystal violet to demonstrate the presence of Heinz bodies (Figure 17.17). The peripheral blood picture depends on the severity of the disease. With severe disease (or during a hemolytic crisis), the blood film usually contains bite cells and irregularly contracted cells (IRCs). Other nonspecific findings, such as basophilic stippling, may also be present. In the presence of large numbers of Heinz bodies, exposure to oxidant drugs/chemicals and unstable hemoglobins must be considered.

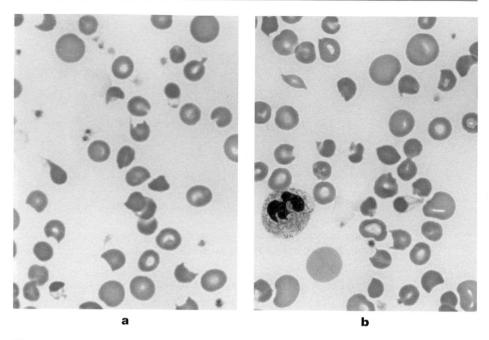

a   b

Figure 17.16 G6PD deficiency during an oxidative attack. (a) Numerous bite cells. (b) Frequent irregularly contracted cells – an occasional one has a 'blister' cell appearance

17.2.8.1 Exposure to oxidant drugs/chemicals

Oxidant drugs and chemicals can cause Heinz body formation. This may be due to chronic exposure, or to an underlying deficiency of either G6PD or another enzyme affecting the pentose-phosphate shunt. Dapsone, which is used most often in HIV-positive patients, is one of the most common offending drugs.

There are about 400 variants of G6PD deficiency, some of which cause chronic hemolysis even in the absence of stress. The most prevalent variants are G6PD A– (in black patients) and G6PD Mediterranean. In these two variants, infection

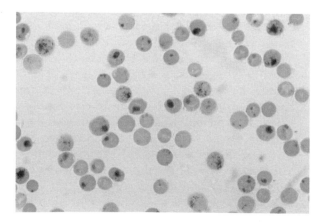

Figure 17.17 Supravital stain: Heinz bodies from a case of G6PD deficiency

or drug exposure (antimalarials, sulfonamides, sulfones and fava beans) can precipitate hemolysis. The onset of hemolysis is within 1–3 days after exposure. Heinz bodies appear at the same time but they are quickly removed from the circulation. The acute hemolysis is followed by reticulocytosis. Since the newly released reticulocytes contain higher G6PD activity, the hemolytic process ends spontaneously after 1–2 weeks.

The fluorescent spot test is a simple and reliable screening test for G6PD deficiency. This test is based on the fluorescence of NADPH generated by G6PD present in an RBC lysate. Because reticulocytes and young RBCs contain higher G6PD activity, reticulocytosis during a hemolytic episode in a G6PD deficient patient may cause a false 'normal' result. If G6PD deficiency is suspected, a negative fluorescent spot test should be followed up by a quantitative G6PD assay, usually performed as part of a battery of RBC enzyme assays. It is preferable to perform the quantitative assay on blood that has been depleted of reticulocytes.

17.2.8.2 Unstable hemoglobins

Unstable hemoglobins are rare despite the large number of variants that have been identified. The most common type is Hgb Köln, which has a worldwide distribution. In variants with a low affinity for oxygen, the patients may have a low hemoglobin level and yet no symptoms of anemia. In variants that have a high oxygen affinity, patients are unusually susceptible to tissue hypoxia and are 'physiologically anemic' despite normal or even high hemoglobin levels. The clinical and hematological manifestations vary greatly in severity, ranging from no anemia to severe hemolysis. Most variants produce mild disease with at most a mild anemia and no appreciable RBC morphologic abnormalities. Any febrile illness, however mild, can precipitate a hemolytic crisis. In addition, drug exposure (especially sulfonamides) may cause hemolysis in some patients.

With unstable hemoglobins, Heinz bodies are usually not seen unless the patient has undergone splenectomy. In rare instances, hemoglobin precipitates may be visible on routine Romanovsky-stained blood films (Figure 17.18). The

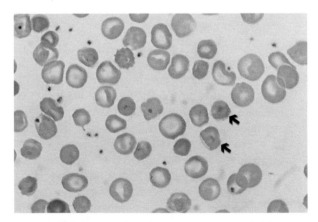

Figure 17.18   Unstable hemoglobin. Hemoglobin precipitates are visible in several RBCs (arrow)

diagnosis is based on demonstrating that the patient's hemoglobin is unstable either by the heat stability test or the simpler isopropanol precipitation test. A false-positive isopropanol precipitation test can occur if the sample contains high levels of Hgb F (> 5%) or when the hemolysate has undergone prolonged storage. Precise identification of the unstable hemoglobin (not necessary for treatment) requires globin chain analysis.

17.2.9 Irregularly contracted cells (IRCs)

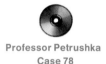

Professor Petrushka
Case 78

On peripheral blood films, IRCs appear densely stained with a diameter smaller than normal RBCs, an irregular contour, and no central pallor (Figure 17.16). When the cell contour is only slightly irregular, IRCs can be easily confused with spherocytes. Identification of IRCs is easier when the hemoglobin is seen as retracting away from the RBC membrane. This type of change has also been referred to as 'ghost' or 'semighost' RBCs, and 'blister' cells. It is preferable to designate this spectrum of changes as IRCs since the various morphological appearances represent the same underlying abnormality, i.e. the presence of altered hemoglobin molecules.

The irregular cell margins presumably result from Heinz bodies having been extracted by the spleen. Appreciable numbers of IRCs are thus seen in the same conditions that feature bite cells (see Section 17.2.8). Small numbers of IRCs, along with more specific RBC abnormalities, may occur in other disorders such as thalassemia, Hgb E disease, and CDA.

The combination of many IRCs and numerous target cells is suggestive of Hgb C disease. Hemoglobin electrophoresis is necessary for diagnosis, however.

17.2.10 Teardrop cells

In the context of an NCNC anemia, the presence of an appreciable number of teardrop cells suggests bone marrow infiltrative disorders, particularly those which result in bone marrow fibrosis (AMM, metastatic solid tumors and extensive granulomata) and/or severe dyserythropoiesis. Frequent teardrop cells, basophilic stippling, and anisocytosis occur in CDA (see Section 12.2.1). Depending on the extent/stage of the bone marrow infiltration, the blood may demonstrate a leukoerythroblastic pattern. Polychromasia and basophilic stippling may also be seen.

A similar peripheral blood picture may be encountered, although infrequently, in thalassemias (usually thalassemia intermedia) in which the high numbers of polychromatophilic RBCs bring the MCV into the normal range. Such cases can be distinguished from bone marrow infiltration based on the absolute reticulocyte count. The reticulocyte count is increased in thalassemia, and decreased or within the normal range in bone marrow infiltration.

If teardrop cells are accompanied by significant numbers of schistocytes, the main differential diagnosis is bone marrow infiltration (especially metastases) and MAHA. A leukoerythroblastic picture may be seen in either disorder.

17.2.11 Dimorphic RBC population

Dimorphism refers to a mixture of RBCs of different cell volumes. The possible mixtures of RBC populations include macrocytes with normocytes, microcytes with normocytes, macrocytes with microcytes and a mixture of all three cell types. The MCV can be low, normal or high.

The most common conditions exhibiting dimorphism include: (1) a response to iron or vitamin therapy; (2) blood transfusion in a patient with either microcytic or macrocytic anemia; (3) hematopoietic malignancies (MDS, acute leukemias and LPDs); and (4) congenital sideroblastic anemia (which presents with a low MCV). If other more specific findings are present, such as blasts or hyposegmented neutrophils, they may give a clue to the underlying disorder.

17.2.12 Basophilic stippling

Basophilic stippling represents abnormally aggregated ribosomes. The ease of detecting basophilic stippling depends on how long the blood has been left in EDTA anticoagulant. With prolonged storage, this finding can be lost. This is one of many reasons to process peripheral blood samples without undue delay.

Basophilic stippling is most pronounced in pyrimidine 5′ nucleotidase deficiency, a rare autosomal recessive disease manifesting with moderate anemia and splenomegaly. Detection of basophilic stippling is often easier after splenectomy (Figure 17.19). The role of pyrimidine 5′ nucleotidase is to rid maturing

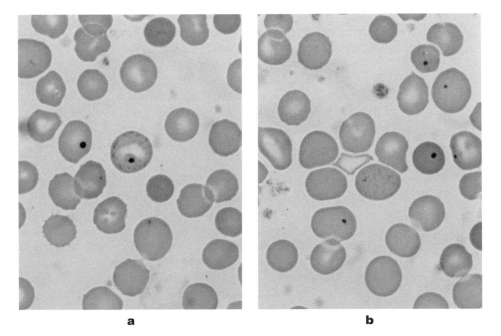

a   b

Figure 17.19 (a), (b) Basophilic stippling in a case of pyrimidine 5′ nucleotidase deficiency. The spleen had been previously removed. One RBC contains both basophilic stippling and a Howell-Jolly body (a)

reticulocytes of ribosomal RNA degradation products (aggregates of which are visible as basophilic stippling). Because of the inhibitory effect of lead on pyrimidine 5′ nucleotidase and other enzymes involved in heme synthesis, lead poisoning results in an 'acquired' enzyme deficiency. This causes pronounced basophilic stippling and NCNC anemia. Hypochromic, microcytic anemias also occur in lead poisoning, usually because of existing iron deficiency which has not been previously detected.

A variable degree of basophilic stippling can be also seen in other conditions in which there is abnormal erythropoiesis and/or stressed erythropoiesis. Examples include CDA, severe B_{12}/folate deficiency, stem cell disorders, thalassemia, unstable hemoglobins, and various severe hemolytic anemias. In these other disorders, the clinical setting, RBC indices and other morphologic abnormalities are helpful to indicate the appropriate work-up.

17.3 Additional laboratory tests for the work-up of anemia with anisocytosis

The laboratory tests discussed below can be carried out in a routine hematology laboratory for the identification of the underlying causes of anemia. The complex serological tests to investigate various immune hemolytic anemias (performed in the blood bank) and tests performed in reference or research laboratories (e.g. RBC enzyme assays and molecular diagnosis) are not discussed.

If a patient is suspected of having a hemoglobinopathy or thalassemia on the basis of their ethnic background, family history, clinical history, peripheral blood manifestations, or the results of the screening tests mentioned above, then hemoglobin electrophoresis and the quantitation of Hgb A_2 and Hgb F are necessary. Ion-exchange high-performance liquid chromatography is an alternative to hemoglobin electrophoresis. Chromatography gives a quick presumptive identification of abnormal hemoglobins. The order of elution of the various hemoglobins depends on the type of column used.

17.3.1 Hemoglobin electrophoresis

Hemoglobin electrophoresis is based on the different relative mobility of the various hemoglobins in an electric field under a given set of conditions relating to pH, ionic strength of the buffer, and the nature of the supporting medium. Electrophoresis on cellulose acetate in an alkaline buffer (pH 8.6) is usually the initial procedure, except during the neonatal period. At alkaline pH, Hgb is a negatively charged molecule that moves from the cathode (−) to the anode (+). The relative mobility of the major Hgb variants, from slow (i.e. near the application point) to fast, are shown in Figure 17.20.

At pH 8.6, Hgb A_2, C, E, and O share the same electrophoretic mobility. The same is true for Hgb S and Hgb D. Further separation requires citrate-agar gel electrophoresis at acid pH (pH 6.2). Rapid quantitation of the major bands of hemoglobin can be done by scanning with a densitometer. More precise methods are required for quantitation of Hgb A_2, however.

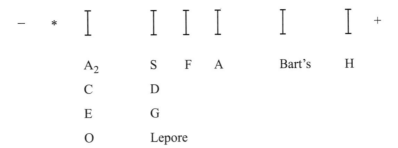

Figure 17.20 Mobility of hemoglobin variants on cellulose acetate in an alkaline buffer (pH 8.6). *= origin

Outside the neonatal period, the level of Hgb F may be so low that a band may not be detected. In contrast, in the newborn, Hgb A_2 is not detectable and Hgb F forms a heavy band overlapping the adjacent bands of Hgb A and Hgb S. This can potentially mask the detection of Hgb S. For this reason, citrate-agar gel electrophoresis at acid pH is the method of choice in patients less than 3 months of age. At acid pH, the relative mobility of the major hemoglobin variants, from cathode to anode, are shown in Figure 17.21. This method is useful when investigating double heterozygotes such as S-D, or S-G, and to distinguish between Hgb C, Hgb E, and Hgb O. Isoelectric focusing can also distinguish between hemoglobins C, E, and O.

17.3.2 Quantitation of Hgb A_2

An increase in Hgb A_2 is characteristic of heterozygous β-thalassemia (including β-thalassemia trait). Quantitation can be done by elution from cellulose acetate after electrophoresis, except in the presence of Hgb S which is incompletely separated by this method. When Hgb S is present, Hgb A_2 can be quantitated by DEAE (diethylaminoethyl) cellulose chromatography. Neither method allows the quantitation of Hgb A_2 in the presence of Hgb C, Hgb E, or Hgb O

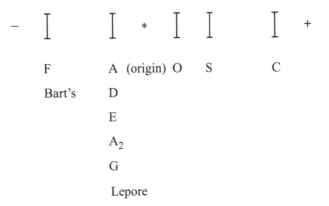

Figure 17.21 Mobility of hemoglobin variants on citrate-agar gel at pH 6.2

(since they elute with Hgb A_2 in a DEAE column). The normal range of A_2 is usually considered to be 1.5–3.5%. Hgb A_2 is in the range of 4–7% in most types of β-thalassemia. Levels greater than 10% suggest the presence of another hemoglobin variant that migrates with A_2.

17.3.3 Quantitation of Hgb F

The simple and reliable modified Betke method for quantitating Hgb F is based on its resistance to denaturation by alkali. In normal subjects beyond 1 year of age, Hgb F levels do not exceed 1% (range 0.2–1.0%). Slightly increased levels of Hgb F (2–5%) can be found in about 50% of patients with β-thalassemia trait, hematopoietic malignancies, severe B_{12} deficiency, aplastic anemia and PNH. Hgb F levels above 15% are seen in β-thalassemias which manifest as either thalassemia major or intermedia, HPFH, and infants below the age of 3 months. High levels of Hgb F can also be seen in juvenile CMMoL, but the peripheral blood picture of juvenile CMMoL is distinctive enough not to cause confusion. In S-S anemia, serial quantitation of Hgb F can be useful in assessing the effectiveness of hydroxyurea therapy.

17.3.4 Approach to electrophoretic interpretation in the major hemoglobinopathies

The three most common abnormal hemoglobins are (in decreasing order of frequency) Hgb S, Hgb E, and Hgb C. Hgb S and Hgb C are most prevalent in people of African descent. There is a lower frequency of Hgb S in Saudi Arabia, parts of India, and the Mediterranean. Hgb E is found mainly among South-East Asians.

Less common abnormal hemoglobins, but still important, are Hgb D_{Punjab}, Hgb O_{Arab}, and Hgb $G_{Philadelphia}$. Hgb G is unusual in that the amino acid substitution is on the α chain. In the other five common variants, the substitution is on the β chain.

17.3.4.1 Electrophoretic patterns in hemoglobinopathies affecting the β chain

There are five possible scenarios involving the β chain:

1. Patients homozygous for a given β chain variant (e.g. S-S or C-C). The abnormal hemoglobin is present in the highest proportion. In addition, Hgb A is absent and the percentage of Hgb F (and/or Hgb A_2) is usually slightly increased. A virtually identical picture is seen if the patient is doubly heterozygous for a β chain variant and either HPFH or a β-thalassemia in which no β chain is produced. Therefore, S $β^0$-thalassemia and S-HPFH are in the differential diagnosis of S-S anemia when the electrophoretic pattern has two distinct bands, S and F (with S being the more prominent band).

2. Double heterozygotes for two different β chain variants (e.g. S-C, S-O). The two abnormal hemoglobins are present in roughly equal amounts. A

slight compensatory increase in Hgb F may be seen. In S-D disease, since Hgb S and Hgb D share the same electrophoretic mobility on cellulose acetate, the findings mimic those of S-S disease. The diagnosis is resolved using citrate-agar electrophoresis.

3. Double heterozygotes for a β chain mutant and a thalassemia in which there is a reduction of β chain synthesis. In this condition, the abnormal hemoglobin predominates over Hgb A with a compensatory increase in Hgb A_2 and Hgb F.

4. Heterozygotes for β chain variants (e.g. Hgb S trait, Hgb C trait). Hgb A predominates and the abnormal hemoglobin comprises less than 50% of the total. In Hgb E trait, the point mutation on the β gene that results in a substitution of lysine for glutamic acid leads to decreased production of the corresponding mRNA (similar to the mechanism operating in the β-thalassemias). Consequently, the level of Hgb E is in the range of 20–35%. In contrast, patients with A-S or A-C have a relative percentage of Hgb S or Hgb C in the 30–45% range.

5. Concurrent inheritance of a homozygous β chain mutant and α-thalassemia. The main example is co-inheritance of homozygous Hgb S along with the deletion of two α genes (S-S with α-thalassemia). The reduction in α chain synthesis results in a decreased intracellular concentration of Hgb S. Patients have a mild anemia with fewer sickle cells on the peripheral blood film. The electrophoretic findings mimic those of S-S disease. It is therefore important to interpret the patient's hemoglobin electrophoresis in the context of the clinical data, peripheral blood findings and the hemoglobin electrophoresis results of the patient's parents and siblings.

17.3.4.2 Electrophoretic patterns in hemoglobinopathies affecting the α chain

The electrophoretic pattern in α chain mutants is complex since there are four α genes (in contrast to two β genes) and the mutation may involve any number of α genes. In most cases, only one or two α genes are affected. Since the α chain is present in other hemoglobins (Hgb F and Hgb A_2), mutations in α genes always cause extra bands, corresponding to the altered Hgb F and/or Hgb A_2, to appear on hemoglobin electrophoresis. The electrophoretic mobility of the extra bands can overlap with that of Hgb C. As a rule of thumb, if the electrophoretic pattern shows more than two prominent bands, then an α chain mutation should be suspected.

A common α chain mutant of clinical importance is Hgb G, the third most common abnormal hemoglobin (after Hgb S and Hgb C) among those of African descent. The presence of Hgb G can lead to diagnostic confusion on cellulose acetate electrophoresis because it has the same mobility as Hgb S. Hgb G can cause confusion in at least three scenarios:

1. Hgb A plus Hgb G in clinically normal individuals can result in a pattern similar to sickle cell trait (A-S) with two prominent bands in the position of Hgb A and Hgb S.

2. In clinically and hematologically normal individuals with sickle cell trait (A-S) plus Hgb G, three major bands in the positions of Hgb A, Hgb S, and Hgb C can be seen.
3. In patients with S-S disease plus Hgb G, two major bands in the positions of Hgb S and Hgb C (the pattern of S-C disease) can be found. The peripheral blood picture will be that of S-S anemia since the α chain variant does not alter the expression of S-S disease.

Leukemoid pattern

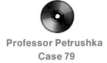

The hallmark of the leukemoid pattern is a marked granulocytic leukocytosis (WBC count $\geqslant 50 \times 10^9/l$). The main differential diagnoses are MPDs, in particular CML, and non-neoplastic leukemoid reactions such as those seen in severe infections, widespread carcinomatosis and G-CSF administration.

In general, the higher the WBC count and the proportion of intermediate myeloid precursors, the higher the index of suspicion for a malignant process, especially if the blood picture remains sustained over several weeks. At times, however, differentiating benign from malignant leukemoid reactions can be extremely difficult, particularly in infants with Down's syndrome.

18.1 Peripheral blood picture in CML

Chronic myeloid leukemia is a stem cell disorder characterized by the (9;22) (q34;q11) translocation (i.e. the Philadelphia chromosome), which can be identified by either standard cytogenetics or molecular probes for the *bcr-abl* fusion.

The peripheral blood picture in CML can be variable, depending on the WBC count and whether or not blasts and/or NRBCs are detected. The blood picture can be a leukemoid pattern, a leukoerythroblastic pattern, an abnormal mononuclear cell pattern, a thrombocytosis pattern and, occasionally, a neutrophilia pattern. Careful examination of the blood film in CML reveals that NRBCs, circulating blasts and immature myeloid precursors are present in virtually all cases. When blasts or NRBCs are present in low numbers (1–3% range), they can easily be missed on a manual differential.

Initially, the morphologic diagnosis of CML is made in the peripheral blood rather than the bone marrow, since the blood findings are typical in the great majority of cases. The blood picture can be thought of as a spillage of marrow elements into the periphery with the following typical findings:

- A WBC count of at least $50 \times 10^9/l$ (often $> 100 \times 10^9/l$).
- An absolute basophilia, greater than $0.2 \times 10^9/l$. Basophils may appear hypogranulated (Figure 18.1).
- A marked granulocytic leukocytosis with increased numbers of myeloid precursors, predominantly myelocytes. The WBC manual differential typically shows two 'peaks', myelocytes and neutrophils. All stages of the myeloid series can be found on a manual differential, including blasts.

The high WBC count in CML is sufficient to bring the lymphocyte and monocyte counts beyond the thresholds established for absolute lymphocytosis and

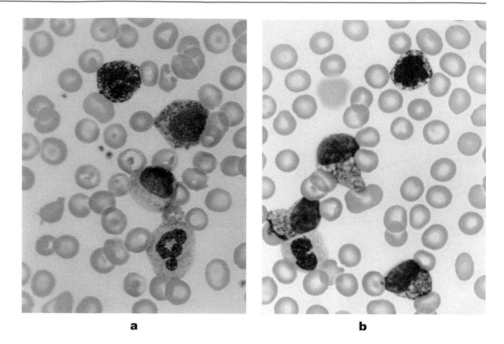

a   b

Figure 18.1   Blood films from two different patients with CML. (a) Intermediate myeloid precursors, a neutrophil and a basophil. The WBC count was 55×10^9/l. (b) Hypogranulated basophils in the accelerated phase of CML. The manual differential revealed 27% basophils in this patient

monocytosis, respectively. These are of no diagnostic relevance in CML, however.

Other frequent findings in CML include absolute eosinophilia, mild anemia, moderate thrombocytosis, and mild qualitative abnormalities. Thrombocytosis may be severe ($> 1000 \times 10^9$/l) with levels overlapping those seen in ET. Qualitative abnormalities are frequent in long-standing disease or exposure to cytoreductive therapy. Common RBC and WBC abnormalities include macrocytosis, stomatocytes, hypersegmented neutrophils and hypogranulated myeloid cells. Circulating megakaryocytes, most often seen as naked nuclei, NRBCs, and occasional giant platelets complete the picture. These features also occur in other MPDs.

Cytogenetics and molecular studies are the most reliable confirmatory tests for CML. The authors do not advocate using leukocyte alkaline phosphatase (LAP) scoring. Although the LAP score is low in most cases of CML, it can be normal or increased in CML under therapy, or CML associated with pregnancy or infection.

18.2 Disease progression in CML

Progression of CML to the accelerated phase can be suspected when any of the following features develop:

- Basophil percentage greater than 20%.
- Platelet count less than $100 \times 10^9/l$ unrelated to therapy.
- Peripheral blood blasts greater than 10% (but less than 20%).
- Bone marrow blasts greater than 10% (but less than 30%).
- Additional chromosomal abnormalities (e.g. $+8$ or a second Philadelphia chromosome).

In the accelerated phase, CML may involve extramedullary sites other than the spleen ('granulocytic sarcomas').

18.3 Other causes of a leukemoid reaction

The differential diagnosis of CML with a leukemoid presentation includes CMMoL, reactive conditions, other MPDs and the condition known as 'transient proliferation of hematopoietic precursors' in Down's syndrome.

18.3.1 Neoplastic leukemoid reactions

A substantial number of MPDs are morphologically indistinguishable from CML. Most, but not all, patients with CML demonstrate basophilia. In CML-like MPDs, however, basophilia is absent to minimal ($<2\%$ basophils in the peripheral blood differential). In addition, the proportion of monocytes may be higher than CML, i.e. in the 10–20% range. The definitive distinction between CML and CML-like MPDs (referred to in the literature as 'atypical' CML) rests on cytogenetics and molecular genetics. In MPDs other than CML, the t(9;22) abnormality and *bcr-abl* rearrangements within the major and minor breakpoint cluster regions are not present. Chromosomal gains (e.g. trisomy 8, trisomy 21) are usually observed in CML-like MPDs.

Agnogenic myeloid metaplasia and ET can mimic CML on rare occasions when they present with a WBC count in the leukemoid range. The WBC count will increase steadily in CML when the patient is observed untreated over weeks to months, whereas it usually does not change significantly in other MPDs. In ET, the platelet count increases continuously over time. In CML presenting with thrombocytosis, the platelet count remains relatively stable. In some patients, the peripheral blood and bone marrow findings at presentation do not allow a definite subclassification of the MPD.

Absolute monocytosis (i.e. $>1 \times 10^9/l$) is a required criterion for CMMoL. This degree of monocytosis is commonly seen in CML. In addition, an increased number of granulocytes can be seen in CMMoL, therefore resulting in potential diagnostic confusion. In the absence of basophilia, the relative percentage of intermediate myeloid precursors and the percentage of monocytes may suggest the correct diagnosis. In CML, the percentage of monocytes is typically less then 5%, while in CMMoL it is usually much higher. In CMMoL, there are usually less than 15% intermediate myeloid precursors in the peripheral blood. In CML, intermediate myeloid precursors predominate.

Chronic neutrophilic leukemia (Figure 18.2) is a rare entity, unlikely to be confused with CML and other MPDs. The WBC is greater than $50 \times 10^9/l$, composed predominantly of mature neutrophils, which may demonstrate hyper-segmentation and/or hypogranulation. Chronic neutrophilic leukemia is a diagnosis of exclusion, however, since patients with underlying solid tumors can develop an identical, sustained blood picture. Bone marrow studies are often not helpful in differentiating this disease from other causes of neutrophilic leukemoid reactions, unless the cellularity is essentially packed and the M:E ratio is excessively increased. The definitive diagnosis rests ultimately on the presence of chromosomal abnormalities (e.g. trisomy 8).

18.3.2 Reactive/transient leukemoid reactions

A leukemoid pattern with a left shift may occur in severe infections, HDN, solid tumors and, rarely, in the recovery phase of a previous agranulocytosis. In solid tumors, the leukemoid reaction can be the result of either bone marrow metastases or tumor production of growth factors. The key hematological parameter that separates a reactive leukemoid picture from CML is absolute basophilia. A marked left shift and the presence of Döhle bodies, toxic granulation or hypergranulation are less discriminatory since they can occur in MPDs and patients receiving G-CSF. It is unusual to see blasts on the manual differential in reactive conditions.

A transient proliferation of hematopoietic precursors (also known as 'transient myeloproliferative disorder') occurs occasionally in infants less than 6 months of age with Down's syndrome and infants with trisomy 21 mosaicism who are phenotypically normal. The WBC count is markedly elevated with increased numbers of circulating immature cells. In many cases, there is a high percentage of circulating blasts, making the picture indistinguishable from an acute leukemia. The disorder undergoes spontaneous resolution within a few weeks, however. Since

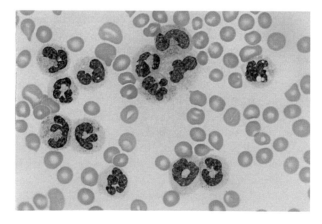

Figure 18.2 Chronic neutrophilic leukemia in a 67-year-old female (WBC 64.4 × 10⁹/l, 90% mature granulocytes). Note one neutrophil with a ring-shaped nucleus. Cytogenetics revealed trisomy 21

patients with Down's syndrome have a high incidence of acute leukemia, the differential diagnosis between leukemia and a transient proliferation of hemato-poietic precursors can be problematic. In the transient condition, the blasts are often of heterogeneous lineage and do not have Auer rods. There are no additional chromosomal abnormalities besides the constitutional trisomy 21. The diagnostic work-up should include cytogenetics and immunophenotyping to rule out acute leukemia.

18.4 Molecular genetics of the Philadelphia chromosome

A diagnostic requirement for CML is the presence of either the Philadelphia chromosome or a *bcr-abl* gene rearrangement. The abnormality is present on all hematopoietic cells except T lymphocytes. Molecular studies (RT-PCR, FISH) are also useful for monitoring response to α-interferon therapy or allogeneic bone marrow transplant.

The (9;22)(q34.1;q11.21) transposition juxtaposes the *c-abl* proto-oncogene on chromosome 9 to the *bcr* gene on chromosome 22. The breakpoints in *c-abl* vary widely over one large region of 100–200 kilobases (kb). In contrast, the breakpoints on the *bcr* gene occur in one of three different regions:

1. The major breakpoint cluster region (M-bcr), a 5.8 kb region located in the middle of the *bcr* gene. Rearrangements within the M-bcr, which occur in most CMLs and a substantial number of Philadelphia chromosome-positive acute leukemias, result in the transcription of an 8.5 kb chimeric mRNA bcr-abl instead of the normal 6–7 kb abl mRNA. A protein of 210 kilodaltons (kd) with increased tyrosine kinase activity is produced, instead of the normal 145 kd abl protein.
2. The minor breakpoint cluster region (m-bcr), upstream from the M-bcr. This rearrangement, which produces a 7 kb chimeric mRNA and a 190 kd fusion protein, occurs in most Philadelphia chromosome-positive ALLs. Occasional CMLs do not contain an M-bcr rearrangement, but an m-bcr rearrangement instead. CML with m-bcr often has a higher proportion of monocytes in the peripheral blood (usually in the 10–20% range), in contrast to the low proportion of monocytes in CML with M-bcr.
3. A third breakpoint region, μ-bcr, downstream from the M-bcr. In this rare rearrangement, described in some cases of chronic neutrophilic leukemia, nearly the entire *bcr* gene is conserved. The resulting large hybrid *bcr-abl* gene produces a 230 kd fusion protein.

Nonspecific pattern

The nonspecific pattern covers all cases with parameters that do not fit the definitions of any of the previously discussed peripheral blood patterns. Most such cases demonstrate a normal hemogram except for a single parameter outside of the reference range. In most instances, examination of the peripheral blood film is not necessary, except where indicated below. Commonly encountered isolated abnormalities that trigger the nonspecific pattern are:

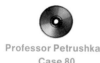

Professor Petrushka
Case 80

1. **An increased RDW.** This is more frequent if the upper range of 'normal' for RDW is set too low (e.g. 13–14). In the context of otherwise normal RBC parameters, a possible explanation for a slightly increased RDW (i.e. 15–16) is replacement therapy for B_{12} or folate deficiency.
2. **An increased MCHC.** This isolated abnormality calls for examination of the peripheral blood film. An increased MCHC is seen in about 50% of patients with HS. The MCHC may be the only hemogram abnormality in well compensated non-anemic patients with HS.
3. **An NRBC suspect flag** in the presence of normal hemoglobin and normal RBC parameters. Outside of the newborn period, where the presence of a few NRBCs can be considered normal, an isolated NRBC suspect flag is often a false-positive. It can be caused by platelet clumps (which may also be flagged) or Howell-Jolly bodies. A quick scan of the peripheral blood film will confirm the abnormalities.
4. **Lymphopenia with a normal WBC count.** Although lymphopenia is commonly associated with AIDS, it can be seen as an incidental finding in otherwise normal/asymptomatic subjects. Possible underlying causes include a mild (or early) infection and the use of steroids.
5. **A mildly increased WBC count** with the absolute number of neutrophils, lymphocytes, monocytes, eosinophils and basophils within the reference range. This condition may be encountered in either the early or resolution phases of an infection. An active (and possibly severe) infection can exist without the patient's WBC count being markedly elevated. In such cases, it is helpful to scan the peripheral blood film to estimate the number of bands. In the absence of neutrophilia, an increased number of bands (i.e. > 20%) may provide the only clue to an underlying infection.
6. **Basophilia**, often due to delayed processing of specimens. If basophilia persists after corrective measures have been attempted, it is helpful to scan the peripheral blood film. True basophilia, in an otherwise normal hemogram, can be seen in treated CML, after the chemotherapy has lowered the WBC count to within the reference range.

7. **An immature granulocyte/band flag** in the context of a normal WBC count. A quick scan of the peripheral blood film may be helpful to estimate the percentage of bands, metamyelocytes, or myelocytes, especially if the patient is known to have an infection or has treated CML. Congenital Pelger-Huët anomaly can also be picked up by scanning the film.

Flow Cytometry

Approach to
flow cytometry

Flow cytometry immunophenotyping provides valuable information in the reproducible diagnosis and classification of acute leukemias, chronic lymphoid leukemias and non-Hodgkin's lymphomas. In order to take maximum advantage of the technique, however, one must pay particular attention to issues of data analysis, interpretation and reporting. Since most samples are not homogeneous, but contain a mixture of cell populations, it is important to perform a multiparameter analysis correlating forward and right angle light scatter with multiple colors of fluorescence. For example, three-color analysis offers high sensitivity and specificity to detect and characterize abnormal populations in heterogeneous samples.

DNA ploidy and cell cycle analysis can also be extremely useful in the work-up of certain lymphoid neoplasms. Aneuploidy is essentially diagnostic of malignancy. In addition, the percentage of cells in the S-phase of the cell cycle has been shown to be an effective indicator of the grade of non-Hodgkin's lymphomas.

Many of our suggestions regarding the technical aspects of FCM are based on the recommendations of the US-Canadian Consensus Conference on the Use of Flow Cytometry Immunophenotyping in Leukemia and Lymphoma, held in Bethesda, Maryland, on 16–17 November 1995. The authors were among the invited participants at this conference.

20.1 Medical indications

One can no longer rely solely on morphology for reproducible diagnosis of hematopoietic malignancies. Therefore, it is important to obtain appropriate specimens for potential FCM immunophenotyping and other ancillary studies (e.g. DNA ploidy, cell cycle analysis, cytogenetics and molecular biology) in every suspected case of acute leukemia, blast transformation of an MPD or lymphoid malignancy. Flow cytometry immunophenotyping can be performed on peripheral blood, bone marrow, body fluids and fresh tissue obtained from lymph node biopsies, spleen or extranodal tumors. The specific indications for different disease categories are summarized below.

20.1.1 Lymphoproliferative disorders (LPDs)

The term 'LPD' is employed to designate a mature lymphoid neoplasm that manifests initially or primarily in the liquid compartment of the hematopoietic and lymphoid systems (peripheral blood and bone marrow) rather than in the solid compartment (lymph node, spleen and extranodal sites). Most, but not all, LPDs have a chronic course. Examples of entities falling under this category include CLL, PLL, HCL, and disorders of LGLs and NK cells.

When properly performed, FCM immunophenotyping is one of the most reliable methods of distinguishing CLL from other morphologically similar LPDs and NHL in leukemic phase (e.g. MCL). In addition, the high degree of sensitivity allows the detection of low levels of circulating hairy cells that can easily be missed on morphologic evaluation. It is now possible, in an experienced laboratory, to detect less than 1% hairy cells in the peripheral blood.

Peripheral blood FCM immunophenotyping should be performed for all unexplained absolute lymphocytosis in adults prior to performing more invasive diagnostic techniques such as bone marrow studies and/or a lymph node biopsy. The peripheral blood is often the specimen of choice whenever sufficient numbers of circulating neoplastic cells are present.

20.1.2 Malignant lymphomas

To improve diagnostic accuracy, FCM immunophenotyping is recommended on all lymph node biopsies in patients with a suspected malignant lymphoma. Although the diagnosis of Hodgkin's disease is not based on FCM immunophenotyping, the procedure is valuable for distinguishing NHL from Hodgkin's disease. When the clinical suspicion is Hodgkin's disease, FCM immunophenotyping should still be performed since the clinical impression may be incorrect.

20.1.2.1 Advantages of FCM immunophenotyping

In many institutions, the diagnosis and subclassification of lymphoid malignancies is still heavily based on morphology and immunohistochemistry on paraffin-embedded fixed tissue. Although immunohistochemistry provides morphologic visualization of 'what is being stained', the technique is no substitute for FCM immunophenotyping for the following reasons:

1. A wider range of monoclonal antibodies can be applied in FCM analysis. In many cases, this allows a specific classification of the disease.
2. Surface immunoglobulins cannot be reliably studied by immunohistochemistry since there is often false-negative staining or high background staining, making interpretation impossible.
3. Many antibodies reacting on fixed tissue have a lower degree of sensitivity and specificity than those used in FCM immunophenotyping. Furthermore, tissue fixation and processing can easily alter immune reactivity leading to a false-negative result. These factors can lead to discrepancies between the results obtained by immunohistochemistry and the FCM immunophenotype. Examples of discrepancies that the authors have frequently encountered include:

   - Cases of SLL and MCL which are CD5$^-$ on paraffin-embedded lymph nodes but are CD5$^+$ by FCM.

- Acute leukemias that are CD34$^-$ and/or TdT$^-$ on paraffin-embedded bone marrow biopsies but are positive for these markers of immaturity by FCM.

4. Well-performed FCM immunophenotyping provides better sensitivity, more rapid availability of results, and reduces interpretative subjectivity. The high sensitivity is most useful in detecting low levels of bone marrow involvement by NHL. Routine integration of FCM immunophenotyping in bone marrow NHL staging will increase the yield of positive bone marrow diagnoses by 10–20%. Furthermore, FCM is extremely useful when the bone marrow morphologic findings do not allow a clear-cut separation of a benign from a malignant process (e.g. when there is a mild degree of lymphocytosis in the aspirate and/or a focal lymphoid aggregate on the biopsy). Identification of circulating malignant cells in the peripheral blood of patients with documented NHL can obviate the need for an additional bone marrow procedure.

5. The current state of the art in FCM analysis is based on a multicolor technique, which allows accurate characterization of the cells of interest. In contrast, immunohistochemistry is essentially a single color technique. Attempts at two-color immunostaining, one color for a nuclear antigen (e.g. PCNA) and a second color for a cytoplasmic antigen (e.g. L26), have not been routinely applied since the technique is quite labor-intensive.

6. With careful study, FCM histograms provide many useful diagnostic clues in the form of visual patterns of antibody reactivity which are not available on microscopic review of immunohistochemistry sections.

FCM immunophenotyping is also preferable to immunohistochemistry on cryostat sections, since the staining intensity can be assessed more easily and reproducibly. The presence of immunoglobulins in the intercellular fluid on frozen sections often results in high background staining which may obscure the true staining of heavy and/or light chains.

When immunostaining is performed on tissue sections or smears, it may not be possible to determine if the antigen detected is located on the surface, in the cytoplasm, or within the cell membrane. The location of the antigen can be an important diagnostic feature. An example of this is CD3 in the diagnostic work-up of mature lymphoid disorders. An aberrant mature T-cell phenotype (e.g. loss of surface CD3) is an important diagnostic clue for T-cell LPD/NHL. When CD3 staining is performed on tissue sections or smears, it may be unclear if the phenotype is normal or aberrant since a positive result may represent either:

- Positive surface CD3 as seen in normal mature T cells.
- Positive cytoplasmic CD3 as seen in T-cell malignancies that exhibit lack of surface CD3 by FCM analysis.

In general, immunostaining on smears is best reserved for the detection of cytoplasmic antigens such as cCD3, cCD22, cmu and myeloperoxidase as part of the diagnostic work-up for acute leukemias.

Flow cytometry and immunohistochemistry are actually two complementary techniques. A useful feature of immunohistochemistry is that the traditional morphologic findings, e.g. the 'pattern of infiltration', can be evaluated on the immunostained sections. On the other hand, properly performed FCM data analysis, taking into account the light scatter and relative staining intensity between multiple clusters, is a powerful tool to separate the malignant population from the benign cells.

There are instances when immunohistochemistry has a higher diagnostic yield than FCM immunophenotyping. For example, immunohistochemistry is the procedure of choice for identifying metastatic tumor and Reed-Sternberg/Hodgkin's cells and variants. For reasons not well understood, a variable proportion of large cells can be lost during the FCM processing. This can lead to false-negative results when the tissue submitted for FCM is small or the large malignant cells are embedded in a fibrous background. In such instances, immunohistochemical staining, using a panel of antibodies, such as L26, CD3, CD30, ALK-1, and Ki-67, is helpful. It is important to note, however, that L26 positivity in large cells does not necessarily indicate a B-cell lymphoma. In some cases of nonlymphocyte predominant Hodgkin's disease (including those with a syncytial pattern), the malignant cells can be L26-positive, leading to possible misinterpretation as large cell lymphoma.

Immunophenotyping is a quick and easy way to monitor disease progression in previously diagnosed malignant lymphoma. Flow cytometry can be performed on either a follow-up biopsy or an adequate fine needle aspirate. In addition, cell cycle analysis provides objective grading of LPD/NHL.

20.1.2.2 Handling of lymph node specimens

Proper handling of lymph nodes and other 'solid' specimens is critical, since a second specimen is not easily obtained if the first sample is mishandled. The following approach for a routine thorough lymph node work-up is suggested:

1. Cell suspensions should be prepared from a generous and representative portion of fresh tissue. Studies that can be performed include FCM immunophenotyping, cytospins, cell kinetic analysis, cytogenetics and molecular analysis. Cytospin preparations of the cell suspension are a required morphologic quality control for FCM analysis and can be used for cytochemical stains.
2. A portion of the lymph node should be snap frozen and saved for potential molecular genetics. Frozen tissue can also be used for immunohistochemistry.
3. Touch imprints provide the possibility of comparing the cytology of the neoplastic cells in the solid tissue with the cytology in the bone marrow, peripheral blood or body fluids. It is easier to compare the cytology between two air-dried, Romanovsky-stained preparations, than to compare an air-dried bone marrow/blood smear with an H&E tissue section.
4. A portion of the lymph node should be fixed and processed for morphologic examination. Fixatives with a heavy metal component (e.g. mercury chloride or barium chloride) yield better fixation than formalin, with crisper cytological details and improved immunostaining reactivity.

20.1.3 Multiple myeloma

Plasma cells are easily identified morphologically. In addition, the diagnosis of multiple myeloma rests on clinical features and routine laboratory findings, such as lytic bone lesions and the presence of monoclonal immunoglobulin in the serum and/or urine. Monoclonal cytoplasmic immunoglobulin can be detected using:

- Flow cytometry, with a combination of antibodies to CD38, CD45 and cytoplasmic light chains.
- Immunostaining on bone marrow aspirate smears.
- Immunohistochemistry performed on the bone marrow biopsy.

Cell cycle analysis is quite useful in multiple myeloma since DNA ploidy and proliferative activity in malignant plasma cells has been shown to be of prognostic value. Cell cycle analysis is most useful if the tumor population is substantial or can easily be separated from the granulocytic elements in the bone marrow by appropriate gating techniques.

20.1.4 Acute leukemia

Current therapy in acute leukemia is influenced by the lineage of the neoplastic cells. Flow cytometry immunophenotyping is a primary modality for distinguishing AML from ALL. Immunophenotyping also forms the basis for the subclassification of ALL. DNA ploidy analysis of pediatric ALL provides information useful for assessing prognosis. When present, aneuploidy also serves as a useful marker to detect early relapse.

With multicolor FCM analysis, it is possible to discriminate between leukemic blasts and their benign counterparts. For example, the presence of asynchronous or aberrant antigen expression allows one to differentiate neoplastic myeloblasts from normal myeloblasts. In addition, benign precursor B cells and precursor B-ALL, despite sharing a similar antigenic profile, can be distinguished by the differences in fluorescence intensity of some of the antigens.

Flow cytometry is useful not only for diagnostic purposes, but also for the accurate detection of residual/early relapsed leukemia and the emergence of new leukemic clones post-therapy. When applied to peripheral blood specimens, a positive analysis can alleviate the need for bone marrow studies.

20.1.5 Myelodysplastic syndromes/myeloproliferative disorders

Flow cytometry immunophenotyping is not recommended in the chronic phase of CML and other chronic MPDs but is useful for any patient suspected of entering a 'blast crisis'. Ongoing studies of altered expression of myeloid antigens (e.g. CD16, CD11b) are being used to determine the clinical value of FCM immunophenotyping in myelodysplastic syndromes.

20.1.6 Minimal residual disease detection

Flow cytometry immunophenotyping can identify minimal residual disease in acute leukemia in the range of one target cell for every 10^3–10^4 cells when the study consists of a multicolor analysis, including permeabilization for cytoplasmic antigen detection and DNA ploidy measurement. While the presence of minimal residual disease in acute leukemias (by FCM, PCR or FISH) is strongly suggestive of a near future relapse, the therapeutic implications remain to be established.

Similarly, detection of minimal residual disease in LPD/NHL can be achieved by multiparameter FCM analysis. However, the clinical significance of a positive result (whether obtained by FCM or other methodologies) in low-grade LPD/NHL is questionable in view of the lack of truly curative therapeutic approaches.

20.1.7 Transplantation

The utility of FCM in transplantation is twofold:

1. To measure the regenerative capacity of the blood/bone marrow to be used as the source of CD34$^+$ hematopoietic stem cells (HSCs).
2. To assess the purity of the cells being transplanted (i.e. no evidence of tumor cell contamination).

A threshold number of 1.2×10^6 CD34$^+$ cells per kg of body weight is considered adequate for engraftment. The quick enumeration of CD34$^+$ cells by FCM influences subsequent medical decisions regarding the need for additional harvesting of HSCs. To ensure the purity of the HSC product, a highly complex FCM analysis, similar to that used for the detection of minimal residual disease, is required.

20.2 Laboratory procedures

The technical aspects of FCM analysis include specimen handling, sample preparation, instrument quality control, and data acquisition. Practical recommendations regarding each of these components of FCM analysis in hematopoietic malignancies are given below. No attempt is made here to provide a comprehensive treatise on the principles and use of FCM.

20.2.1 Specimen acquisition and transport to the laboratory

Specimens obtained for FCM analysis should be transported to the laboratory and processed immediately after collection. Each specimen must be properly identified (specimen source, patient ID number) and all pertinent clinical and/or laboratory information concerning the patient should be included on the requisition form. Specimens that can be processed within an hour of collection should be maintained at room temperature prior to processing. Addition of a small amount of sterile isotonic fluid to solid tissue samples (e.g. normal saline or tissue culture media) is useful to prevent dehydration.

Although the upper limit of storage before processing for FCM analysis is not well defined, 48–72 hours may be acceptable for peripheral blood and bone marrow aspirates collected in sodium heparin. Storage is to be avoided, however, if a high-grade malignancy (e.g. Burkitt's lymphoma-leukemia) is suspected. Because of the high metabolic activity of such tumors, any storage will only worsen the yield of viable cells. Theoretically, if blood or bone marrow is collected in EDTA, the sample should be stored for no more than 12–24 hours before processing to avoid potential depletion of myeloid cells.

20.2.2 Sample preparation

A crucial step in FCM analysis is the preparation of a single-cell suspension. For peripheral blood and bone marrow aspirates, this is not an issue unless the specimen is partially clotted. If clots are present, they should be removed by filtration through a 50 µm nylon mesh prior to further processing.

For tissue samples, including fine-needle aspirates, the goal is to dissociate the cells to obtain a single-cell suspension, maximizing the yield and at the same time maintaining the integrity and antigenicity of the sample. The preferred method is mechanical dissociation (as opposed to enzymatic dissociation). Most lymphoid tissues are rapidly and easily dissociated in a buffered isotonic solution using mild mechanical pressure applied with wire mesh screens or perhaps a needle and syringe.

For specimens containing abundant RBCs (blood, bone marrow and body fluids), the red cell lysis approach is preferred rather than Ficoll-Hypaque separation, which causes more cell loss. Avoiding cell loss can be crucial when the number of the critical cells in the sample is low. In the case of bone marrow specimens, Ficoll separation precludes the availability of an internal control for myeloid antibody staining since granulocytes are selectively removed.

A cytospin (i.e. morphologic quality control) should be prepared from the single-cell suspension and examined to ensure there has not been significant loss of the cells of interest. A cell count is necessary prior to antibody staining.

20.2.3 Color compensation and calibration of fluorescence intensity

The Consensus Conference recommended that five-parameter (three-color) analysis (i.e. forward scatter, side scatter, and three fluorescent probes) is optimal for FCM immunophenotyping. One of the fluorescence parameters may be used for exclusion of nonviable cells (e.g. propidium iodide) or for gating purposes (e.g. gating on CD45 to further characterize a leukemic blast population). Single-color analysis is not an appropriate procedure, except as an immunocytochemical method to detect intracellular antigen. It should be noted that six-parameter (four-color) analysis is now feasible and will become routine in the near future.

20.2.3.1 Fluorochrome selection

Typical multiparameter immunofluorescence protocols use a combination of fluorochromes. Propidium iodide is commonly used for DNA analysis. FITC and PE have been widely used for routine dual-color immunophenotyping. Because of its exceptional quantum yield, PE should be used to detect weakly expressed antigens, thereby maximizing the separation of positive cells. When three-color analysis is performed, PerCP (peridinium-chlorophyll-protein complex) is the third fluorochrome of choice since it requires little color compensation when used with FITC and PE. Because of its low quantum yield, PerCP is best utilized for the detection of brightly expressed antigens. Other available color reagents (often used in four-color analysis) include APC, Cy-5, and tandem conjugates such as PE-Cy5 or PE-Texas red. Tandem conjugates may result in nonspecific signals by one of two mechanisms: (1) inefficient energy transfer between the donor dye and the acceptor molecule; and (2) in the case of PE-Cy5, nonspecific binding of the conjugate to high-affinity Fc receptors for IgG (CD64) expressed by monocytes and stimulated granulocytes.

There can be a variable degree of overlap in the emission spectrum of these dyes when they are used in combination. For this reason, color compensation is required to ensure that the fluorescent signal from a cell labeled with one fluorochrome can be distinguished from the signals of cells labeled with another fluorochrome.

The correct use of color compensation protocols is critical in the analysis of hematopoietic malignancies. Overcompensation can lead to false-negative results, i.e. lack of detection of weakly expressed antigen(s) present on cells co-stained with other markers. Conversely, undercompensation can yield false-positive signals, i.e. apparent weak expression of an antigen that is not, in reality, expressed.

The usual method for removing the unwanted contribution of fluorescent light from a fluorochrome with an overlapping emission spectrum is electronic hardware subtraction from the detector picking up the overlapping emission. Once a set of fluorescence detectors have been appropriately adjusted, the compensation factor is only valid if the photomultiplier tube voltage remains constant and the optical filters in use are not changed. If these factors have changed on the instrument, color compensation must be performed again.

20.2.3.2 Fluorescence intensity determinations

In contrast to T-cell and B-cell subset analysis, in which well-characterized normal lymphoid populations are enumerated, identifying and characterizing a hematological malignancy necessitates the detection of abnormal expression of cell surface antigens. For that reason, fluorescence intensity (an indirect measurement of the amount of antigen on the cell surface) is an important diagnostic parameter. For example, weak expression of surface light chains and CD20 (along with coexpression of CD5) is virtually diagnostic of CLL. In addition, while CD20 and CD5 are present in MCL, the disease can, in part, be differentiated from CLL by a higher intensity of immunoglobulin and CD20 expression. Despite its diagnostic utility, inexperienced laboratories performing FCM immunophenotyping analysis often overlook fluorescence intensity.

The measurement of absolute fluorescence intensity was expected to improve the comparability of immunophenotyping data obtained from different instruments at multiple sites. However, the process is far from straightforward, requiring, in addition to careful instrument calibration, standards with the same excitation and emission spectra as the fluorochromes used on the samples. Furthermore, the calibrating standard must demonstrate a rather uniform signal, and be calibrated in meaningful fluorescence units, e.g. 'antibody-binding capacity' or 'molecules of equivalent soluble fluorochrome'. Quantitative measurements of fluorescence intensity do not resolve the difficulty of separating the negative population from a population that expresses a given marker very weakly.

For diagnostic purposes, a qualitative determination of fluorescence intensity using a two-part scale (i.e. weak vs. strong, dim vs. bright) or, preferably, a three-part scale (i.e. weak/dim vs. moderate vs. strong, represented as +, + +, and + + + respectively) is sufficient. To avoid interpretative confusion, it is preferable not to represent fluorescence data using the symbols '−/+' or '+/−'. For instance, +/− means an equivocal result in one laboratory, but the same symbol is used to describe weak fluorescence in other institutions.

20.2.4 Data acquisition on the flow cytometer

Since diagnostic samples almost always contain heterogeneous cell populations, with variability in cell size and granularity, it is recommended that the collection of list mode data be performed ungated. This is no different from the microscopic evaluation of hematological samples where all elements are examined although only the abnormal component is stressed in the report. Ungated list mode data are especially critical when the nature of the abnormal population is not known, thus ensuring that all abnormal cells are included in the collected data. Using a live light scatter gate at the initial stage may cause a diagnostically important population to be missed. For instance, large cells present in minute proportion (e.g. circulating hairy cells) are missed when the analysis is gated on cells with the light scatter characteristics of normal lymphoid cells. Another advantage of the ungated approach is that the presence of other cells serves as internal positive and negative controls. After the initial collection of ungated data, appropriate gated list mode data can be collected to further confirm the coexpression of specific antigens on the abnormal cells.

Collecting only gated data may seem appropriate when the specimen is a follow-up sample and the light scatter properties and phenotypic profile of the abnormal cells are known from a previous analysis. Even in this situation, it is judicious that ungated list mode data are acquired prior to any gating strategies. The purpose for gating is to enrich the population being searched for. The following are well-accepted gating strategies, which can be performed in addition to the acquisition of ungated data:

1. Gating on B cells to determine clonality and the presence of certain specific markers, using an antibody cocktail with a pan-B antibody as a common marker in several tubes.
2. Use of a pan-T marker in combination with other markers to characterize the phenotype of mature T-cell malignancies.

3. A combination of CD45 and side scatter (SSC) to identify blast cells in acute leukemia. This approach is more sensitive than the approach based on SSC and forward scatter (FSC).

20.2.4.1 SSC/CD45 dot plot

The FSC/SSC characteristics of leukemic blasts can overlap with those of lymphocytes and monocytes. In contrast, the intensity of CD45 expression is invariably lower on blasts than on lymphocytes and monocytes. By visualizing the SSC/CD45 dot plot (with CD45 conjugated to a third fluorochrome such as PerCP), the blast cluster can be discriminated from other cellular components (Figure 20.1). Immunophenotypic characterization for CD34, CD13, CD33 and CD19 can be carried out by gating on the blast cluster.

Small percentages of blasts can be easily detected by specific gating using the SSC/CD45 dot plot. Using this approach will reduce the number of false positives for biphenotypic leukemias and acute leukemias with 'aberrant' markers, caused by the inclusion of other cells in a light scatter gate. In addition, false negatives caused by an arbitrary 20% threshold for calling a marker positive can also be eliminated. Furthermore, the pattern of the blast cluster on SSC/CD45 can be virtually pathognomonic for some subtypes of AML (Figure 20.2). Note that normal myeloblasts and their malignant counterparts can share similar SSC/CD45 characteristics.

In addition to the above advantages, it is also possible to estimate a bone marrow differential based on the distribution pattern of the various cell clusters seen on the SSC/CD45 display, provided that the sample submitted for FCM analysis is not hemodilute. The pattern may differ with the type of scale used for SSC, i.e. linear versus logarithmic. In the following discussion and illustra-

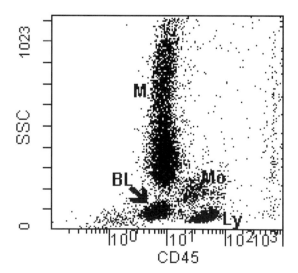

Figure 20.1 Visualization of different cell populations on the SSC/CD45 dot plot from a peripheral blood sample with acute leukemia. BL, blast cluster; Ly, lymphocytes; Mo, monocytes; M, maturing granulocytes

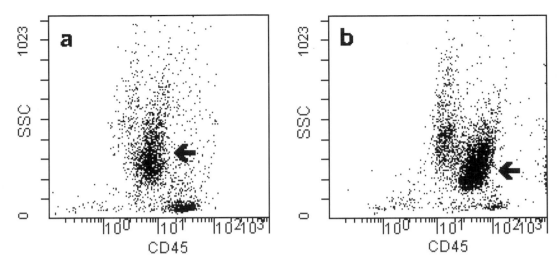

Figure 20.2 SSC/CD45 dot plot from bone marrow samples with acute leukemia. (a) Blast cluster with moderately high SSC (arrow) in AML-M3, hypogranular variant. (b) Blast population (arrow) in the 'monocyte' region, a typical feature in AML with monocytic differentiation (AML-M5)

tions, a linear scale for SSC is employed. The linear scale is preferred since it allows a better separation of the various cell clusters. The characteristics of the different cell types on an SSC/CD45 dot plot are as follows:

1. **Lymphocytes**: highest CD45, lowest SSC.
2. **Monocytes**: slightly lower CD45 expression than lymphocytes, and higher SSC.
3. **Myeloid precursors**: lower CD45 expression than in monocytes, and much higher SSC. This population may be seen as two clusters. The cluster on the right with CD45 of medium intensity corresponds to the more mature elements; the cluster on the left with low CD45 represents the more immature myeloid precursors (Figure 20.3). Eosinophilia, when present, manifests as a cluster with very high SSC, located to the right of the myeloid cluster (Figure 20.4).
4. **Erythroid precursors** fall in the CD45-negative region with low SSC (Figure 20.5).
5. **Blasts**: low SSC, and lower CD45 intensity than monocytes and lymphocytes. Lymphoblasts may be negative for CD45, in which case the cluster will appear in the 'erythroid' region.

20.3 Antibody panel selection

The Consensus Committee recognized that each individual laboratory has their own preferences for reagents, either commercially available or 'home-grown' for research purposes. For this reason, no final recommendations were made as to which antibody combinations constitute the ideal immunophenotyping panel

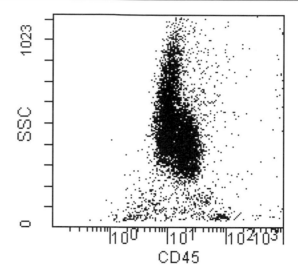

Figure 20.3   SSC/CD45 dot plot from a bone marrow sample. The myeloid cells are seen as two merging clusters. The cluster on the left with lower CD45 and higher SSC represents the more immature elements

for malignant lymphomas and leukemias. However, there was strong agreement on a number of important issues that are summarized here.

1. The use of isotype controls is optional. With a panel of sufficient size, there will always be cells that serve adequately as negative controls. There is no need for normal peripheral blood as a control. However, isotype controls are especially useful in the case of nonspecific staining. An example is the nonspecific pick-up of PE by platelet clumps (Figure 20.6). This phenom-

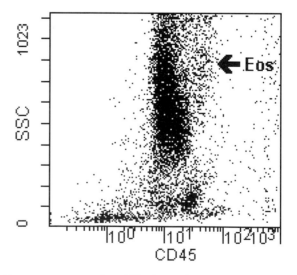

Figure 20.4   Bone marrow eosinophilia (arrow) seen on the SSC/CD45 dot plot from a bone marrow sample with CML

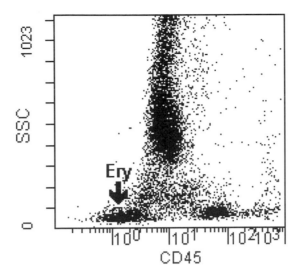

Figure 20.5 SSC/CD45 dot plot from a bone marrow with increased erythroid precursors (arrow)

enon should be suspected if an unknown cluster with low FSC demonstrates reactivity with all of the antibodies conjugated to PE.

2. Antibody cocktails created by individual laboratories need to be validated internally. The mixed reagents should give the same results as those obtained when cells are stained with the individual reagents alone.

3. The purpose of FCM immunophenotyping is to identify hematopoietic neoplasms by the presence and absence of cellular antigens. Therefore, the

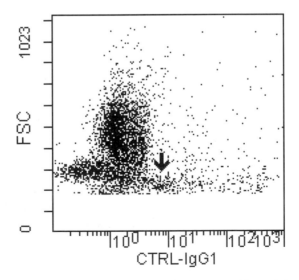

Figure 20.6 Isotype control sample, showing nonspecific staining with PE by platelet clumps, seen as a cluster with low FSC

development of 'normal ranges' for the percentage of positive cells for each antibody used in a panel is neither relevant nor useful.

4. The following markers are important for the diagnosis and characterization of malignant lymphomas and leukemias:

CD2, CD3, CD4, CD5, CD7, CD8, CD10, CD11c, CD13, CD14, CD19, CD20, CD22, CD23, CD25, CD33, CD34, CD56, kappa, lambda, TdT, HLA-DR and myeloperoxidase (MPO).

When appropriate, both surface and cytoplasmic staining should be performed for CD3, CD22, kappa and lambda.

5. Although complete consensus was not reached, the following antibodies were also highly recommended:

CD16, CD38, CD41, CD45, CD57, CD61, CD71, CD79a, CD103, CD117, glycophorin A and IgM.

6. The rationale for antibody combinations is to increase the sensitivity of FCM in the detection and characterization of abnormal populations. Therefore, in addition to a sufficiently large antibody panel, a certain degree of antibody redundancy between different tubes is necessary. For example, in acute leukemias CD45 can be used as an anchor in several tubes to gate the blast population on the SSC/CD45 dot plot (see Section 20.2.4.1), and the combinations CD34/CD13, CD34/CD33 and CD34/19 should all be examined.

If for any reason (e.g. economic constraints, remote location), a laboratory cannot afford to perform a large, comprehensive FCM panel for the study of hematopoietic malignancies then a minimum panel, e.g. TdT, CD34, CD3, CD5, CD7, CD19, MPO antibody and surface light chains, may be employed. Staining for cCD3 and cCD22 is also invaluable in the characterization of acute leukemias. This minimum number of tests establishes the maturity and lineage of the abnormal cells in most cases, thereby identifying the most common major categories of lymphoma and leukemia. If the cells are morphologically mature-appearing, TdT, CD34 and MPO antibody may be omitted. If a minimal panel cannot be performed locally, then an acceptable alternative is to expedite (via an overnight delivery service) the fresh sample to a hematopathology center with experience in multiparameter FCM analysis, where an appropriate comprehensive panel can be performed.

A controversial subject is whether FCM analysis should be performed as a one-step analysis using a large comprehensive panel in which all of the necessary antibodies are included initially, or as a two-step process (i.e. the first step to determine the lineage and maturity status, and the second step using additional antibodies for further subclassification). Given the cost of antibodies, a laboratory may opt for the second approach. However, the second round of testing can be ultimately more costly in terms of technologist time. Also, the added time delay can lead to cellular alterations or a decrease in cell viability, which may render the subsequent FCM results uninterpretable. Using microtiter-plates for cell staining, a one-step approach becomes more cost-effective since the amount of antibody required in the microtiter-plate is a fraction of that used in standard test tubes.

20.4 DNA ploidy and cell cycle analysis

A multiparameter approach to the diagnosis and classification of lymphomas and lymphoid leukemias should include DNA ploidy and cell cycle analysis. DNA ploidy has prognostic value in pediatric ALL. In LPD/NHL, the S-phase fraction of the neoplastic cells provides objective information on the grade of the tumor. Although the role of DNA ploidy as a prognostic factor in NHL is unclear, the finding of clear-cut aneuploidy is essentially diagnostic of malignancy.

A basic prerequisite for the proper interpretation of any of these studies is a technically optimal specimen. The following recommendations apply to specimens for flow cytometric DNA ploidy and cell cycle analysis:

1. DNA flow cytometry should be performed on fresh, unfixed tissue in order to reduce debris and obtain the best possible coefficient of variation (CV) of the G_0/G_1 peak. Many non-Hodgkin's lymphomas show only minor degrees of aneuploidy (i.e. a DNA index between 1.01 and 1.15). For single-parameter DNA histograms, it is essential to have low CVs in order to demonstrate distinct peaks for the DNA aneuploid cells and the residual DNA diploid cells which are always present in the background. If Ficoll-separated peripheral blood lymphocytes are used as a control to ensure proper functioning of the flow cytometer, the CV of the G_0/G_1 peak in the lymphocyte control should be less than 2.5%.

2. An attempt should be made to quantitate the percentage of neoplastic cells in the specimen before interpreting DNA histograms. The best method is the technique of dual-parameter DNA analysis where the cells are simultaneously stained for DNA and a surface antigen specific for the individual tumor. In a B-cell NHL, for example, dual-parameter staining for the expressed monoclonal light chain and DNA will allow specific gating for the tumor cells. In a large B-cell lymphoma which is negative for surface immunoglobulins, DNA analysis can be gated on the CD20-positive cells with high FSC. With correlated dual-parameter analysis, the S-phase fraction of the tumor can be calculated without contamination from benign cells. If dual-parameter staining is not possible, then the DNA content results should be compared with the immunophenotyping results and morphologic controls (e.g. cytocentrifuge preparations of the cell suspensions used for DNA analysis).

20.5 Data analysis and interpretation

In order to systematically evaluate immunophenotyping data, one must first determine if there are malignant cells in the population being studied. If so, these cells become the cells of interest and further interpretation should be restricted to this population. As previously mentioned, the initial evaluation of the sample should include investigation of all viable cells. Limiting the analysis to gated populations should only be employed after it has been determined that the gated population is exclusively composed of the cells of interest. Generic gating strategies that employ forward versus right angle scatter are not appropriate when phenotyping is performed for the diagnosis and classification of leukemias and lymphomas.

Data analysis and interpretation should only be carried out by qualified laboratory physicians with experience in FCM and neoplastic hematopathology. Proper identification of the abnormal cell population requires examination of the visual displays of multiparameter list mode data. This is a more logical approach than the use of an arbitrary cut-off value (e.g. 20% positive cells) for determining antigen expression. Expressing FCM data as percentage values is only acceptable if abnormalities consist of altered levels of the normal components in the specimen, e.g. altered CD4 and CD8 subpopulations in immunocompromised patients. This practice is inappropriate and even misleading, however, when studying hematological malignancies where it is critical to determine which antigens are present and which are absent. Visualization of the list mode data is also necessary to qualitatively evaluate fluorescence intensity. For some disorders, fluorescence intensity of specific antigens and/or the pattern of the FCM histograms are crucial to precise diagnosis and classification.

If malignant cells are present, then the following steps should be taken:

1. Determine if the malignant population has a mature or an immature phenotype.
2. Identify the lineage of the malignant cells.
3. Establish a diagnosis if the FCM data, along with clinical history, other laboratory tests, and known morphology, are characteristic of a given disease. In many cases, the immunophenotype, without further data, supports only a differential diagnosis rather than a specific diagnosis.

In order to carry out all of the above steps, the panel of FCM markers must be sufficiently large to include most possible phenotypes. Immaturity is best proven or excluded by including TdT and CD34 in the panel. This is especially important in the context of a lymphoid lineage. When one of these two markers of immaturity is negative and the other has not been performed, then the maturity of lymphoid cells remains undetermined unless there is evidence of either sIg or cytoplasmic immunoglobulin (cIg) light chain expression. Alternatively, the presence of a significant percentage of blasts (e.g. >30%) can be used as a morphologic indication of immaturity. This use of morphology to determine maturity is acceptable in the context of a myeloid lineage because there are reliable morphologic features to separate blasts from intermediate myeloid precursors. Caution must be exercised, however, when interpreting a lymphoid population as 'immature' based on 'blast' morphology alone for the following reasons:

- Cytologic features, such as a distinct/prominent nucleolus, irregular nuclei, increased nuclear/cytoplasmic ratio, and scant to moderate pale blue cytoplasm, have been described in both blasts and the mature, transformed lymphoid cells of high-grade NHL. None of these morphologic features is a pathognomonic indicator of immaturity. A prominent nucleolus reflects increased RNA production, which occurs in activated benign cells as well as malignant cells, irrespective of maturity. The authors have seen NHL in leukemic phase (e.g. MCL and large cell lymphoma) misdiagnosed as ALL when the initial FCM panel did not include CD34, TdT or sIg.

- In our current understanding of the maturation of hematopoietic cells, blasts are clearly identified as immature cells. In many institutions, however, particularly in Europe where the Kiel classification of NHL is popular, the term 'blast' is still being used in a morphologic sense for any transformed cell with a distinct nucleolus, including the mononuclear cells in Hodgkin's disease and the lymphoma cells of high-grade NHL. Many laboratories have different FCM panels for different subgroups of diseases, for example, a 'lymphoproliferative' panel (for LPD/NHL) and an 'acute leukemia' panel, which often does not include sIg light chains. The authors have witnessed many instances where the term 'blasts' was used inappropriately for large NHL cells in leukemic phase, and the 'acute leukemia' panel was erroneously applied. Subsequently, the FCM results (with sIg light chains not done) were interpreted based on 'blasts' as the morphologic arbitrator of immaturity. In such cases, the indiscriminate use of the term 'blast' can lead to incorrect diagnosis and therapy.

20.6 Flow cytometry data reporting

To communicate the results of FCM immunophenotyping and DNA content analysis meaningfully, careful attention should be given to the format for data reporting. Hematopathologists/laboratory hematologists use FCM data for diagnosis, but the ultimate consumer of diagnostic reports are clinicians responsible for therapeutic decisions and patient management. A wealth of information, much of which is technical, is generated by FCM immunophenotyping. For clinicians to understand the relevance of the analysis, it is vital to report only essential diagnostic information. Experience has shown that most clinicians do not comprehend (nor care for) the technical details of FCM analysis. To include such details in the reports only dilutes the important diagnostic information. The technical details of the analysis should be saved in the laboratory.

There is a wide range of FCM reporting formats. Many FCM laboratories feel compelled to report immunophenotyping results as 'per cent positives' for each antibody in a manner analogous to reporting the numerical results of chemistry tests. Per cent positives and absolute values of T cells and B cells are only relevant when reporting the results of T-subset analysis on peripheral blood samples in immunodeficiency states.

It should be remembered that proper interpretation of FCM immunophenotyping in hematopoietic neoplasia requires an approach closer to the practice of anatomic pathology (i.e. a qualitative description of patterns) than clinical pathology. In addition, it is important to keep in mind that FCM results must be correlated with the clinical information, morphology and other laboratory tests.

One of the goals of the Consensus Conference was to address the variable and often deficient reporting of flow cytometric analysis of leukemias and lymphomas.

A standard reporting approach was recommended to provide useful information to both diagnosticians and clinicians. The relevant steps for FCM reporting in hematopoietic malignancies are described below.

20.6.1 Patient information

The report should include patient demographics, history and clinical findings, prior therapy (if relevant to the results), and the reason for requesting the analysis (e.g. a presumptive clinical diagnosis). Correlation of the findings with those of previous flow cytometric analyses should be reported, if applicable. It is recognized that sufficient clinical information is not often provided to the FCM laboratory on the requisition form. Every effort must be made to obtain the pertinent data for appropriate interpretation and reporting of results, however.

20.6.2 Sample information

Every report should include a sample identification number, an indication of the sample source/type, and the date of collection. If the reporting laboratory is a referral center located some distance from the patient, the date of arrival of the specimen to the laboratory should also be noted.

20.6.3 Specimen preparation and staining

The final report should include a listing of the antibodies used (as CDs) and an indication of whether the staining was for surface or intracellular antigens. The antibody trade name may be relevant when antibodies with an identical CD designation display different specificities (e.g. CD14, CD103). Fluorochrome conjugates and the two-color or three-color antibody combinations usually do not need to be reported. Information of a strictly technical nature (e.g. cell suspension preparation, cell yield and viability, cell staining, testing of negative/positive controls, instrument quality control and the number of cells analyzed) should not be included in the report, but kept in the laboratory's records.

20.6.4 Data analysis

When abnormal (neoplastic) cells are present in the population, it is important to report a textual description of the phenotype of the abnormal cells. The description should include:

- The percentage of abnormal cells as determined by multiparameter analysis.
- The cell size (often determined by forward light scatter).
- The positive markers and salient negative results (i.e. the antigenic profile).
- The fluorescence intensity of the antigens expressed.

As discussed above, reporting a list of numerical values for antibody reactivity (i.e. per cent positives) is unsatisfactory. Numerical values do not describe in sufficient detail the phenotype of the relevant cells.

The fraction of neoplastic cells in the population being studied is often relevant (i.e. the percentage of abnormal cells with the indicated phenotype) and should be included whenever possible. If a well-defined gating procedure was performed (e.g. gating on CD19 or CD20 for kappa and lambda expression), this may be indicated in the report.

If no abnormal cells are detected (e.g. reactive conditions), then the relative fractions of normal cells may be reported along with frequently used values such as the kappa/lambda and CD4/CD8 ratios. In the presence of an abnormal population, however, information on the normal residual cells is irrelevant and should be omitted from the report so that the important diagnostic information is not diluted.

20.6.5 Interpretation of results

Optimal reporting of FCM results requires professionals with adequate knowledge of both flow cytometry and hematopathology. If a single individual lacks sufficient experience in both disciplines, he or she should actively seek out other laboratory professionals with complementary qualifications and the final report should reflect this combined expertise. The optimal report reflects the integration of the FCM data with as much clinical and laboratory data as can be obtained.

A 'stand alone' report limited to a simple description of the phenotype is discouraged since such a report is often inadequate for patient management. Reports of FCM immunophenotyping should always include a written interpretation of the results along with an explanation of their significance. The interpretation should include the following:

- A statement indicating whether an abnormal population was identified.
- A qualitative description of the phenotype of the abnormal population(s).
- A differential diagnosis consistent with the FCM results.
- If clinical, morphologic, or other laboratory information is available, a definite diagnosis should be rendered whenever possible.
- If no abnormal population is identified, a statement of the relative proportion of the normal cells in the sample should be made.

CHAPTER 4

Stem cell
pattern

The immunophenotype of a cell population fits the stem cell pattern when the sole markers present are TdT or CD34. To be absolutely certain that the proliferation is indeed composed of stem cells, the FCM panel should include an adequate number of B-cell, T-cell, myeloid, erythroid and megakaryocytic markers. In this context, the myeloperoxidase cytochemistry results (using a sensitive substrate) should also be taken into consideration. Therefore, a true stem cell phenotype is TdT$^+$ and/or CD34$^+$ but negative for B-cell antigens (especially cCD22, cCD79), T-cell antigens (especially cCD3), myeloid markers (mainly CD13, CD33, CD14, myeloperoxidase antigen/cytochemistry) and megakaryocytic markers (CD41, CD61). Since there may be variations between batches of antibody reagents, it is helpful to repeat the FCM analysis on the bone marrow if the original study was done on the blood, and vice versa. Follow-up studies at the time of any leukemic relapse may be necessary to confirm the stem cell phenotype. Subsequent study often discloses the expression of a myeloid antigen.

The next diagnostic step for a 'stem cell' acute leukemia may include MPO and platelet-peroxidase cytochemistries by electron microscopy. A positive result for MPO ultracytochemistry identifies the case as AML-M0. A positive result for the platelet-peroxidase reaction indicates AML-M7 (megakaryoblastic leukemia).

The phenotype TdT$^+$, CD34$^+$, HLA-DR$^+$, with or without CD10 expression, is also considered to be a stem cell pattern. Certain authors believe that cells with this profile represent the earliest B-cell precursors, despite the fact that HLA-DR and CD10 are not lineage specific.

On blasts, a positive MPO reaction by cytochemistry is a very specific identifier of myeloid differentiation and the MPO stain is the basis of the FAB subclassification of AML. Using FCM immunophenotyping, the primary antibodies that identify a myeloid phenotype in acute leukemias include anti-myeloperoxidase (MPO antibody), CD13 and CD33. Rare AMLs are negative for CD13 and CD33, but positive for MPO cytochemistry or MPO antibody.

Other determinants, e.g. CD11b, CD14, CD15 and CD16, being less specific and less sensitive, are not sufficient to define the myeloid phenotype when present without one of the primary markers. The significance of altered expression of some of these antigens is being evaluated in MDS and MPD. Although the presence of CD14 in the context of a myeloid pattern is suggestive of a monocytic component, there is no correlation between CD14 positivity and the FAB classification of AML. It has been shown that a substantial number of cases of AML-M4 (acute myelomonocytic leukemia) and AML-M5 (acute monocytic leukemia) lack CD14 expression, and that AML-M1 and AML-M2 can be CD14-positive. Furthermore, there are marked variations between different CD14 reagents. For these reasons, if CD14 is included in the panel, it should be analyzed together with CD64. In general, CD64 is more sensitive and specific than CD14. Strong CD64 staining is seen with monocytic differentiation. CD64 staining in intermediate myeloid precursors is less intense. Another visual clue to monocytic differentiation can be the pattern of the SSC/CD45 dot plot (Figure 20.2b). The NSE stain, preferably ANBE, is still the defining criterion of monocytic differentiation. Further details regarding the use of special stains in the diagnosis of acute leukemia can be found in Section 32.5.5.

A considerable number of myeloid leukemias do not express the markers of immaturity, CD34 and/or TdT. Furthermore, myeloblasts are present not only in AML, but also in MPDs (e.g. CML), MDS and in normal bone marrow. Therefore, a myeloid phenotype does not necessarily indicate an AML, unless the percentage of blasts in the corresponding specimen (peripheral blood, bone marrow) is known. Because of the tendency to allocate the better portion of bone marrow aspirate for routine morphologic evaluation, the aspirate specimen sent to the FCM laboratory is often hemodilute. Consequently, the proportion of blasts as determined by FCM or seen on the cytospin morphologic control may be significantly lower than the percentage on the bone marrow manual differential. Correlation of the myeloid pattern with the percentage of blasts in the bone marrow differential is necessary to interpret the data properly and 'narrow the diagnostic possibilities.

Professor Fidelio
Cases 1–4

Professor Fidelio
Case 5

22.1 Myeloid maturation

The expression of myeloid-related antigens corresponds to pathways of normal differentiation (Figure 22.1). Within the normal hematopoietic compartment, CD13 and CD33 are present on nonlymphoid progenitor cells. CD13 persists into the late stages of myeloid maturation, whereas CD33 is lost or expressed only weakly by neutrophils. During granulocytic maturation, the cells lose HLA-DR at the promyelocyte stage and gradually acquire CD11b and CD14. In the monocytic lineage, the expression of CD13, CD33 and HLA-DR is maintained throughout the differentiation process. CD14 expression on monocytes is stronger than that on granulocytes.

22.2 Pure myeloid phenotype

In general, a 'pure' myeloid phenotype is established when at least one of the primary markers (MPO cytochemistry/antibody, CD13, and/or CD33) is expressed and other lineage-associated markers are absent.

If the blast percentage in the specimen is diagnostic of an acute leukemia (by World Health Organization or FAB criteria) the constellation of marker results and clinical history may indicate a specific subtype of AML. For example:

**Professor Fidelio
Case 6**

1. MPO cytochemistry negative but positive staining for CD13 and CD33 (or MPO antibody). This profile is seen in AML-M0. If MPO antibody is negative and only one marker from the CD13/CD33 group is positive, AML-M7 (acute megakaryoblastic leukemia) is also in the differential diagnosis unless CD41 and CD61 are negative.

2. $CD13^+$, $CD33^+$, $HLA-DR^-$ and $CD34^-$. This combination is highly consistent with a diagnosis of AML-M3. This profile correlates with a typical AML-M3 blast morphology and a uniformly dense MPO cytochemistry reaction. The pattern of the SSC/CD45 dot plot is often a diagnostic fingerprint for AML-M3 and AML-M3v (Figures 22.2 and 20.2a). Rarely, HLA-DR may be positive in AML-M3v, yielding a 'nondescript' myeloid phenotype. HLA-DR expression in these cases is markedly down-regulated when compared to other AMLs, however.

**Professor Fidelio
Cases 7–8**

For prognostic and therapeutic purposes, the diagnosis of APL should be confirmed by either the t(15;17) translocation or promyelocytic/retinoic acid receptor alpha mRNA transcripts. Cases of AML-M3 with abnormalities of chromosome 17 other than t(15;17), e.g. t(11;17), are not responsive to all-trans-retinoic acid therapy.

3. A 'nondescript' myeloid phenotype (i.e. MPO cytochemistry positive, $CD13^+$, $CD33^+$, $HLA-DR^+$). This phenotype can occur in any AML subtype other than AML-M0, AML-M7 or typical AML-M3. The subclassification of AML with a nondescript myeloid phenotype requires a thorough evaluation of bone marrow aspirates, including a manual differential to assess the proportion of hematopoietic precursors other than blasts. Although the presence of CD14 is only suggestive of monocytic differentia-

**Professor Fidelio
Case 9**

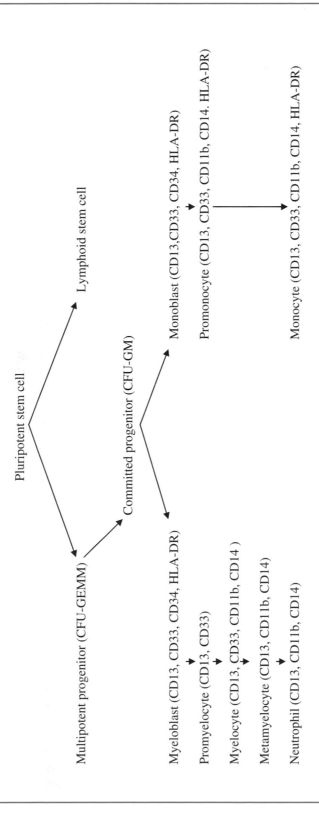

The CD14 intensity in granulocytes is weaker than that in monocytes.
CFU-GEMM: progenitor cell capable of producing colony-forming-unit of granulocytes, monocytes, erythroid cells and megakaryocytes.
CFU-GM: progenitor of the granulocyte/monocyte lineage.
The surface antigenic determinants on CFU-GEMM and CFU-GM are the same as those on myeloblasts.

Figure 22.1 Stages of myeloid maturation

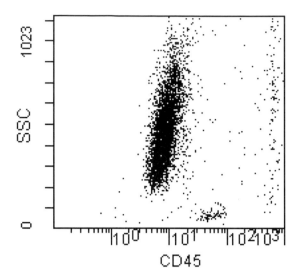

Figure 22.2 Bone marrow sample: blast cluster with high SSC in typical AML-M3

tion, the patterns of the SSC/CD45 and CD64/CD14 dot plots are of value in determining the presence or absence of monocytic differentiation (Figures 20.2b and 22.3). Monocytic differentiation can be further confirmed with an NSE stain.

4. An 'aberrant' myeloid phenotype (i.e. CD13⁻, CD33⁺, CD41⁻, CD61⁻). CD13 is normally present throughout myeloid ontogeny. Therefore, when AML-M7 has been excluded, loss of CD13 is considered an aberrancy. In the follow-up of AML, an aberrant myeloid profile can be a useful 'finger-

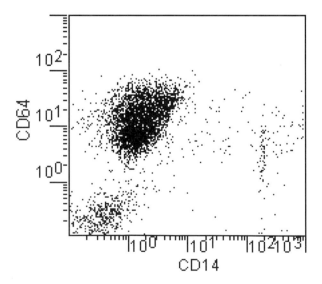

Figure 22.3 Coexpression of CD14 and CD64 in the blast population of a case of AML-M5

print' to identify a small number of neoplastic myeloblasts (i.e. minimal residual disease) in an apparently negative (remission) bone marrow.

A subset of CD13$^-$, CD33$^+$ AML are negative for HLA-DR, with or without CD34 (Figure 22.4). Some may coexpress CD56. Such cases should not be interpreted as AML-M3, as they do not have the (15;17) translocation. The blast morphology in most of those cases is nondescript (i.e. regular nuclear contour, scant to moderate and agranular cytoplasm). Rare cases have blasts with some fine cytoplasmic granules and a round nucleus (Figure 22.5), and care should be taken not to mistake them for AML-M3v. These cases do not demonstrate the characteristic cluster with high SSC.

Professor Fidelio
Case 10

5. A myeloid phenotype does not differentiate an AML from a myeloblastic crisis of an MPD. Therefore, knowledge of the clinical antecedents is necessary for diagnosis. The clinical course of the latter, as a rule, is worse than that of an AML.

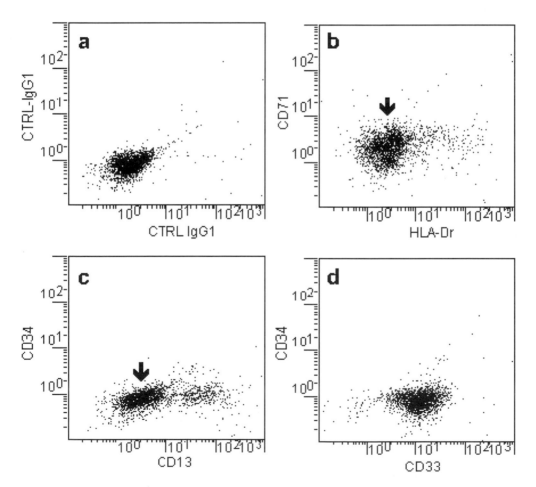

Figure 22.4 AML-M1: CD33$^+$, CD13$^-$ and HLA-DR negative (compare with the isotype control in (a))

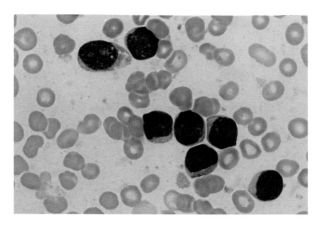

Figure 22.5 AML-M1 with the phenotypic profile shown in Figure 22.4, exhibiting blasts with a few cytoplasmic granules

22.3 Data interpretation when myeloid and lymphoid markers coexist

If a multiparameter analysis is performed and the FCM data are expressed in a format which clearly indicates whether or not the malignant cells are positive, then it is reasonable to conclude that the neoplastic cells truly express both myeloid and lymphoid determinants.

If only single-color FCM analysis is performed, or when the FCM data are expressed as numerical values only, the apparent coexpression of myeloid and lymphoid markers can be the result of any of the possibilities listed below.

1. True coexpression of both myeloid and lymphoid antigenic determinants on the surface of the malignant cells.
2. The coexistence of two separate cell populations within the 'gate', which can represent either:

   - Two malignant clones, one myeloid and one lymphoid (i.e. a biclonal acute leukemia). Biclonal acute leukemia (Figure 22.6) is a very rare occurrence, mainly associated with t(9:22).
   - A mixture of malignant cells and benign reactive cells. A common scenario is the combination of neoplastic myeloid precursors and benign T lymphocytes. One should avoid erroneously labeling such cases 'biphenotypic' or 'AML with aberrant lymphoid expression'. Expressing FCM data as percentage values and using a numerical threshold (20%) can easily lead to this pitfall.

Example. The FCM data on a bone marrow case were reported as follows:

CD2	45%
CD7	42%
CD13	77%
CD33	71%

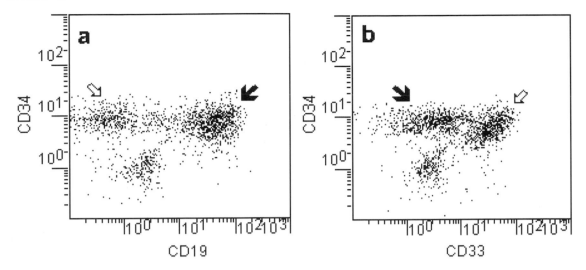

Figure 22.6 Biclonal leukemia. (a), (b) There are two blast populations. One is CD34$^+$, CD19$^+$ and CD33$^-$ (solid arrow). This blast population is also negative for CD13 (not shown). The second blast population (open arrow) is CD34$^+$, CD19$^-$ and CD33$^+$ (CD13 also positive). The monocyte cluster (no arrow) serves as an internal negative control

CD19	13%
CD20	2%
HLA-DR	76%

TdT: Positive by fluorescence microscopy.
Cytochemical stains: MPO cytochemistry negative, NSE negative.
Per cent blasts on a bone marrow manual differential: 55%.

This case was submitted with the diagnosis of biphenotypic leukemia. Repeat FCM analysis, using a multiparameter technique and specific gating by SSC/CD45, yielded the following data on the blasts:

CD13	++
CD33	++
CD34	++
HLA-DR	++
CD2	–
CD7	–
Other T-cell markers	–
B-cell markers	–
Megakaryocytic markers	–

TdT and cytochemical stains as reported above.
    With the FCM data properly reported, it became evident that the case was AML-M0 and not a biphenotypic acute leukemia. The T-cell markers were positive on benign lymphocytes.

22.3.1 Leukemias with both myeloid and lymphoid markers

Acute leukemias with both myeloid and lymphoid markers include biphenotypic acute leukemia, AML with aberrant lymphoid marker(s), and ALL with aberrant myeloid expression. The last group is discussed in Chapters 25 and 26.

Consensus criteria to define these subgroups of leukemia have not been established and the clinical significance of aberrant marker expression remains a subject of controversy. Some institutions refute the concept of biphenotypic leukemia. Others record a significant number of cases as biphenotypic and an even higher number as AML with aberrant lymphoid marker(s) or ALL with aberrant myeloid expression. Besides the lack of established criteria, some of the factors underlying this controversy include:

• The technique (multiparameter vs. single-color analysis).
• The number of antibodies included in the FCM panel.
• The reagents used in a given laboratory.

Conceptually, the term 'AML with aberrant lymphoid expression' should be limited to those AMLs that also express a reliable lymphoid surface marker (e.g. CD19). There is a strong association between aberrant CD19 expression in AML and the (8;21) translocation (Figure 22.7).

When two or more aberrant features occur, the possibility of a biphenotypic leukemia needs to be considered. Note that the presence of TdT does not imply lymphoid differentiation, since many straightforward AMLs (in which the lymphoid determinants are negative) are TdT$^+$.

22.3.1.1 Relative specificity of markers

In the work-up of acute leukemias, the markers considered most specific for lineage differentiation are MPO for myeloid differentiation, cCD22 for B-lymphoid differentiation and cCD3 for T-lymphoid differentiation. The lineage-associated antigens (e.g. CD13, CD33, and CD19) do not share the same degree of specificity as MPO, cCD22 and cCD3. Therefore, interpretation of immunophenotyping data needs to take into account the 'weight' of the markers. The relative value of a given marker also depends on 'the company it keeps' (e.g. CD14 can be considered as a 'full' myeloid marker when present together with CD13 or CD33). On this basis, an interpretation of AML with aberrant lymphoid expression can be made when there is evidence of immaturity, the cells are positive for one or more primary myeloid markers, and there is also expression of one lymphoid-associated surface marker (e.g. CD19, CD20, CD10, CD2, or CD5). Because CD4 is found both in T cells and, with less intensity, on monocytes (Figure 22.8), the presence of CD4 in an AML is not a sufficient indicator of lymphoid coexpression. Similarly, expression of CD56 or CD57 (natural killer cell markers) is not counted as lymphoid differentiation in this context.

The presence of CD7 in an AML also raises questions as to whether the case can be classified as AML with an aberrant lymphoid marker. The FAB definition

**Professor Fidelio
Cases 11 and 12**

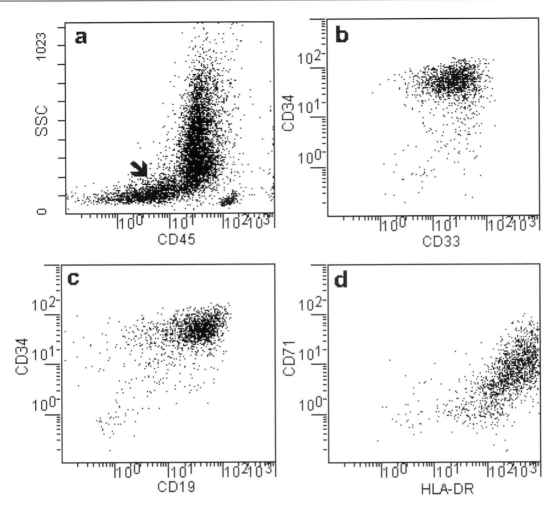

Figure 22.7 Bone marrow sample from a case of AML-M2Eo. (a) A sizable blast cluster (arrow) with low SSC and weak CD45. Graphics (b)–(d) are gated on the blast cluster. (b), (c) Blasts coexpress CD34, CD33 and CD19. CD13 is also positive (not shown). (d) Blasts are positive for CD71 and HLA-DR (strong)

of AML-M0 includes cases positive for CD7, implying that CD7 positivity in AML does not signify aberrant lymphoid expression. It should be noted, however, that the data leading to this conclusion were obtained from multiple institutions with different immunophenotyping techniques, and the number of lymphoid markers tested was not uniform among the cases included in the study group. Until better criteria are established, the 'weight' of CD7 in the context of AML is presumed to be dependent on the presence of TdT, as shown by the following example cases, each of which had 70% blasts on a bone marrow differential.

Case 1: Positive staining for myeloid markers, CD7 and TdT. This case may be considered as an AML with aberrant lymphoid expression.

Case 2: Positive staining for myeloid markers and CD7, but CD34 and TdT were not done. Since there is presumptive evidence of immaturity by morphology

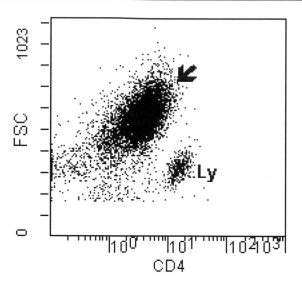

Figure 22.8   CD4 expression in the blasts (arrow) of a case of AML-M5

(70% blasts), this case may also be considered as an AML with an aberrant lymphoid marker.

Case 3: Positive staining for myeloid markers, CD7 and CD34, but TdT was negative. This case shows no definite evidence of aberrant CD7 expression, because TdT is negative.

Case 4: Positive staining for myeloid markers and CD7, but negative staining for both CD34 and TdT. This case is considered a straightforward AML (without aberrant lymphoid expression).

22.3.1.2 Biphenotypic leukemias

Professor Fidelio Case 13

True biphenotypic leukemia with myeloid and lymphoid antigens is an uncommon occurrence. Its prognostic significance (independent of the cytogenetics findings) is still unknown. Biphenotypic blasts should coexpress at least two reliable surface markers (or one cytoplasmic marker) from each lineage. Most cases of biphenotypic leukemia demonstrate a combination of myeloid and immature-B patterns, as shown in the following examples.

Case 1: CD13$^+$, CD33$^+$, CD10$^+$, CD19$^+$, CD34$^+$, TdT$^+$.

Case 2: CD13$^+$, CD33$^+$, cCD22$^+$, CD34$^+$.

Biphenotypic leukemia is mainly associated with the (9;22) translocation, irrespective of a previous history of CML.

In those cases with a combination of the myeloid and 'immature-T' patterns, one should ensure that the data were not obtained from single-color analysis. As previously noted, with single-color analysis one may not be able to rule out a mixture of reactive lymphoid cells and leukemic myeloid blasts. Biphenotypic leukemia with myeloid and T-cell markers is rare (Figure 22.9). If the surface-marker results suggest such a diagnosis, it is judicious to repeat the analysis with cCD3 for confirmation.

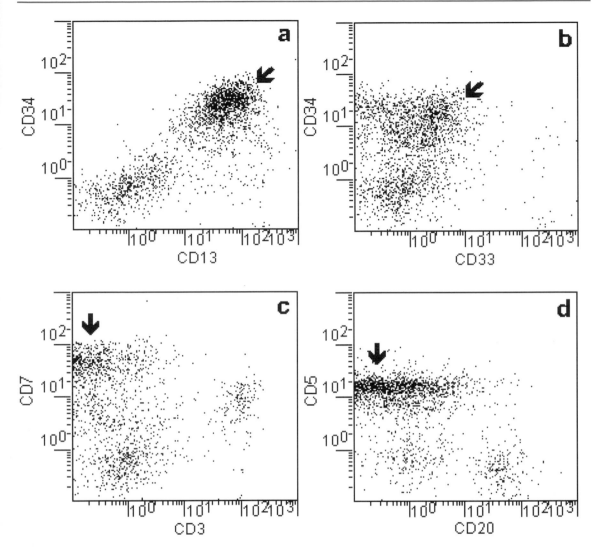

Figure 22.9 Biphenotypic leukemia with coexpression of myeloid and T-cell antigens. (a)–(d) The blast population (arrow) is CD34$^+$, CD13$^+$, CD33^{weak}, CD7$^+$, CD5$^+$. CD2 is also positive (not shown). CD3 is not expressed

Professor Fidelio
Case 14

A false impression of biphenotypic leukemia can also be the result of 'stickiness' of the leukemic cells, e.g. nonspecific binding of lymphoid markers via Fc receptors on cells with monocytic differentiation. If isotype controls are used, they may also demonstrate nonspecific staining. Improper FCM data analysis in such instances can lead to an erroneous combination of myeloid, immature-B and immature-T phenotypes. For these reasons, careful visual assessment of the FCM histograms is necessary to establish true antigenic expression as opposed to nonspecific binding.

22.3.2 Cases with CD13 or CD33 and one lymphoid marker

When the immature cells express only CD13 or CD33 and just one lymphoid marker (e.g. CD19), the findings do not allow a definite classification of the acute leukemia. The diagnostic possibilities include an AML with aberrant lymphoid expression or an ALL with an aberrant myeloid marker. This diagnostic dilemma can be resolved by testing for the most specific lineage markers, i.e. MPO antibody, MPO cytochemistry, cCD22, and/or cCD3, as necessary. If these are inconclusive, then myeloperoxidase ultracytochemistry may need to be performed.

Anti-glycophorin A (anti-GpA) is specific to the erythroid lineage. It detects mainly maturing erythroid precursors, readily identifiable on Romanovsky-stained preparations. The transferrin receptor is strongly expressed in erythroid precursors. Therefore, the pattern of the FSC/CD71 dot plot is very useful in recognizing erythroid hyperplasia. Other determinants present on erythroid precursors are CD36 and the H antigen (the backbone component of the ABO blood group antigens). These markers lack specificity, however, since CD36 is also associated with monocytic and megakaryocytic differentiation and the H antigen is found on megakaryocytes and platelets.

The existence of leukemias composed solely of proerythroblasts (these early erythroid precursors do not react with anti-GpA) is questionable. In erythroleukemia (AML-M6) where erythroid precursors feature prominently, the leukemic blasts are actually myeloblasts based on their cytochemical and/or antigenic characteristics. The FCM data rarely if ever yield an erythroid pattern alone. The bone marrow samples in AML-M6 contain subpopulations reacting with myeloid antibodies and GpA separately, resulting in concomitant myeloid and erythroid patterns. On visual inspection of the FCM raw data, findings strongly suspicious for AML-M6 include: (1) increased erythroid precursors on the FSC/CD71 dot plot; and (2) a large cluster of cells in the 'erythroid' region of the SSC/CD45 dot plot in addition to a cluster of blasts (Figure 23.1).

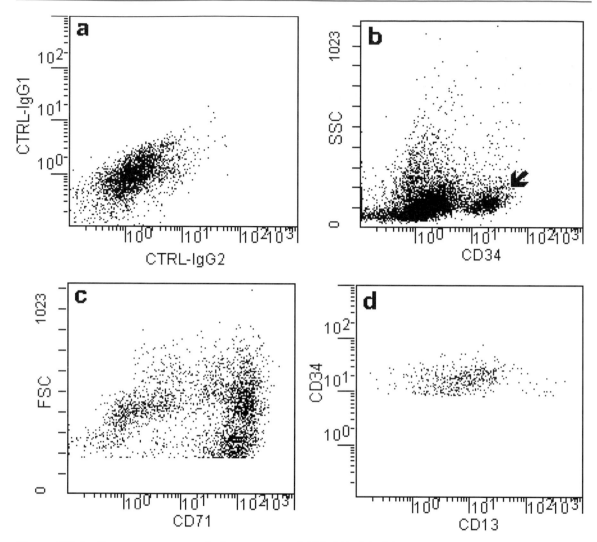

Figure 23.1 Bone marrow sample from a case of AML-M6. (a), (b) Blast cluster (arrow) with low SSC and CD34 expression. The predominant cluster, which lacks CD34 (compare with the isotype control in (a)), consists of erythroid precursors. (c) The pattern of the cell cluster on the FSC/CD71 dot plot indicates increased erythroid precursors. (d) Gated on the blast cluster: blasts coexpress CD34 and CD13. CD33 is also positive (not shown)

Supportive evidence of megakaryocytic differentiation is based on the expression of platelet glycoproteins (Gp). These include mainly CD41/CD61 (Gp IIb/IIIa) and CD42. CD41 represents the integrin α-IIb chain of Gp IIb, and is associated with CD61, which corresponds to the integrin β-3 chain of Gp IIIa. CD42 is itself composed of four subunits: CD42a (Gp IX), CD42b (Gp Ib α), CD42c (Gp Ib β), and CD42d (Gp V). CD42 appears late in megakaryocytic maturation and is therefore of limited diagnostic utility. It is helpful to ensure that a positive reaction with anti-platelet Gp is actually on the cell population studied, rather than on the platelets which may have contaminated the specimen or coated the cells of interest.

The proposed stages of megakaryocytic maturation are as follows:

1. **Immature megakaryoblast**: $CD34^+$, $CD33^+$, $HLA-DR^+$. The expression of CD33 and HLA-DR is variable. It appears that the most immature megakaryoblasts are $HLA-DR^+$ and $CD33^-$, and subsequently lose HLA-DR as CD33 appears. CD41/CD61 and CD42 are not always expressed on immature megakaryoblasts.
2. **Megakaryoblast**: $CD41/CD61^+$, $CD42^+$. CD36 is also present. CD42 expression occurs late.
3. **Megakaryocyte and platelets**: Antigen expression is identical to that on megakaryoblasts. They are also factor VIII-positive, which can be demonstrated on tissue sections by immunohistochemistry.

All stages contain platelet peroxidase activity.

It is presumed that acute megakaryoblastic leukemia (AML-M7) is composed of cells arrested at various steps of maturation, including the megakaryoblast stage and more immature stages. Depending on the level of differentiation of the leukemic cells, the phenotype encountered in AML-M7 and a megakaryoblastic crisis of myeloproliferative disorders can be any of the following patterns:

Professor Fidelio
Case 16

- **Stem cell pattern**: $CD34^+$, $HLA-DR^+$.
- **Myeloid pattern**: $CD34^+$, either CD13 or CD33 positive (expression of both CD13 and CD33 is uncommon), $CD14^-$, $HLA-DR^+$, MPO antigen negative, MPO cytochemistry negative.
- **Megakaryocytic pattern**: expression of platelet Gp, most often CD41/CD61 (Figure 24.1), and no other detectable determinants. The expression of CD34 and HLA-DR can be variable.
- **A combination of myeloid and megakaryocytic patterns**: Note that MPO (antigen and cytochemistry) must be negative.

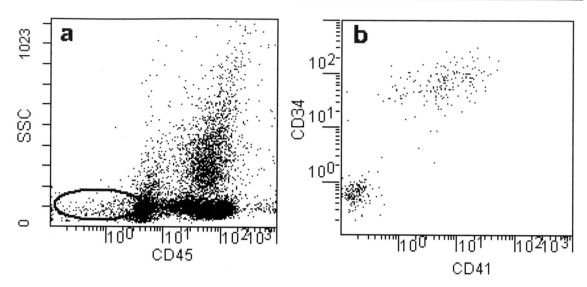

Figure 24.1 Peripheral blood sample with a small number of circulating megakaryoblasts. (a) A small cluster of megakaryoblasts (ellipse) with low SSC and absent CD45. (b) Gated on the CD45 negative cluster: megakaryoblasts are CD34$^+$ and CD41$^+$

In the absence of detectable platelet Gp on the leukemic cells, the megakaryoblastic lineage can only be established by positive platelet peroxidase ultracytochemistry.

Immature
B-cell pattern

A cell population meets the definition of the immature B-cell pattern when there is evidence of immaturity (TdT$^+$ and/or CD34$^+$) along with expression of one or more B-cell lineage-associated markers. During normal B-cell development, the earliest progenitors express CD19 and accumulate molecules of CD22 and CD79 in the cytoplasm. CD79 is the heterodimer mb-1/B29 molecule that is noncovalently bound to sIg. This molecule is presumed to allow stable insertion of sIg within the cytoplasmic membrane. Its pattern of expression parallels that of CD19. The two main antibodies available for the detection of cCD79 are HM57 (cCD79a) directed against mb-1, and B29/123 (cCD79b). Because of their appearance in the earliest B cells, CD19, cCD22 and cCD79 are considered the most reliable B-cell markers. Virtually all precursor-B ALLs are cCD22 positive. Another specific cytoplasmic marker is cytoplasmic mu heavy chain (cmu). This marker is usually included in the immunophenotyping panel for identifying pre-B ALL.

By itself, CD10 is not sufficient to establish lineage differentiation. As discussed under the myeloid pattern, the relative value of a given marker depends on 'the company it keeps'. Because CD10 is mostly associated with B-cell neoplasms (ALL and follicular center cell lymphoma), it can be considered a B-cell marker when present in the company of a reliable B-lineage determinant. Testing for CD10 and cmu are useful for the subclassification of precursor-B ALL.

In addition to immunological markers, DNA analysis by FCM can be of prognostic value in childhood ALL. A DNA index (i.e. the ratio between the DNA content in leukemic G_0/G_1 cells and the DNA content of normal diploid cells) of less than or equal to 1.16 (which corresponds roughly to 53 chromosomes) is associated with an unfavorable outcome. Cases with higher DNA indices have a more favorable prognosis.

25.1 B-cell differentiation

It has been suggested that the phenotypes of malignant immature B cells reflect the various steps of normal B-cell differentiation. B lymphocytes are derived from pluripotent stem cells (TdT$^+$, HLA-DR$^+$) present in the embryonic yolk sac, fetal liver, and postnatal/adult bone marrow. The number of B-cell precursors is much higher in regenerative bone marrows and pediatric samples than in adult samples. The current subclassification of precursor-B ALL is based on the proposed sequence of CD19, CD10, CD20 and cmu appearance during B-cell ontogeny. Recent studies have shown that there is actually overlap in the expression of CD10, CD20 and cmu during the differentiation and maturation of normal B-cell precursors. As B-cell precursors mature, the intensity of CD10 expression decreases while that of CD20 and cmu increases. The earliest precursors appear to be CD19$^-$.

During normal B-cell maturation, detectable surface expression of CD22 does not occur until the resting mature B-cell stage (TdT$^-$, CD34$^-$). However, membrane expression of CD22 has been reported in precursor-B ALLs, suggesting that the phenotypes of malignant immature B cells do not always reflect the stages of normal B-cell differentiation. CD22 expression can be seen in any subtype of precursor-B ALL.

25.2 Immunophenotypic subclassification of precursor-B ALL

Professor Fidelio
Case 17

Most cases of B-lineage ALL demonstrate the immature B-cell pattern alone, with no evidence of myeloid antigen expression. A lymphoid blast crisis of CML may also present with this phenotype. The leukemic manifestation of Burkitt's lymphoma is a high-grade mature B-cell malignancy and is therefore discussed in Chapter 27. As stated previously, it is important to include both CD34 and TdT in the FCM panel to confirm immaturity in the neoplastic cell population. 'Blast' morphology should not be used as the sole evidence of immaturity.

Morphologic subclassification of ALL is no longer considered necessary since immunophenotyping, cytogenetics and molecular genetics allow better characterization of these leukemias. The FAB subtypes L1 and L2 do not reflect immunologic phenotypes. The leukemic cells in ALL L1 or L2 can be immature B cells, immature T cells or, in rare cases of pediatric ALL, mature B cells. These rare cases of 'monoclonal sIg$^+$ non-L3 ALL' in children differ from Burkitt's leukemia since they lack both the high S-phase and the t(8;14) translocation.

In childhood, precursor-B ALL phenotypes are associated with age. There is a correlation between some immunophenotypic subgroups and certain specific cytogenetic abnormalities. The immunophenotypic subgroups, which are identified on the basis of certain antigenic combinations, include:

1. **Null ALL**: HLA-DR$^+$, CD19$^+$, CD10$^-$, cmu$^-$. This phenotype, which accounts for 15% of B-lineage ALL, occurs mainly in infants. In patients less than 1 year of age, the 'null' phenotype is associated with t(4;11)(q21;q23) and other poor prognostic factors (hyperleukocytosis, DNA index <1.16, pseudodiploidy). In older patients, the lack of CD10 expression does not appear to be of prognostic importance.

2. **Common ALL**: HLA-DR$^+$, CD19$^+$, CD10$^+$, cmu$^-$. This phenotype is seen in the majority of childhood ALL (Figure 25.1). CD20 may be absent or present.

3. **Pre-B ALL**: cmu$^+$. This phenotype, defined by cmu expression, occurs in approximately 20% of childhood ALL. This subgroup of ALL, seen more often in blacks, is associated with adverse prognostic features including hyperleukocytosis, high serum LDH levels, a DNA index <1.16 and

Professor Fidelio
Case 18

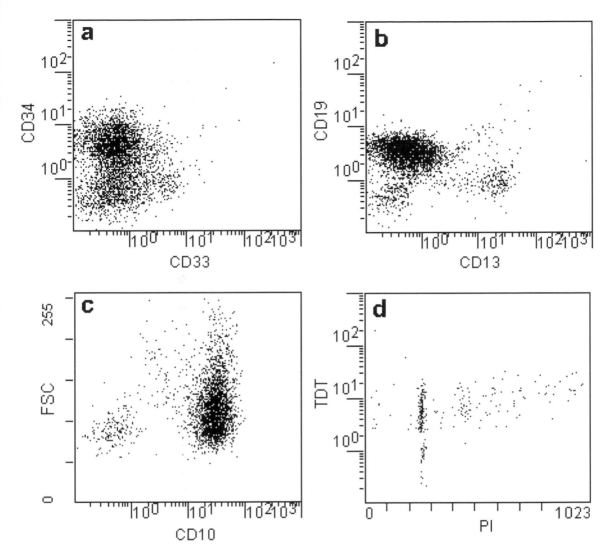

Figure 25.1 Precursor-B ALL. (a)–(d) Blasts are medium-sized and coexpress TdT, CD19, CD10 and CD34. CD34 expression is heterogeneous. CD13 and CD33 are negative

Professor Fidelio
Case 19

pseudodiploidy. These poor prognostic factors are actually linked to the presence of t(1;19)(q23;p13), found in approximately one-third of pre-B ALL cases. Patients without the translocation have a similar prognosis to patients with common ALL.

4. **Transitional pre-B-cell ALL** is a recently recognized ALL subtype which accounts for less than 1% of precursor-B ALL. This subtype is 'transitional' between pre-B ALL and Burkitt's lymphoma-leukemia (monoclonal surface light chain positive). Leukemic blasts of the transitional pre-B ALL

subtype do not have Burkitt's morphology. The immunological characteristics are expression of immature markers (TdT and/or CD34), B-cell markers (including CD10), cytoplasmic and surface IgM, but no demonstrable surface light chains. This subgroup is associated with favorable prognostic features, namely a lower WBC count at presentation, no CNS involvement, and a DNA index >1.16. There is no association with any particular cytogenetic abnormality.

Transitional pre-B-cell ALL can only be identified if the FCM panel systematically includes TdT, CD34, cmu, sIgM and surface light chains, in addition to the routine B-cell antibodies. If the FCM panel is incomplete, the following results may be obtained: TdT not done, CD34$^-$, B-cell markers positive, cmu$^+$, sIgM$^+$, kappa$^-$, lambda$^-$. This set of data is insufficient to differentiate transitional pre-B-cell ALL from a mature B-cell LPD/NHL which lacks surface light chain expression.

5. **Precursor-B ALL with T-lineage associated markers**: a small number of precursor-B ALLs express CD2 (e.g. CD34$^+$, TdT$^+$, CD2$^+$, CD19$^+$, CD10$^+$, CD20$^-$, cmu$^-$). Some authors have named these 'biphenotypic ALLs'. Studies using *in vitro* cultures have demonstrated that the lymphoblasts in such cases could be induced to acquire CD20 and cmu, whereas acquisition of CD3 was not observed. Based on this evidence of B-lineage differentiation, it is more logical to include CD2$^+$, CD19$^+$ ALLs within the group of precursor-B ALL than to consider these as 'biphenotypic' ALL. Normal lymphoid progenitor cells with this phenotype have been found in fetal liver and bone marrow. The example given above can be considered a common ALL.

The phenotype TdT$^+$, CD34$^+$, CD7$^+$, CD19$^+$ is found in rare cases of ALL, raising the question of the lineage differentiation of the leukemic cells. This question can be resolved by testing for cCD3 and cCD22.

25.3 ALL with aberrant myeloid antigens

The number of ALLs with aberrant myeloid antigens reported in the literature is high, especially among adults. Many of the studies were based on single-color FCM analysis, however. When single-color analysis is performed on bone marrow specimens, apparent myeloid antigen expression may be due to residual myeloid precursors within the 'gate'. Furthermore, some studies included 'myeloid-associated' markers of rather low specificity (e.g. CD14, CD11b, CD15). It is preferable to restrict the category 'precursor-B ALL with aberrant myeloid antigens' to those cases with either CD13 or CD33 expression. Such cases meet the definition of both the immature B-cell and myeloid patterns.

The prognostic importance of myeloid antigens in ALL has been a subject of controversy. There may be no prognostic significance if highly effective therapy is applied. From studies that correlate immunophenotyping and cytogenetic data, there appears to be an association between myeloid antigen expression and certain karyotypic abnormalities. Myeloid antigens are often seen in ALL with the (9;22) translocation (Philadelphia chromosome) or 11q23 rearrangements, including t(4;11)(q21;q23).

25.4 Hematogones (precursor B cells)

Bone marrow samples in normal children are known to contain a high number of 'lymphocytes', many of which are actually precursor B cells. Increased numbers of hematogones have been observed in children with various hematological disorders, including ITP, congenital neutropenia and congenital red cell aplasia, and with solid tumors and during continued remission after chemotherapy or bone marrow transplantation for ALL. A confusing array of terms (e.g. post-therapeutic stem cells, CALLA$^+$ cells, TdT$^+$ cells, and residual blasts) has been used to designate hematogones. Phenotypically, hematogones are comprised of heterogeneous populations of precursor B cells.

Precursor B cells have been reported to comprise 4–21% of the bone marrow of normal children, in contrast to 0.2–3.5% observed in adult samples. This finding is presumed to be due to repetitive antigenic stimulation during childhood. A marked increase in hematogones has been misinterpreted as ALL, malignant lymphoma and metastatic tumor. Because of the potential confusion between hematogones and ALL in children, both morphologically and immunologically, it is important to pay attention to the clinical setting, DNA content analysis and karyotypic studies. Hematogones have normal, diploid DNA content, low S-phase and no cytogenetic abnormalities. Visual inspection of the FCM list mode data can allow the detection of subtle immunophenotypic differences between hematogones and ALL blasts. Hematogones may be recognized by:

- Low FSC and low SSC.
- Heterogeneous CD20 intensity spanning from the negative range into the first decalog.

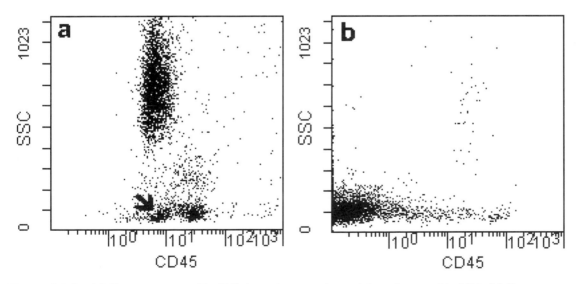

Figure 25.2 (a) Bone marrow with 20% hematogones (arrow) in a 5-year-old child. (b) Bone marrow with precursor-B ALL. CD45 on the blast cells is markedly down-regulated

- Usually absent CD34.
- CD10 that is often less bright than that expressed by ALL blasts.

In contrast, the blast population in ALL has higher FSC with absent CD20 and down-regulated CD45 in most cases (Figure 25.2). If the pattern of the FCM histograms does not allow a clear-cut distinction between benign precursor B cells and precursor-B ALL, DNA content analysis and review of the peripheral blood film can be helpful, since the presence of aneuploidy or circulating immature cells are features of a malignant process.

Immature
T-cell pattern

An immature T-cell phenotype is defined by the presence of either TdT or CD34 together with expression of T-cell lineage-associated markers (CD2, CD3, CD5, CD7). The expression of the surface epitopes of CD3 requires the presence of the TCRαβ heterodimer. CD3 molecules are present in immature T cells, but surface expression of CD3 is not detectable because the TCR molecules are not fully assembled. Therefore, cytoplasmic CD3 (cCD3) is considered the most specific marker for identifying a T-cell lineage in immature cells. The immature T-cell phenotype is seen in normal thymocytes and precursor-T ALL/ lymphoblastic lymphoma.

26.1 T-cell differentiation

Substantial immunological data exist to suggest that malignant immature T cells mimic the phenotype of normal thymocytes at different stages of differentiation. Normal T cells arise during embryonic and early postnatal life, when bone marrow progenitor cells migrate to the thymus. The thymus provides the necessary microenvironment for the development of functionally competent T cells. The various stages of intrathymic differentiation are accompanied by changes in cell surface antigenic expression (Figure 26.1).

TdT is present in thymocytes and a small number of bone marrow progenitor cells, but not in mature lymphoid cells. Approximately 10% of thymocytes are stage I and 70% are stage II.

Stage III thymocytes are immune competent, as indicated by the expression of the CD3/TCR complex. They are further segregated into helper (CD4$^+$) and suppressor (CD8$^+$) subgroups.

CD38 is no longer present on 'resting' mature (post-thymic) T cells. CD38 reappears again on activated T cells, along with other activation markers such as CD25 and HLA-DR.

26.2 Features of precursor-T ALL/lymphoblastic lymphoma

In general, precursor-T ALL has a poorer prognosis than precursor-B ALL because of the association with adverse prognostic features including an older age (15 years and older), hyperleukocytosis (WBC $>50 \times 10^9$/l), central nervous involvement and a mediastinal mass. Approximately 15% of childhood ALL are precursor-T ALL.

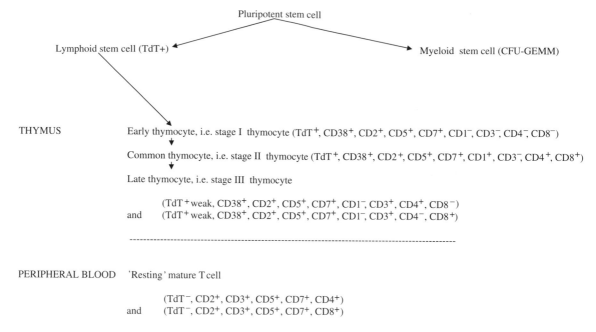

Figure 26.1 Stages of intrathymic T-cell differentiation

In some studies, a stage I thymocyte phenotype is seen in the majority of T ALLs. Other studies have demonstrated that T ALL cells can correspond to any of the three stages of intrathymic differentiation, however. In lymphoblastic lymphomas (most of which are of T-cell lineage), about half express a phenotype consistent with a stage II thymocyte and the remaining are roughly equally divided between stages I and III. Subclassification of T ALL and lymphoblastic lymphoma according to the three intrathymic stages of differentiation is not widely advocated, since no clinical differences among the subgroups are known to exist.

In addition to the lack of surface expression of CD3 in most cases of T ALL and lymphoblastic lymphoma, the immature T cells in these diseases may fail to express other pan-T markers. Since the lack of one or more pan-T antigens is also a feature of mature T-cell malignancies, and CD4/CD8 restriction is not an absolute indicator of maturity, it is important to include both CD34 and TdT in the FCM panel.

Although CD34 is expressed in only a small number of T ALLs, virtually all immature T-cell malignancies are TdT$^+$. Because TdT is extremely labile, it is best to perform the analysis on fresh specimens to avoid false-negative results. This is especially true if testing for TdT is done by the APAAP procedure on smears/cytospins. If the procedure is to be delayed, then deep-freeze the slides quickly. Leaving the smears/cytospins at room temperature for a few hours can easily result in a false-negative result (Figure 26.2). The expression of CD1 cannot be relied upon as proof of immaturity since CD1 positivity has been reported in mature T-cell malignancies (see Section 28.6).

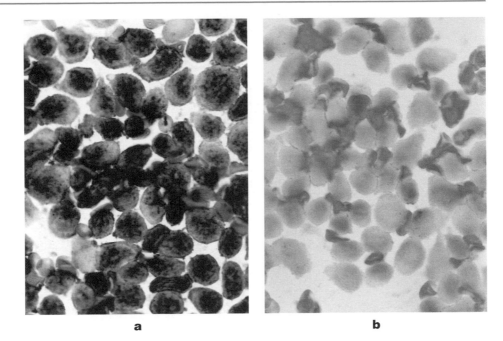

a   b

Figure 26.2   Smears from the same patient: immunostaining for TdT (APAAP procedure). (a) Positive TdT seen as strong nuclear reactivity. (b) False-negative result when the smear was left on the bench at room temperature for 2 hours before the staining procedure was performed

T ALL and lymphoblastic lymphoma can also express CD10 in up to 40% of cases. It appears that the lack of CD10 expression in T ALL is associated with a poor clinical outcome. Occasionally, activation markers such as CD25 and HLA-DR may be present.

26.3 Examples of the immature T-cell phenotype

Professor Fidelio
Case 20

In many laboratories, the 'acute leukemia FCM panel' contains only a few T-cell-associated antibodies (e.g. CD2 and either CD7 or CD5). In such situations, FCM analysis on T ALL/lymphoblastic lymphoma often yields results such as: CD2$^-$, CD7$^+$, TdT$^+$, or CD2$^+$, CD5$^+$, TdT$^+$. While these data are suggestive of immature T-cell malignancies, it would be helpful to confirm a T-cell phenotype with testing for cCD3.

As shown in the examples below, neoplastic immature T cells in ALL/LL can demonstrate CD4/CD8 restriction. Without testing for TdT and CD34, the results could be easily misinterpreted as a mature T-cell pattern.

A comprehensive lymphoma-leukemia panel was employed in these four examples of T-ALL and lymphoblastic lymphoma:

1. Lymph node cell suspension: TdT$^+$, CD34$^+$, CD2$^+$, CD3$^+$, CD4$^+$, CD5$^+$, CD7$^+$ and CD8$^+$.

2. Lymph node cell suspension: TdT⁺, CD34⁻, CD2⁺, CD3⁻, CD4⁺, CD5⁺, CD7⁺, CD8⁻, CD10⁺, CD25⁺, CD56⁺ and HLA-DR⁺. Note the presence of CD25 and an NK-associated antigen. This does not necessarily indicate that the precursor-T lymphoblastic lymphoma is of NK lineage.

3. Bone marrow aspirate: TdT⁻, CD34⁺, CD2⁻, CD3⁺, CD4⁺, CD5⁺, CD7⁺ and CD8⁻. Note the importance of including both markers of immaturity in the immunophenotyping panel. TdT was negative in this case but the positive CD34 established the immaturity of the leukemic population.

4. Bone marrow aspirate: TdT⁺, CD34⁻, CD2⁺, CD3⁻, CD4⁺, CD5⁺, CD7⁺, CD8⁺ and CD10⁺.

Professor Fidelio
Case 21

It should be noted that the immunophenotype in T ALL does not correlate with the morphologic classification of L1 and L2 ALL. With the increased understanding of the biology of leukemias gained by FCM analysis, the FAB morphologic subclassification of ALL is no longer necessary. DNA content analysis in ALL has been shown to be a useful prognostic indicator in ALL (see Chapter 25).

26.4 Aberrant myeloid expression in T ALL/LL

Professor Fidelio
Case 22

A small number of T ALL/lymphoblastic lymphoma demonstrate aberrant expression of a myeloid marker (either CD13 or CD33) on multiparameter analysis. Such cases meet the definition of both the immature-T and myeloid patterns. With single-color analysis on bone marrow aspirates, apparent myeloid antigen expression can be due to residual myeloid precursors within the 'gate'. In such instances, multicolor analysis is necessary to confirm true coexpression.

Since the myeloid-associated determinants are not equally specific, the occurrence of a myeloid marker with low specificity such as CD14, CD11b or CD15 in T ALL/lymphoblastic lymphoma does not necessarily indicate aberrant myeloid antigen expression. The prognostic significance of aberrant myeloid markers in ALL remains uncertain. Cumulative evidence from multiple studies appears to indicate that the presence of a myeloid antigen in ALL does not confer an adverse prognosis when highly effective therapy is administered, particularly in childhood ALL.

Mature
B-cell pattern

Surface immunoglobulin light chain expression is the hallmark of mature B cells. Accurate identification of surface light chains requires careful reagent selection and proper technique. It is important to ensure that the anti-light chain reagent is specific with an optimal fluorochrome to protein ratio. The reagent should be free of soluble aggregates as these can yield false-positive staining caused by nonspecific binding to the cell membrane. Nonspecific binding can also occur via the Fc receptors present on hematopoietic cells, especially monocytes and activated T cells. To reduce this occurrence ensure that the antibodies employed are F(ab'2) reagents. Another cause of cytophilic immunoglobulin bound to the cell surface is hypergammaglobulinemia, either polyclonal, as in abnormal immune conditions (including HIV), or monoclonal, as in multiple myeloma or Waldenstrom's macroglobulinemia. A solution to this problem is warming the cell suspension in a water bath at $37°C$ for 30 minutes prior to the analysis.

The most commonly used pan-B markers include CD19, CD20, CD22, and FMC-7. The reactivity pattern of FMC-7 parallels that of CD22 and CD20. Pan-B markers alone do not provide adequate information on the maturity of B cells. In general, immature B-cell malignancies are $CD20^-$, whereas mature B-cell disorders are $CD20^+$. However, the expression of CD20 can be lost in some NHLs, especially those with plasmacytoid differentiation (Figure 27.1).

If the phenotype of a population is $CD19^+$, $CD20^-$, $kappa^-$, $lambda^-$, with CD34 and TdT not done, it is not possible to determine whether the critical cells are precursor-B lymphoblasts or mature neoplastic B cells. In addition, since aberrant expression of one myeloid antigen (e.g. CD13 or CD33) can occasionally occur in mature B-cell neoplasms, this feature cannot be relied upon to favor an immature process.

The identification of surface heavy chain isotopes does not provide information on clonality. However, in those cases of NHL that are negative for both kappa and lambda, expression of one or more surface heavy chains suggests that the abnormal cells are mature B cells. One exception to this rule is the presence of surface IgM alone. Since ALL of the transitional pre-B-cell subtype is sIgM-positive (see Section 25.2), this finding does not prove that B cells which lack surface light chains are mature.

Indirect evidence of maturity can be obtained morphologically if the proliferation is composed of small cells with clumped chromatin (e.g. CLL or FCC lymphoma in leukemic phase). There are, however, cases of ALL composed of small blasts with coarse chromatin, simulating the appearance of mature cells.

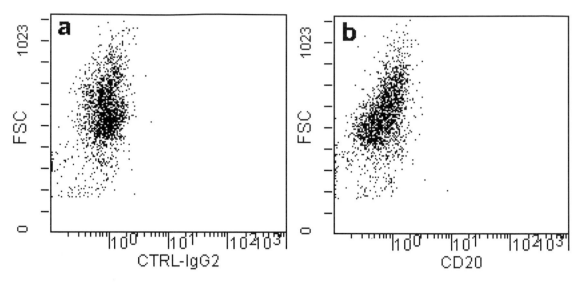

Figure 27.1 (a), (b) A large B-cell NHL with loss of CD20, compared with the isotype control

27.1 Clonality

Professor Fidelio
Case 23

In reactive conditions, the mature B cells are polyclonal, composed of a mixture of kappa and lambda B cells, in a roughly 2:1 ratio. In peripheral blood, bone marrow and body fluids, polyclonal B cells are part of a reactive lymphoid population composed predominantly of mature T cells. In lymph nodes, tonsils, and spleen, polyclonal B cells may predominate in florid reactive follicular hyperplasia (FRFH). In cases with marked FRFH (e.g. HIV-positive patients), CD10 is present in a subset of polyclonal B cells which also express bright CD20. These cells correspond to benign reactive follicular center cells. The pattern of CD20/CD10 expression in such cases is distinctly different from that seen in follicular lymphoma (Figure 27.2).

To detect monoclonality, it is recommended that analysis of surface kappa and lambda light chains is restricted to B cells. This requires a multiparameter FCM technique, at least dual-color staining, using the combination of a pan-B antibody and anti-light chain antibodies. It may be helpful if the FCM panel includes more than one set of kappa/lambda reagents. One set can be combined with CD19 (CD19/kappa and CD19/lambda) and the second to CD20 (CD20/kappa and CD20/lambda). If only one type of kappa/lambda reagent is employed, then the preferred antibody combination is CD20/light chain as CD20 has a wider dynamic range than other B-cell markers. The intensity of CD20 expression is different between malignant and benign cells and is typically down-regulated in CLL/SLL (Figure 27.3). The intensity of CD19 expression is not as useful a discriminator between different B-cell populations as CD20.

It is not appropriate to study surface light chains by single-color FCM. When the sample is analyzed by a single-color technique, determinations of kappa and lambda are derived from the entire population in the gate, including irrelevant cells, causing a 'dilution' of the relevant FCM data. This can result in apparent

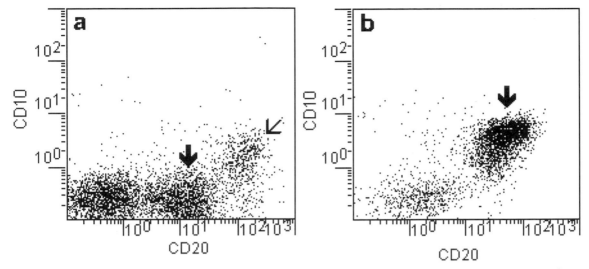

Figure 27.2 (a) Lymph node with florid reactive follicular hyperplasia. There are two distinct CD20$^+$ cell clusters. The population which coexpresses very bright CD20 and weak CD10 (thin arrow) represents reactive follicular center cells. The CD10-negative B-cell population (thick arrow) consists mostly of nonfollicular center cells. (b) Lymph node with FCC lymphoma. All the malignant B cells coexpress CD10 and bright CD20. There is slight nonspecific staining with CD20 on the benign T cells in the background due to the presence of cytophilic CD20

polyclonality, especially when the number of monoclonal neoplastic B cells in the sample is low. The multiparameter FCM approach has been shown to be superior to the various single-parameter immunofluorescence clonal excess assays.

Detecting monoclonal surface light chain in a substantial B-cell population is virtually pathognomonic of a mature malignant B-cell proliferation (i.e. B-NHL or B-LPD). As noted above, a small number of mature B-cell neoplasms may present with the following phenotype: CD19$^+$, CD20$^+$, CD34$^-$, TdT$^-$, kappa$^-$, lambda$^-$ (i.e. no detectable surface light chains). This phenotype indicates an abnormal/malignant B-cell proliferation (a plasma cell dyscrasia cannot be excluded). In some cases, the apparent absence of light chains may be a false-negative result since the cells may have light chain epitopes that were not recognized by the anti-light chain reagents. In many such cases, down-regulation of one or more pan-B-cell antigens is a further clue to the malignant nature of the B-cell proliferation.

Professor Fidelio
Case 24

27.2 Mature B-cell differentiation

The following scheme of B-cell maturation and differentiation has been proposed. Mature, resting B lymphocytes generated from pre-B cells in the bone marrow are quickly exported to the peripheral blood and primary follicles of the lymph nodes and spleen. Immunoglobulins produced by these cells are of

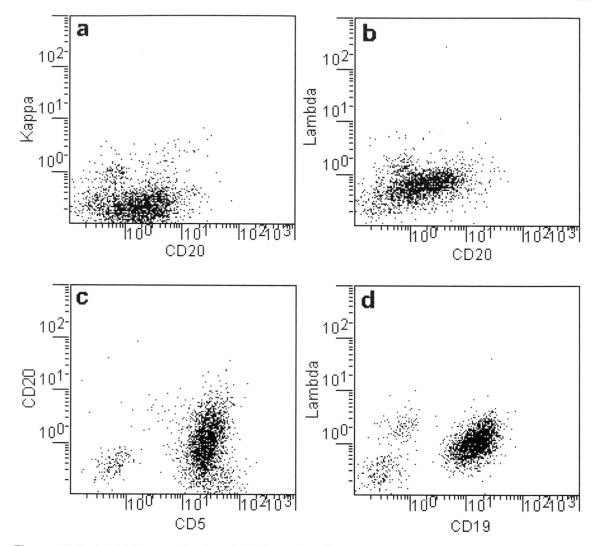

Figure 27.3 (a)–(d) The profile of weak CD20, weak surface monoclonal light chain and CD5 expression is typical of CLL/SLL

the IgD and IgM classes. A small number of the resting B cells are CD5 positive and are therefore hypothesized to be the normal counterpart of the neoplastic lymphocytes of CLL/SLL. With rearrangement of the constant region of the immunoglobulin heavy chain genes during antigen-induced B-cell activation and maturation, IgG is produced. Presumably, the cells are then transformed into B immunoblasts, plasmacytoid lymphocytes and ultimately plasma cells.

In ALL, it is possible to assign the phenotype of a given case to a particular differentiation stage of precursor B cells or precursor T cells, based on the speculation that neoplastic cells attempt to recapitulate the ontogeny of normal precursor cells. In mature B-cell malignancies this approach is not feasible, since for many of these disorders the putative normal counterparts remain to be proven.

27.3 Grading of non-Hodgkin's lymphomas

Some NHLs/LPDs can be diagnosed solely on the basis of immunophenotyping results, especially if the data are interpreted in conjunction with cell cycle analysis. The combination of cell size (by FSC), S-phase fraction, and CD71 (transferrin receptor) expression can be used to determine if a monoclonal B-cell proliferation is low grade or intermediate/high grade. Small cell size, an S-phase fraction below 5%, and negative CD71 expression are all features of low-grade B-cell neoplasms. Conversely, large cell size, S-phase above 5%, and bright CD71 expression are features of intermediate/high-grade tumors (Figure 27.4).

At least two pieces of corroborating evidence and no contradicting evidence should be used to grade a tumor. For example:

1. A monoclonal B-cell neoplasm with small cell size, S-phase fraction 2.3%, and CD71 not done is considered low grade because the cell size and low S-phase fraction are in agreement. If CD71 is strongly positive, however, it would be inappropriate to comment on the grade because bright CD71 expression does not agree with the other data.
2. It is difficult to comment on the grade of a monoclonal B-cell neoplasm with variable cell size, S-phase fraction 8%, and CD71 not done. Although the S-phase fraction is consistent with an intermediate/high-grade neoplasm, a second piece of corroborating evidence is needed. If the cell size was large or the CD71 was bright, then an intermediate/high-grade neoplasm could be confirmed.

**Professor Fidelio
Cases 25–26**

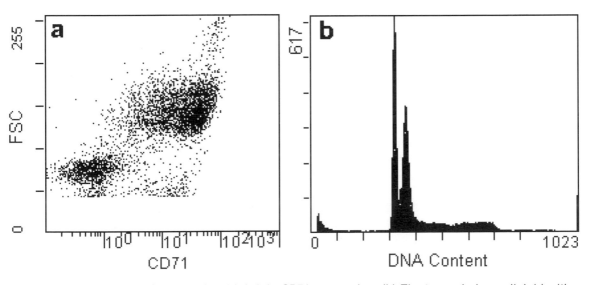

Figure 27.4   (a) A large B-cell NHL with bright CD71 expression. (b) The tumor is hyperdiploid with a high S-phase fraction

27.4 Diagnostic B-cell profiles

Immunophenotyping and cell cycle analysis can be essentially diagnostic in some B-cell malignancies. Table 27.1 lists the key immunophenotypic features in CLL/SLL, FCC lymphoma and hairy cell leukemia.

Table 27.1 Key features in low-grade B-cell neoplasms with diagnostic immunophenotypes

Key features in the immunophenotypic profile	Diagnosis
CD5$^+$, CD23$^+$, weak monoclonal sIg, CD20^{weak}, low S-phase	CLL/SLL
CD10$^+$, monoclonal sIg, low S-phase	FCC NHL
CD25$^+$, CD11c^{bright}, CD103$^+$, bright monoclonal sIg	HCL

27.5 CD5$^+$ B-cell neoplasms

Professor Fidelio
Case 27

CD5$^+$ B-cell malignancies encompass several entities which need to be distinguished from each other. In particular, the distinction of MCL from the family of CLL/SLL and closely related disorders is important for therapeutic and prognostic reasons. Evaluating the expression of CD23 in the context of CD5 positivity helps to establish the diagnosis. When CD23 is not performed, it may not be possible to achieve a more precise interpretation than 'low-grade LPD' when faced with a small mature B-cell, CD5$^+$ lymphoid tumor.

27.5.1 Chronic lymphocytic leukemia, small lymphocytic lymphoma and related disorders

Professor Fidelio
Cases 28–31

Chronic lymphocytic leukemia and SLL are but one disease. The term CLL is used when the disease is found in the bone marrow and peripheral blood. The disease is designated SLL when it manifests in the lymph nodes or spleen without evidence of an absolute peripheral lymphocytosis. The difference in anatomic distribution may be related to the differences in the expression of adhesion molecules. The phenotypic profile is otherwise identical between SLL and CLL (Figure 27.5). In some cases, the low level of sIg expression may not be detectable, particularly when only one set of anti-light chain reagents is employed. About 20% of cases express CD14 (especially if the antibody tested is MY4). Note that CD23 positivity is only diagnostically meaningful when CD5 is also positive.

Several FCM studies on 'CLL' have included cases (presumably diagnosed morphologically) which are either CD5$^-$, CD23$^-$, CD22/FMC-7^{bright}, or monoclonal sIg^{bright}. Overall, it has been shown that such cases have a poorer clinical course than typical CLL. They have been referred to under the vague term 'atypical CLL'. Because of their different biological behavior, it is preferable that such cases are set apart from CLL and further characterized by other laboratory parameters. Immunoelectrophoresis and correlation with morphologic features

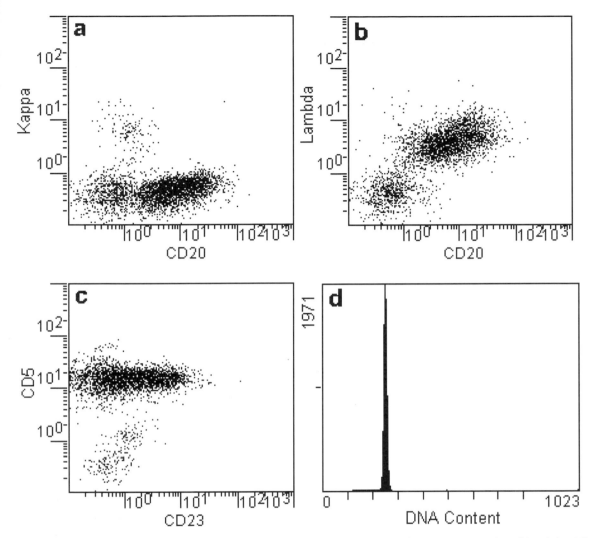

Figure 27.5　CLL/SLL. (a)–(c) The tumor cells coexpress CD5, CD23, CD20 and monoclonal lambda. (d) The tumor is diploid with a very low S-phase fraction

should be performed in such cases. Data from clinical/morphological studies (which invariably lack detailed FCM information) appear to indicate that CLL with an increased percentage of prolymphocytes (i.e. CLL/PL) is associated with a poorer prognosis (see Section 5.5.2). Similarly, so-called 'CLL' composed mainly of plasmacytoid lymphocytes (a more appropriate name is LPC leukemia) with a detectable monoclonal IgM paraprotein also appears to behave more aggressively. It is unclear whether CLL/PL and LPC leukemia (according to the clinical/morphological studies) correspond to 'atypical CLL' from the FCM investigations.

To gain a better understanding of disorders considered to be 'atypical CLL', the minimum diagnostic work-up for all cases designated CLL should include the following:

1. Peripheral blood analysis with morphologic assessment (e.g. an estimate of the percentage of prolymphocytes).
2. Multiparameter FCM analysis on the appropriate sample(s).
3. Serum protein immunoelectrophoresis. If the initial results are normal, then follow-up studies can be done at 6–12 month intervals. CLL patients should not develop an IgM or IgA monoclonal protein.

Other studies (lymph node biopsy, cytogenetics and molecular genetics) may also be helpful.

Dual expression of a pan-B antigen (i.e. CD19 or CD20) and CD5 does not identify CLL/SLL since similar results can be seen in MCL and a subset of DLCL, some of which cases may have plasmacytoid differentiation. Furthermore, CD5 expression is found in a fraction (20–30%) of normal B cells in the peripheral blood, spleen, lymph node and tonsils. Presumably, these CD5$^+$ cells are involved in autoimmunity.

27.5.2 CD5$^+$ diffuse large cell lymphoma (DLCL)

CD5$^+$ DLCL (either *de novo* or arising in the setting of CLL/SLL, i.e. Richter's syndrome) is easily distinguished from CLL/SLL based on FCM immunophenotyping and DNA content/cell cycle data as follows:

- CLL and SLL demonstrate a very low S-phase and no overt DNA aneuploidy, whereas the cell cycle results in *de novo* CD5$^+$ DLCL are typically those of an intermediate/high-grade NHL (i.e. a high S-fraction and frequent aneuploidy).
- CD5$^+$ DLCL normally exhibits a large cell size by light scatter, bright CD20, and absent CD23 (Figure 27.6). However, in some cases, CD20 is down-regulated or nondetectable, and surface light chain expression is weak or absent. Weak expression of CD20 and sIg in large cell NHL often corresponds morphologically to plasmacytoid differentiation, also referred to as immunoblastic lymphoma. Such cases have detectable monoclonal cytoplasmic light chain expression.

27.5.3 Mantle cell lymphoma (MCL)

Professor Fidelio
Cases 32 and 33

It is important to distinguish MCL from CLL/SLL and other subtypes of low-grade NHL, as this disorder behaves differently and responds poorly to current therapeutic regimens. The typical immunophenotype in MCL is CD20^{bright}, CD5$^+$, CD10$^-$, CD23$^-$ (Figure 27.7), with moderate to strong sIg expression. This phenotype is not pathognomonic of MCL, however, since the combination CD5$^+$, CD23$^-$, strong sIg, can be found in a small subset of CLL/PL, B-PLL and LPC lymphoma-leukemia. When CD19 expression is less intense than CD20, it is a helpful clue in identifying MCL. In addition to the morphology and immunophenotype, the current diagnostic criteria for MCL include *bcl*-1 rearrangement, and the (11;14)(q13;q32) translocation. The availability of anti-cyclin D1 antibodies, which can also be applied to paraffin-embedded, fixed tissue, provides an additional parameter to diagnose MCL (see Section 40.4.2).

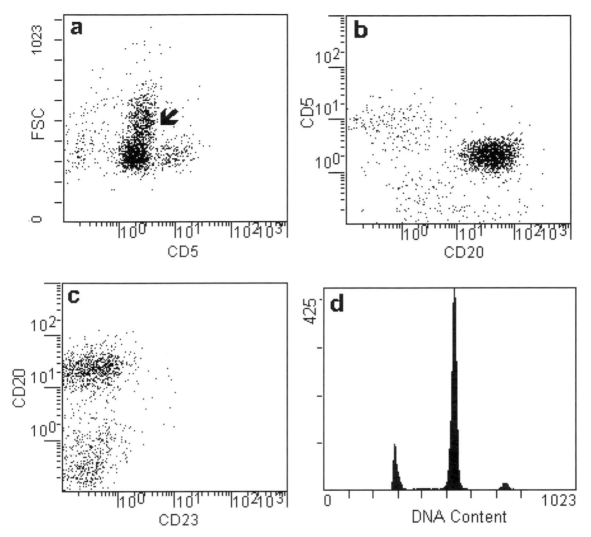

Figure 27.6 CD5$^+$ high-grade B-cell NHL. (a)–(c) The tumor cells coexpress CD5 and bright CD20. CD23 is negative. (d) The tumor is hyperdiploid

The 'blastoid' variant (also known as large cell variant) of MCL, so named because of morphologic similarities to lymphoblastic lymphoma on H&E sections, needs to be differentiated from ALL/lymphoblastic lymphoma for treatment purposes. The distinction is straightforward by FCM immunophenotyping. ALL/lymphoblastic lymphoma expresses immature markers (CD34, TdT) and lacks sIg, whereas the reverse is true in MCL.

27.5.4 B-prolymphocytic leukemia (B-PLL)

The diagnosis of B-PLL requires correlation of the clinical presentation (splenomegaly, minimal lymphadenopathy and marked leukocytosis), the cytology of the neoplastic cells in the peripheral blood (see Section 5.5) and the FCM

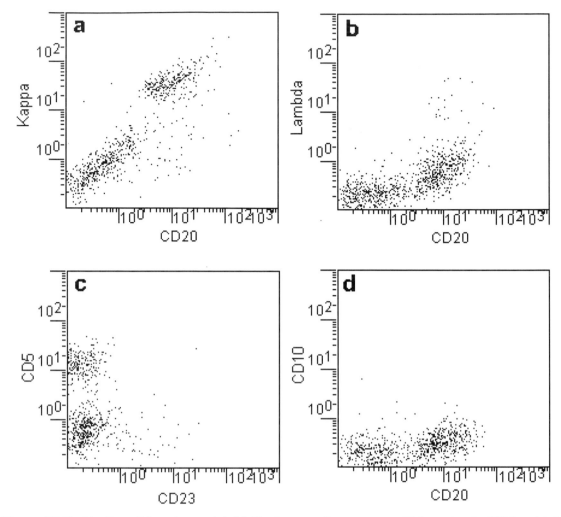

Figure 27.7 Mantle cell lymphoma. (a)–(d) The tumor cells coexpress CD5, moderate CD20 and bright monoclonal kappa. CD10 is negative

Professor Fidelio
Case 34

results. The usual phenotypic profile, CD5$^-$, CD10$^-$, CD23$^-$, CD19/CD20/CD22$^+$, and strong sIg, is confirmatory of a mature B-cell neoplasm. This is a 'nondescript' phenotype, however. The same profile can be seen in large cell lymphoma in leukemic phase. The subset of B-PLL expressing CD5 needs to be distinguished from *de novo* CD5$^+$ DLCL as well. Cell cycle data available in a small number of B-PLL cases have shown low S-phase values similar to CLL.

27.5.5 Lymphoplasmacytoid (LPC) lymphoma-leukemia and Waldenstrom's macroglobulinemia

The recognition of lymphoplasmacytoid disorders can be difficult, both immunophenotypically and morphologically. The many possible phenotypes and the frequent morphological artifacts are the main contributing factors.

27.5.5.1 Immunophenotypes in lymphoplasmacytoid malignancies

There is variability in the expression of CD5 in lymphoplasmacytoid disorders. The majority of cases of Waldenstrom's macroglobulinemia and LPC lymphoma-leukemia exhibit a 'nondescript' immunophenotypic profile (CD5⁻, CD10⁻, CD23⁻, CD11c⁺), with variable expression of the monoclonal sIg depending on the degree of differentiation towards the plasma cell stage. Increasing plasmacytic differentiation is accompanied by decreased sIg intensity, monoclonal cytoplasmic light chain expression, down-regulated CD45 and pan-B cell antigens, and increased CD38 intensity. These features can also occur in high-grade B-cell lymphoma, especially those with a plasmacytoid appearance, and in some cases of multiple myeloma (see Section 29.1). Including CD56 in the panel helps in differentiating LPC lymphoma-leukemia from plasma cell dyscrasias.

If extremely bright sIg is encountered in a lymphoplasmacytoid disorder with high serum levels of M protein, coating of neoplastic cells by cytophilic monoclonal immunoglobulin should be suspected.

A substantial number of LPC lymphoma-leukemias can display a phenotype similar to that of MCL, i.e. CD5⁺, CD23⁻ and bright sIg. Furthermore, cyclin D1 expression and t(11;14) occur in some cases of LPC lymphoma-leukemia. Occasionally, LPC lymphoma-leukemia can also be CD5⁺, CD23⁺. In such cases, the monoclonal sIg is bright, distinguishing them from CLL.

LPC lymphoma-leukemia, CLL, CLL/PL, B-PLL, and intermediate/high-grade NHL can all be positive for CD11c (Figure 27.8). The expression of CD11c in these disorders does not have the characteristic intense fluorescence seen in HCL, however. Similar to CLL, LPC lymphoma-leukemia may express CD14. Rarely, weak CD25 may be present. The unusual case of LPC expressing CD11c and

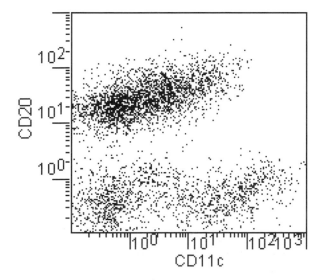

Figure 27.8 Coexpression of CD20 and CD11c (weak) in a case of lymphoplasmacytoid lymphoma-leukemia. The pattern of the tumor cell cluster on the CD20/CD11c dot plot is different from that in hairy cell leukemia

CD25 can be distinguished from HCL based on the pattern of the CD20/CD11c dot plot.

27.5.5.2 Confusion between lymphoplasmacytoid disorders and other diseases

In addition to the variability in the phenotype, morphologic artifacts from specimen processing may lead to overcalling or undercalling of plasmacytoid lymphocytes (see Sections 1.3 and 8.2). In the peripheral blood and bone marrow, because of artifacts associated with poor drying of smears, many cases of LPC lymphoma-leukemia are diagnosed as other entities, such as marginal zone lymphoma or hairy cell leukemia variant. In the authors' experience, there is a tendency to overcall LPC lymphoma-leukemia on lymph node tissue sections (especially in Europe); many are actually SLL with proliferation centers.

These problems can be alleviated if immunophenotyping on suspected LPC lymphoma-leukemia cases includes cytoplasmic light chain analysis, and immuno-electrophoresis (to document a monoclonal IgM or IgA band) is included in the diagnostic work-up and follow-up.

The phenotypic profile of so-called 'splenic lymphoma with villous lymphocytes' (SLVL) is no different from that of LPC lymphoma-leukemia. In the FAB classification, this disorder is grouped under the 'lymphoplasmacytic' category and arbitrarily separated from Waldenstrom's macroglobulinemia when the M-protein level is less than 20 g/l. The M-protein level does not necessarily remain static during the clinical course of the disease, however, especially if the patient is untreated. Aside from the villous/hairy projections (which can easily be induced by suboptimal film preparation), there are no definite features which distinguish SLVL from LPC lymphoma-leukemia.

27.6 Follicular center cell (FCC) lymphoma

Professor Fidelio
Cases 38 and 39

The majority of FCC lymphomas are composed predominantly of small neoplastic cells. The diagnosis can be straightforward by FCM when the following characteristics are present: CD10$^+$, monoclonal sIg, strong CD20, absent/dim CD71 and low S-phase (Figure 27.9). CD10 expression is present in 75–80% of the cases (presumably these correspond morphologically to cases with a high number of small neoplastic cells). The relative proportion of small and large cells varies from case to case. Therefore, the cell size of the malignant population as determined by FSC can be small, variable, bimodal, or, in rare cases, even large. An increased proportion of large cells may be associated with aneuploid DNA content and increased proliferative activity.

A small number of FCC lymphomas lack demonstrable light chains. Detection of bright bcl-2 expression in such cases is helpful to confirm the diagnosis and distinguish these cases from the rare cases of marked FRFH in which light chains are not detectable. Bcl-2 can also be performed by immunohistochemistry on fixed tissue.

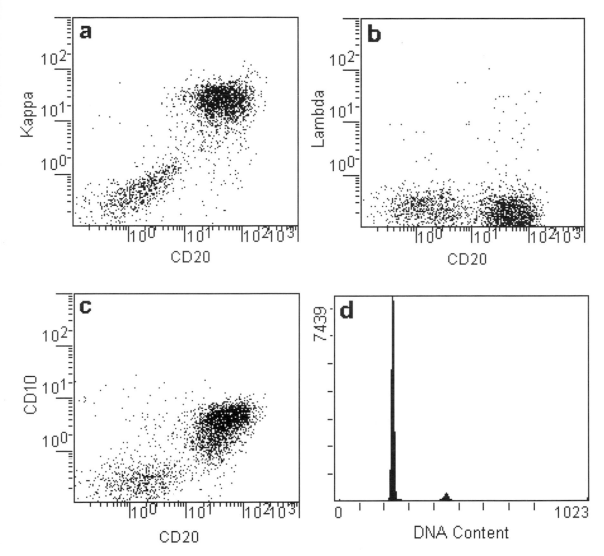

Figure 27.9 FCC lymphoma. (a)–(c) The tumor cells coexpress CD10, bright CD20 and bright monoclonal kappa. (d) The tumor is diploid with a low S-phase fraction

27.7 Hairy cell leukemia (HCL)

Hairy cell leukemia is a well-defined clinicopathological entity characterized by male preponderance, splenomegaly, peripheral blood cytopenias, and a low number of circulating neoplastic cells (circulating hairy cells are more easily detected if the patient has undergone splenectomy). The bone marrow usually yields a 'dry tap'. Hairy cell leukemia responds well to several therapeutic agents (α-interferon, $2'$-deoxycoformycin and 2-chlorodeoxyadenosine). Diffuse TRAP reactivity is a characteristic of hairy cells (see Section 5.4). HCL demonstrates the following specific FCM markers:

- High FSC. The small number of circulating hairy cells in the peripheral blood are easily missed if the FCM analysis is restricted to cells with the light scatter characteristics of lymphocytes (these are normal T cells in the sample).
- Intense expression of CD11c, along with CD25 positivity. The pattern of the CD20/CD11c dot plot is virtually pathognomonic for HCL (Figure 27.10).
- Positive CD103 (Figure 27.11). The particular clone of CD103 is important. Bly-7 has a high degree of specificity for HCL. Other clones of CD103 may be less specific (positive in other types of benign or neoplastic lymphoid cells). Even Bly-7 can be positive in a small number of lymphoplasmacytoid disorders, however.

Professor Fidelio
Case 40

> CD25 is an activation marker present on activated T cells, activated B cells, monocytes and macrophages. It can be expressed in NHL and LPD other than HCL, with or without CD11c. When the FCM results are reported as 'CD19/CD20$^+$, CD11c$^+$, CD25$^+$, CD5$^-$, CD10$^-$', the information is inadequate to distinguish HCL from other NHL/LPD unless the fluorescence intensity of CD11c is specified.

CD2 expression may be found on some hairy cells. This 'aberrancy' is not an indication of T-cell lineage, however.

The entity known as HCL variant (HCL-v) is described as having the following characteristics:

- High WBC count (in the range of that seen in PLL).
- Neoplastic cells with prominent nucleoli (similar to those seen in PLL) and a higher nuclear/cytoplasmic ratio than hairy cells.
- 'Hairy' cytoplasmic projections (which can easily result from slow drying of the blood film).

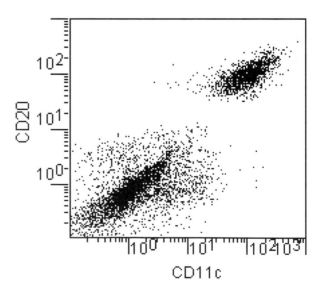

Figure 27.10 Hairy cell leukemia, with the characteristic coexpression of bright CD20 and bright CD11c

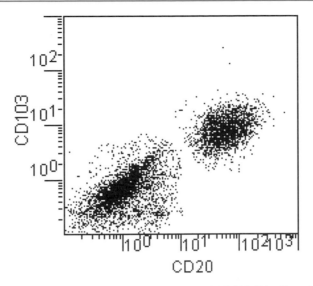

Figure 27.11   Hairy cell leukemia: coexpression of CD103 (Bly-7) and bright CD20

- The TRAP stain results on HCL-v cases are described as either negative or focally positive. Because a true-positive TRAP reaction is defined specifically as diffuse staining, focal or weak staining is actually a negative result.
- An easily aspiratable marrow.
- A poor clinical response to the current therapeutic agents for HCL.

The FCM profile in HCL-v does not have the characteristic features of HCL described above. Although CD103 expression has been reported in some cases of HCL-v, the FCM results in HCL-v are typically that of a nondescript monoclonal B-cell neoplasm. In our opinion, the overall clinicopathological picture of this disorder is too dissimilar from HCL to justify the designation HCL-v. Most of the features described for this entity are actually reminiscent of B-PLL (Figure 5.20), itself characterized by a high WBC count, neoplastic cells with prominent nucleoli, a higher nuclear/cytoplasmic ratio than hairy cells, and a relatively 'nonspecific' immunophenotype. The authors have also reviewed cases of LPC lymphoma/leukemia, which subsequently revealed a small IgM monoclonal band and peripheral lymphadenopathy, originally misinterpreted as HCL-v because of the 'hairy' cytology.

27.8 'Nondescript' monoclonal B-cell profiles

The immunophenotypic profiles in many high-grade and some low-grade NHLs may not display specific features, even when a large number of antibodies are included in the FCM panel.

Examples of 'nondescript' monoclonal B-cell profiles are:

1. CD5⁻, CD10⁻, CD23⁻, CD25⁻, CD103⁻, moderate to strong pan-B-cell markers and monoclonal surface light chain, no cytoplasmic light chain, low S-phase. Such data exclude CLL, MCL and HCL. This nondiagnostic

profile can be seen in multiple disorders such as lymphoplasmacytoid malignancies, B-PLL, monocytoid B-cell lymphoma and some cases of CD10⁻ FCC lymphoma.

2. CD5⁻, CD10⁺, CD23⁻, moderate to strong pan-B-cell markers and sIg, high S-phase (Figure 27.12). This phenotype can be seen in large cell lymphoma and Burkitt's lymphoma. Characteristically, the S-phase fraction in Burkitt's lymphoma (usually in the range of 30–50%) is higher than that seen in DLCL.

Burkitt's lymphoma, when found in the bone marrow and/or peripheral blood, is also known as ALL-L3. While the disease is 'acute' because of its aggressive biology, the neoplastic cells are not blasts (i.e. not immature cells) phenotypically. Because of the relatively distinctive morphology on air-dried Romanovsky-

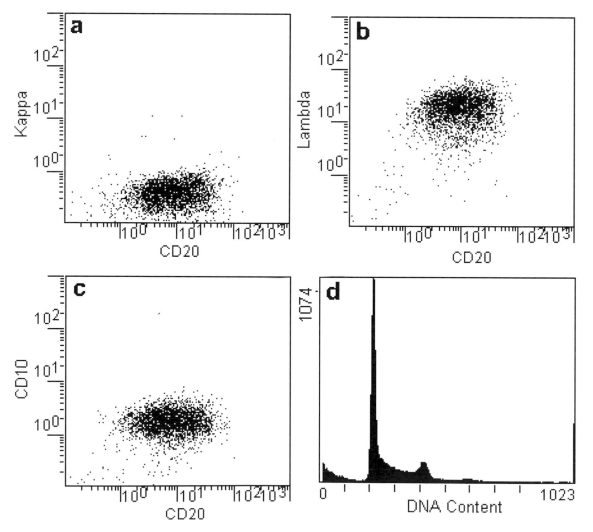

Figure 27.12 Burkitt's lymphoma. (a)–(c) The tumor cells coexpress CD10, moderate CD20 and bright monoclonal lambda. (d) The S-phase fraction is very high

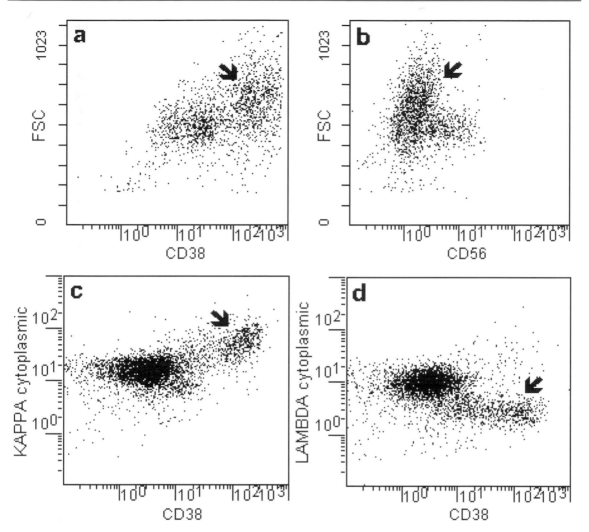

Figure 27.13   Large B-cell lymphoma with plasmacytoid differentiation (arrow). (a)–(d) The tumor cells coexpress very bright CD38, weak CD56 and cytoplasmic kappa

stained preparations, which correlates highly with the phenotype, the term 'acute lymphoblastic' has remained acceptable for this aggressive, mature B-cell malignancy. Virtually all cases of Burkitt's lymphoma-leukemia demonstrate rearrangement of the c-*myc* oncogene. Very high S-phase values are also observed in the HIV-related aggressive NHLs, most of which have either a Burkitt's or immunoblastic/plasmacytoid morphology.

High-grade B-cell NHLs, especially those with plasmacytoid differentiation, can lack one or more pan-B-cell antigens and CD45. Surface light chains may also be nondetectable despite the presence of surface heavy chains. Other common characteristics include very bright CD38, expression of CD56, and the presence of the monoclonal cytoplasmic light chain (Figure 27.13). Rare cases may lack both surface and cytoplasmic light chains.

Mature T-cell pattern

A cell population meets the definition of the mature T-cell pattern if there is expression of the T-cell lineage-associated markers (CD2, CD3, CD5 and CD7) and no evidence of immaturity. The most definite indicator of maturity is the lack of both TdT and CD34. Alternatively, a T-cell proliferation can be presumed to be mature on the basis of helper/suppressor restriction (either $CD4^+$/ $CD8^-$ or $CD4^-$/$CD8^+$) since such restriction is present in the great majority of peripheral T-cell lymphomas. Note that neoplastic immature T cells can have CD4/CD8 restriction (see Section 26.3), however.

Expression of surface CD3 is specific for mature T cells. CD3 is part of the TCR complex involved in the recognition of antigenic determinants. The CD3/ TCR complex is composed of five CD3 chains ($\gamma, \delta, \varepsilon, \eta$ and ζ), associated with either the $\alpha\beta$ or $\gamma\delta$ heterodimer of the T-cell receptor. Most monoclonal antibodies directed against CD3 recognize a conformational epitope of the ε chain which results from the association of the ε chain with either the δ or γ chain. The paraffin-resistant polyclonal anti-CD3 antibodies may have lower sensitivity and specificity, and some may stain myeloid precursors.

Determinants equivalent to surface light chains in mature B cells are not known to exist in T cells. Therefore, it is not always possible to establish the malignant nature of a T-cell proliferation based solely on immunophenotyping data. Neither the CD4/CD8 ratio nor the TCRαβ/TCRγδ ratio can be used to determine clonality. A lack of one or more surface pan-T-cell markers is highly suggestive of malignancy and is seen in a significant number of mature T-cell malignancies. Caution should be exercised, however, if such a profile is seen in young children, since lack of a surface pan-T-cell antigen (especially CD3) is a feature of certain congenital immune deficiencies (e.g. severe combined immunodeficiency).

28.1 Mature T-cell subpopulations and natural killer cells

Benign mature lymphoid cells are divided into three broad categories: B cell, T cell and natural killer (NK) cells. Normal T cells, identified by positive surface CD3, are further categorized based on the expression of one of the two mutually exclusive associated TCR proteins, either TCRαβ or TCRγδ.

28.1.1 Mature T-cell subpopulations

The great majority of $TCR\alpha\beta^+$ T cells can be further subdivided as follows:

1. CD3$^+$, CD4$^+$ cells account for approximately 55–65% of peripheral blood T cells, and encompass several functional subgroups: (a) T-helper cells which induce B-cell proliferation; (b) cells responsible for the activation of suppressor cells (T-inducer/suppressor cells); and (c) a minor subgroup of CD4$^+$ cytotoxic and CD4$^+$ suppressor cells.
2. CD3$^+$, CD8$^+$ cells account for approximately 20–35% of peripheral blood T cells. CD8$^+$ cells are composed of cytotoxic and suppressor cells. The cytotoxic activity of CD3$^+$, CD8$^+$ and CD3$^+$, CD4$^+$ T cells are specific for major histocompatibility (MHC) class II and class I antigens, respectively. A subset of CD8$^+$ cells expresses one or more NK-associated antigens, mainly CD16 and CD57. The proportion of CD8$^+$ cells increases in altered immune conditions, including HIV and other viral infections (Figure 28.1).
3. Populations of CD4$^+$/CD8$^+$ and CD4$^-$/CD8$^-$ cells are present in extremely low proportions (1–2%). A relative increase of double-positive CD4/CD8 cells (usually in the range of 10–20%) can be seen after chemotherapy.

About 4% of T cells are TCRγδ$^+$. Most are CD4$^-$, CD8$^-$. Small subsets of TCRγδ$^+$ cells can express weak CD8 and/or CD56, however.

Overall only a small fraction (< 5%) of T cells express NK-associated antigens, most of which are TCRαβ$^+$. Similar to NK cells, these NK-like T cells are capable of non-MHC restricted cytotoxicity and are preferentially distributed in extranodal sites, e.g. spleen, gastrointestinal tract and skin.

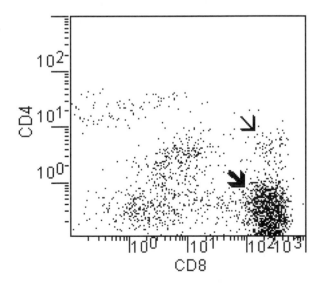

Figure 28.1 Increased number of CD8$^+$ cells (thick arrow) in a case of infectious mononucleosis. Note a small population of CD4$^+$, CD8$^+$ cells (thin arrow)

28.1.2 Natural killer cells

Approximately 10–15% of peripheral blood lymphocytes are NK cells, although the number and activity of NK cells can vary widely among individuals. Because NK-associated antigens can be present on T cells, the current definition of true NK cells requires the absence of CD3, TCRαβ and TCRγδ. In addition, the *TCR* genes must be in germ-line configuration.

Current data suggest that NK cells are derived from bone marrow precursors and that their maturation/differentiation is thymic-independent. The majority of NK cells have the morphology of LGLs. However, NK cells can appear as nondescript, small, round lymphocytes and not all LGLs are NK cells. The LGL morphology encompasses both NK-like T cells and true NK cells.

NK-associated antigens include CD56, CD57 and CD16. None of these antigens are limited to NK cells, however. Most normal NK cells are CD16$^+$, CD56$^+$. Since anti-CD16 monoclonal antibodies differ in epitope specificities, CD16 expression on NK cells may not be detectable with a given reagent. T-cell markers present on true NK cells include CD2, CD7, and CD8; the last at a weaker intensity than that on T cells. CD4$^+$ NK cells are extremely rare. NK cells mostly express the homodimers CD8α/CD8α instead of the heterodimers CD8α/CD8β found on CD8$^+$ T cells. NK cells contain truncated CD3ε mRNA. Paraffin-resistant polyclonal CD3 antibodies can recognize the resulting isolated CD3ε chains in the cytoplasm. Therefore, positive CD3 staining on paraffin sections cannot distinguish T cells (surface CD3$^+$) from NK cells (surface CD3$^-$).

28.2 Recommended diagnostic work-up for mature T-cell and NK-cell malignancies

Mature non-B-cell neoplasms replicate more or less the phenotypes of their benign T-cell and NK-cell counterparts. Neoplastic transformation, however, is often accompanied by down-regulation or loss of one or more pan-T-cell markers and/or TCR determinant(s). This fact, along with the overlapping antigenic features of T cells and NK cells, complicates the task of assigning the correct lineage (NK cell vs. NK-like T cell) to these neoplasms. The difficulties are further compounded if only a limited marker panel is employed. Potential problems can be avoided if the diagnostic work-up for mature non-B lymphoid proliferations routinely includes:

- A large immunophenotyping panel composed of all surface T-cell markers including TCRαβ, TCRγδ, and the NK-associated markers CD16, CD56, CD57.
- Molecular analyses of *TCR*β, δ and γ genes. This is most important to distinguish true NK malignancies from the few cases of NK-like T-cell neoplasms in which CD3 and TCR determinants are not expressed despite the presence of rearranged *TCR* gene(s).

- Cytogenetics. The presence of karyotypic abnormalities may be of prognostic significance and helps to resolve the dilemma of benign vs. malignant in difficult cases.
- Detection of known oncogenic viruses (e.g. EBV, HTLV-I).
- Cytologic assessment of Romanovsky-stained air-dried preparations, in addition to routine H&E sections.

28.3 Diagnostic T-cell profiles

Immunophenotyping and cell kinetic analysis can be essentially diagnostic in some T-cell malignancies. Table 28.1 lists the key immunophenotypic features of ATLL, NK-cell and NK-like T-cell neoplasms.

Table 28.1 Key features in T-cell neoplasms with diagnostic immunophenotypes

Key features in the immunophenotypic profile	Diagnosis
$CD4^+$, $CD8^-$, $CD25^+$ and lack of a pan-T marker	ATLL
$CD2^+$, $CD3^-$, $CD7^+$, $CD4^-$, $CD8^{-/weak}$, $CD16^+$ and $CD56^+$	NK-cell malignancies
$CD3^+$, $CD8^+$ and $CD57^+$	$CD3^+$ LGL leukemia

28.4 Large granular lymphocyte (LGL) disorders

Disorders which share the expression of T cell and NK-associated antigens and an LGL morphology fall into two broad categories: NK-like T-cell ($CD3^+$ LGL) and NK-cell ($CD3^-$ LGL) proliferations. The process can be either reactive or neoplastic.

Morphologically, there is an increased number of circulating LGLs, identifiable on blood films by the presence of azurophilic granules (see Section 8.2.3). NK-cell disorders exist in which the cells do not have the morphology of LGLs, but appear as normal 'resting' lymphocytes.

The proliferation is considered malignant if there is evidence of involvement of bone marrow, spleen or liver. Aneuploidy or cytogenetic abnormalities, if present, are further supportive evidence of malignancy. Lymph node infiltration and skin involvement are unusual. In the case of $CD3^+$ LGL disorders, the presence of clonal T-cell receptor rearrangement (either the *TCRβ* gene or the *TCRγ* gene) confirms a putative neoplastic proliferation. Clonality alone is not sufficient to establish malignancy, however, since clonal populations have been detected in patients with autoimmune processes or following bone marrow transplantation. Conversely, the absence of rearrangement does not necessarily exclude a clonal process since technical artifacts or the use of inappropriate *TCR* gene probes may interfere with the detection of rearrangements. *TCR* rearrangement studies in $CD3^-$ LGL proliferations are noncontributory, since NK cells, whether normal or malignant, do not rearrange *TCRα, β, γ*, or *δ* genes. Clonality studies of $CD3^-$ LGL can be performed, however, on female patients who are heterozygous for certain X-linked loci.

The neoplastic group is further subdivided into indolent/chronic and aggressive disease.

28.4.1 Indolent LGL leukemia

**Professor Fidelio
Case 42**

There is a high association between CD3$^+$ LGL proliferations and autoimmune disorders (especially rheumatoid arthritis). Serologic abnormalities in such patients include rheumatoid factor, antinuclear antibody, anti-neutrophil and/or anti-platelet antibodies, and polyclonal hypergammaglobulinemia. The patients are frequently neutropenic with mild to moderate splenomegaly.

Most cases have an NK-like T-cell phenotype of CD3$^+$, CD4$^-$, CD8$^+$, CD16$^+$, CD56$^-$, CD57$^+$, TCR$\alpha\beta^+$ (Figure 28.2). Cases that are either CD4$^+$/CD8$^-$ or CD4$^+$/CD8$^+$ are rare. Because of differences in the sensitivity and specificity of anti-CD16 monoclonal antibodies, there may be variability in the detection of CD16 expression. A very small number of cases can be CD4$^-$, CD8$^+$, TCR$\gamma\delta^+$ or CD4$^-$, CD8$^-$, TCR$\gamma\delta^+$. A mild to moderate absolute lymphocytosis ($>4 \times 10^9$/l) is present in about 75% of cases. Even in those cases without overt lymphocytosis, the proportion of neutrophils to lymphocytes in the blood is reversed and the absolute number of LGLs (normally $<0.4 \times 10^9$/l) is markedly increased. The neoplastic cells are morphologically similar to benign LGLs, with parallel tubular arrays present ultrastructurally.

The peripheral blood diagnostic criteria are presented in Section 8.2.3.

28.4.2 Aggressive LGL malignancies

Aggressive LGL malignancies are uncommon and include NK and NK-like T-cell lymphoma-leukemias. In contrast to the CD16$^+$, CD57$^+$ phenotype in

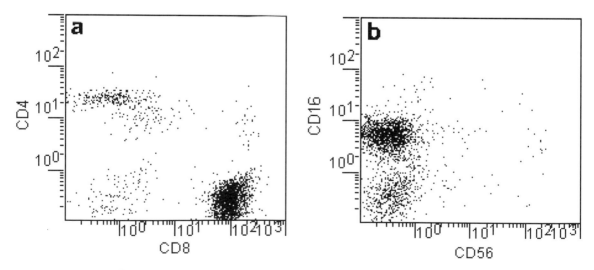

Figure 28.2 CD3$^+$ indolent LGL leukemia. (a)–(b) The tumor cells coexpress CD8, CD16 and CD57 (not shown). CD56 is not expressed

indolent LGL leukemia, the aggressive forms are invariably CD56$^+$, with or without CD16. CD57 expression is infrequent. There is no association with rheumatoid arthritis.

Aggressive NK and NK-like T-cell lymphoma-leukemias exhibit diverse clinical and histological manifestations. The literature on this subject is confusing since a comprehensive characterization has not been applied to all cases, and often the disorder is named after the site of its manifestation. Both groups of disorders are common in young males. Both the NK and NK-like categories share similar sites of extranodal involvement (predominantly liver/spleen, small bowel, bone marrow, peripheral blood and skin), which reflect the fact that both cell types are preferentially distributed in extranodal sites. Infiltration of skin and subcutaneous soft tissue can result in a panniculitis-like picture.

In addition to the above clinical manifestations, the aggressive NK-cell disorders that affect patients native to the Far East and Central/South America have a predilection for the nasal/nasopharyngeal region. These tumors have been previously described as lethal midline granuloma and angiocentric lymphoma. Irrespective of the site of involvement (nasopharyngeal or other extranodal site), the aggressive NK lymphomas in these ethnic groups have a strong association with EBV. Similarly, the leukemic counterparts (known as CD3$^-$ LGL leukemia) in these geographical areas are also EBV-positive. The usual phenotype of NK-cell lymphoma-leukemia is CD3$^-$, CD4$^-$, CD8$^-$, CD16$^+$, CD56$^+$ and CD57$^-$.

The phenotypic subgroups of aggresive NK-like T-cell lymphoma-leukemia reflect those of their benign counterparts. Many are TCRαβ$^+$, CD4$^-$ and CD8$^+$. A substantial number of cases are CD4$^-$, CD8$^-$ and TCRγδ$^+$, a disease known as γδ T-cell lymphoma (Figure 28.3). Most of these have been referred to as hepatosplenic lymphoma. However, γδ T-cell lymphoma can also occur at cutaneous and mucosal sites. NK-like T-cell malignancies can also occur as a

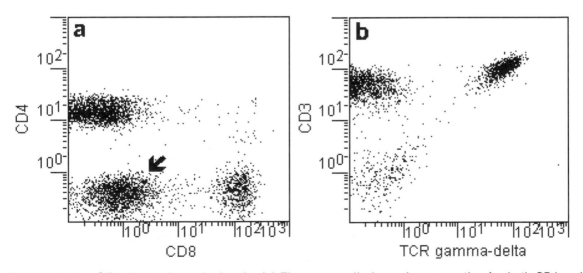

Figure 28.3 γδ T-cell lymphoma-leukemia. (a) The tumor cells (arrow) are negative for both CD4 and CD8. There are residual benign T-helper and suppressor cells. (b) The neoplastic cells coexpress CD3 and TCRγδ

late complication (average latency, 15 years) of solid organ transplantation, and may or may not contain EBV.

Occasional NK-like T-cell lymphoma-leukemias may exhibit loss of T-cell antigen(s) and TCR determinants (presumably from nonproductive rearrangements or post-translational defects of the *TCR* genes), resulting in a phenotype indistinguishable from that of NK malignancies, i.e. CD3$^-$, CD5$^-$, TCR$\alpha\beta^-$, TCR$\gamma\delta^-$, CD2$^+$, CD7$^+$, CD56$^+$ and CD4$^-$/CD8$^+$ or CD4$^-$/CD8$^-$. Lineage determination in such instances requires molecular analyses of the *TCR* genes.

Establishment of NK vs. NK-like T-cell lineage is best done by FCM immunophenotyping. Paraffin immunostaining is less helpful.

It is important to note that the presence of NK markers, especially CD56, does not imply NK differentiation. In addition to its common expression in myeloma, CD56 can also occur in AML and ALL.

28.4.3 Reactive large granular lymphocytes

A transient or chronic increase in the number of cells expressing NK-associated antigens (with or without the morphology of LGLs) can occur in viral infections (e.g. CMV, HIV) and in association with various hematopoietic malignancies, autoimmune diseases and aging. In IM, there are increased numbers of CD8$^+$ cells, but these are not CD57$^+$. The distinction between persistent reactive CD3$^+$ LGLs and neoplastic CD3$^+$ LGLs may necessitate *TCR* rearrangement studies, especially if there is no evidence of an absolute lymphocytosis.

Cases with a presumably reactive CD3$^-$ LGL proliferation have been described. The benign nature of the process can usually only be inferred from its indolent clinical course (in contrast to the acute presentation of CD3$^-$ LGL leukemia). In female patients, the lack of clonality (based on studies of X-linked genes) would support the non-neoplastic nature of the proliferation.

28.5 Adult T-cell leukemia-lymphoma (ATLL)

Professor Fidelio
Case 43

The diagnosis of ATLL can be suspected immunologically when the immunophenotype is that of an aberrant, mature T-helper cell with distinct expression of CD25. The usual phenotypic profile is CD2$^+$, CD3$^+$, CD4$^+$, CD7$^-$, CD8$^-$, CD25$^+$ (Figure 28.4). Expression of CD5 is variable. The phenotypes CD4$^+$/CD8$^+$, CD4$^-$/CD8$^-$, or CD4$^-$/CD8$^+$ are rarely encountered. Although some cases of peripheral T-cell lymphoma and Sezary syndrome may express CD25, the intensity is weaker than that in ATLL.

Most of the post-thymic T-cell malignancies with a helper phenotype demonstrate helper function *in vitro* when studied in a pokeweed mitogen-stimulated B-cell system. The helper phenotype of ATLL cells is not associated with helper function, however. The neoplastic cells act as suppressor cells in mitogen-induced B-cell differentiation and immunoglobulin synthesis.

The lymph node picture of ATLL can mimic other post-thymic T-cell malignancies morphologically. Various histologic subtypes have been described that bear no correlation to the prognosis. In the peripheral blood, ATLL cells (also

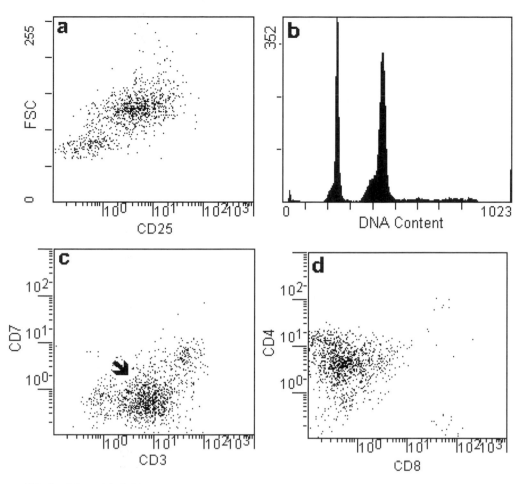

Figure 28.4   ATLL. (a)–(d) The tumor cells are medium-sized and demonstrate an aberrant T-cell phenotype: CD3$^+$, CD7$^-$, CD4$^+$. CD25 is distinctly positive. The tumor is hyperdiploid with a high S-phase fraction

referred to as 'flower' cells) exhibit marked cytologic variation from cell to cell. Confirmation of the patient's HTLV-I status is important to distinguish ATLL from T-PLL and Sezary syndrome (see Section 5.9).

28.6 Aberrant T cells (without NK antigens or distinct CD25 expression)

Large studies have shown that many peripheral T-cell lymphomas (PTCL) demonstrate immunophenotypes different from those seen on normal mature T cells. The incidence of aberrant phenotypes depends on the number of antibodies included in the panel, their respective specificities and sensitivities, and the definition of what constitutes an aberrant phenotype. It is uniformly accepted that the loss of at least one surface pan-T antigen signifies 'aberrancy'.

In general, the observed abnormalities (in decreasing order of frequency) are loss or down-regulation of CD7, CD5, CD2, and CD3 (Figure 28.5). Such aberrancy is highly suggestive of malignancy, except in the pediatric age group where certain immunodeficiencies may result in the loss of a pan-T-cell antigen.

Aberrant phenotypes are seen in approximately 50–70% of post-thymic T-cell malignancies. Most cases are CD4$^+$/CD8$^-$, with variable expression of the activation markers HLA-DR, CD38, CD30 and CD71. CD25 may be present. If CD25 expression is distinct, however, then ATLL needs to be excluded.

There is no correlation between the aberrant mature T-cell phenotypes and the multiple histologic subtypes of PTCL. The number of morphologic subtypes of PTCL and their nomenclature vary with the subclassification scheme in use. It has not been proven that the morphologic subclassification of PTCL is of any therapeutic or prognostic significance.

The following antigenic combinations can also be considered as aberrant, even without the loss of a pan-T marker:

1. Mature cells with loss of both CD4 and CD8 antigens. Such a proliferation is very likely to be abnormal since the number of mature CD3$^+$, CD4$^-$, CD8$^-$ ($\gamma\delta$ T cells) cells is extremely low in normal peripheral blood and reactive lymphoid organs. Clinical correlation is necessary to exclude hepatosplenic $\gamma\delta$ T-cell lymphoma. If the proliferation is CD3$^-$, CD4$^-$, CD8$^-$, then an NK-cell malignancy needs to be considered.

2. Mature cells with coexpression of CD4 and CD8. Under normal reactive conditions, the number of CD4$^+$/CD8$^+$ mature T cells is very low. As mentioned above, a mild relative increase in CD4$^+$/CD8$^+$ cells may occur in reactive conditions.

3. Expression of CD1. CD1 is considered a thymic antigen, normally expressed in stage II thymocytes. Many precursor-T ALLs/lymphoblastic

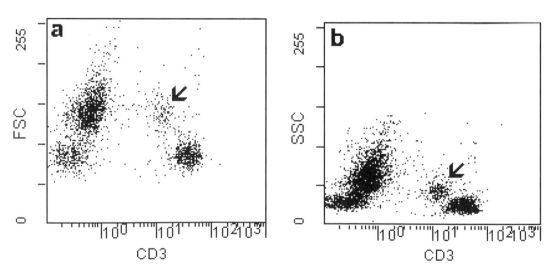

Figure 28.5 (a)–(b) Peripheral blood with 3% circulating malignant T cells. The neoplastic cells are medium-sized with down-regulated CD3

lymphomas exhibit the phenotype of stage II thymocytes, (i.e. TdT$^+$, CD1$^+$, CD2$^+$, CD3$^-$, CD4$^+$, CD7$^+$, CD8$^+$). Expression of CD1 does occur in mature T-cell neoplasms, albeit infrequently. For this reason, CD1 expression cannot be relied upon as proof of immaturity. Morphologically, CD1$^+$ mature T-cell malignancies do not resemble T-ALL/lymphoblastic lymphoma (Figure 28.6).

4. Increased expression of a pan-T-cell marker, usually CD5 (Figure 28.7). Neoplastic T cells with up-regulated CD5 can be separated from coexisting

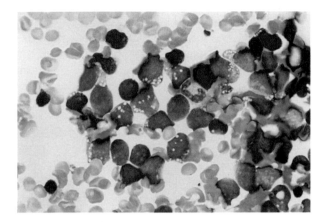

Figure 28.6 CD1$^+$ peripheral T-cell lymphoma (TdT$^-$, CD34$^-$, CD1$^+$, CD2$^+$, CD3$^+$, CD4$^+$, CD5$^+$, CD7$^-$, CD8$^-$), showing large lymphoma cells with abundant sharp cytoplasmic vacuoles. The morphology simulates that of Burkitt's lymphoma

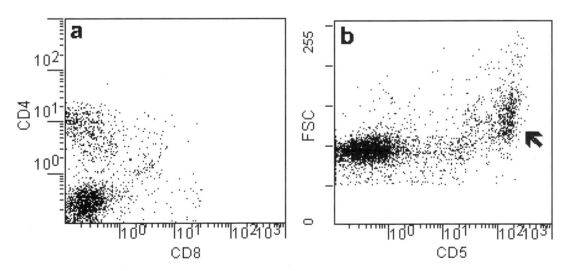

Figure 28.7 Peripheral T-cell lymphoma. (a)–(b) the tumor cells are positive for CD4 and CD5. The intensity of CD5 on the neoplastic cells (arrow) is stronger than that on the benign T cells

Professor Fidelio
Cases 44–46

benign/reactive T cells since normal T cells display a moderate intensity of CD5. The analysis of other T-cell determinants (e.g. CD4) can be 'gated' on the up-regulated CD5 population to further characterize the malignant cells.

28.7 Normal mature T-cell pattern

Professor Fidelio
Case 47

The distinction between a reactive and a malignant process cannot be made immunologically when the FCM data fit a normal T-cell phenotype. The intensity of one of the pan-T markers may be slightly down-regulated (i.e. less intense than that on normal T cells) in post-thymic T-cell malignancies (T-PLL, MF/Sezary syndrome) but this may also occur in other conditions including the reactive background of Hodgkin's disease or the so-called T-cell rich B-cell lymphomas. In the latter condition, the correct interpretation can be made if a multiparameter FCM analysis is performed to identify the small number of malignant B cells. The presence of activation markers (e.g. HLA-DR, CD38 and CD30) cannot be relied upon to distinguish a benign from a malignant process. Although the prevailing tendency in such situations is to leave morphology as the final arbitrator of a diagnosis of malignant lymphoma, care should be taken since certain reactive lymphadenopathies (e.g. IM) can closely simulate malignant lymphoma morphologically. Unless the clinicopathological picture is characteristic for the disorder (e.g. T-PLL), it is judicious to perform molecular genetics (rearrangement of *TCR* gene) using appropriate probes to confirm the diagnosis of malignancy.

Disorders presenting with a normal mature T-cell phenotype, no loss of T-cell associated markers and no evidence of increased expression of any T-cell antigens include T-PLL and MF/Sezary syndrome (early stage). Careful FCM data analysis invariably reveals an overwhelming excess of CD4$^+$ lymphoid cells, with a resulting CD4/CD8 ratio of greater than 10:1. The intensity of CD4 expression on the malignant cells is identical to that of normal helper T cells (Figure 28.8).

Professor Fidelio
Case 48

Correlation with the clinical manifestations and peripheral blood findings is necessary to establish the diagnosis of Sezary syndrome (see Section 5.10) and T-PLL (see Section 5.5.1). CD25 may be weakly expressed. A small number of T-PLL cases are CD4$^+$/CD8$^+$ or CD4$^-$/CD8$^+$. If the NK-associated markers were not initially included in the FCM panel, the subset of CD4$^-$/CD8$^+$ T-PLL needs to be differentiated from CD3$^+$ LGL with agranular lymphocytes.

If the FCM results fit a mature T-suppressor phenotype, a proliferation of CD3$^+$ LGLs needs to be excluded by testing for NK-associated markers. As previously mentioned, the CD4/CD8 ratio cannot be relied upon as an indicator of malignancy. Similarly, when there is no clinical evidence of malignancy, it may be difficult to determine the malignant nature of a relative expansion of CD8$^+$, NK-antigen negative lymphoid cells, since this can occur with chemotherapy, immunodeficiencies and autoimmune disorders. Supportive evidence that a mature CD8$^+$, NK-antigen negative population is clonal includes aberrant antigenic expression (see Section 28.6) and/or *TCR*β rearrangement.

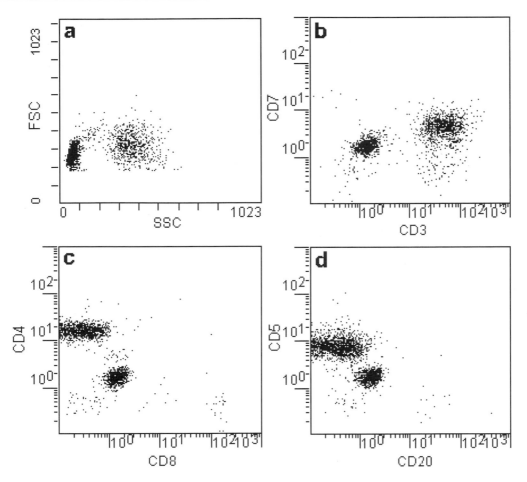

Figure 28.8 Circulating Sezary cells. (a) The cells of interest are in the size range of small lymphoid cells. (b)–(d) Gated on mononuclear cells: the cell cluster positive for CD3, CD7, CD4 and CD5 includes both benign and malignant T cells. The intensity of CD4 on the Sezary cells is identical to that of normal lymphocytes. The marked excess of CD4+ cells (c) is the only subtle clue to suggest a malignant process. There is a cluster of monocytes with slight nonspecific staining with all markers

Plasma cell
pattern

The *sine qua non* of plasma cell differentiation is the presence of cytoplasmic light chains and a concomitant absence of surface light chains. Cytoplasmic immunoglobulins have traditionally been demonstrated by microscopic methods (cytospin preparations and fixed tissue sections). Recently, FCM techniques have been developed for the detection of cytoplasmic antigens. The presence of both cytoplasmic kappa and lambda light chains (cKappa, cLambda) in a population of plasma cells (i.e. polyclonality) indicates a reactive process whereas monoclonal cIg is synonymous with a plasma cell dyscrasia. Note that analysis for cIg should be gated on cells with very bright CD38 (Figure 29.1).

In addition to the absence of surface light chains, the expression of surface pan-B-cell antigens and HLA-DR is attenuated to absent on plasma cells. CD45 may be the only marker expressed and, in many cases, it too may be lost. Therefore, unless testing for cKappa and cLambda are performed, FCM analysis on a plasma cell population may yield negative results (i.e. no pattern), similar to the findings in nonhematopoietic cells. On tissue sections, plasma cells are positive for epithelial membrane antigen (EMA). The combination $CD45^-$, EMA^+ is a feature shared by nonhematopoietic malignancies, plasma cell proliferations, and some high-grade lymphomas with plasmacytoid differentiation.

Plasma cells typically exhibit intense CD38 expression. Neoplastic plasma cells also frequently express CD56. The diagnosis of a plasma cell neoplasm rests on the demonstration of monoclonal cIg in a cell population with strong CD38, or morphologic evidence of plasma cell differentiation. CD10, weak CD14 or, less commonly, weak CD13 or CD33 can also be present. In instances where the malignant plasma cells lack intense CD38 (an infrequent occurrence), analysis for cIg can be gated on such aberrant myeloid markers. There is extreme heterogeneity in the expression of these determinants among plasma cell tumors.

In the majority of plasma cell tumors, the morphology is straightforward. In some cases, the neoplastic cells may be very immature-appearing or have bizarre cytology. This has led to a number of different designations for such tumors (e.g. immunoblastic lymphoma and anaplastic plasmacytoma), especially when they are found at extramedullary sites. It appears that cases with immature/bizarre morphology behave aggressively.

DNA content analysis may be of some benefit in plasma cell tumors. A high tumor S-phase fraction in multiple myeloma at the time of diagnosis is associated with a poorer prognosis.

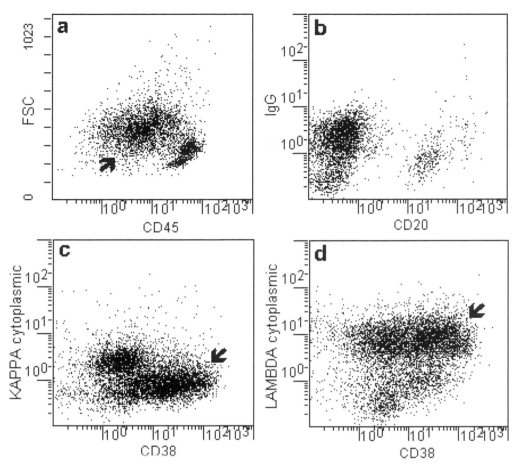

Figure 29.1 Multiple myeloma. (a) The tumor cells are medium-sized with down-regulated CD45. (b) CD20 is not expressed and there is weak surface IgG. (c), (d) The tumor cells coexpress bright CD38 and cytoplasmic lambda

29.1 Phenotypes encountered in plasma cell dyscrasias

The phenotypes encountered in plasma cell dyscrasias are:

Professor Fidelio
Cases 49 and 50

1. Monoclonal cIg, absent sIg, down-regulated or absent B-cell markers, CD56$^+$, and very bright CD38. This is the typical profile (i.e. 'plasma cell' pattern) seen in most cases of multiple myeloma and plasmacytoma.

2. Expression of both cytoplasmic and surface immunoglobulins of the same monoclonal light chain type. This results in a combination of the plasma cell pattern and the mature B-cell pattern. Note that in cases with high levels of serum monoclonal protein, nonspecific coating of the M protein on the surface of leukocytes can result in an artifactual monoclonal B-cell population. This artifact can be identified by paying attention to the lineage-associated antigens of the cells that appear to express monoclonal sIg. In monoclonal B-cell populations, a pan-B antigen is coexpressed. The

intensity of pan-B-cell markers is often weak when the plasma cell and mature-B patterns coexist.

The diagnostic possibilities include:

Professor Fidelio
Case 51

- Multiple myeloma, plasma cell leukemia, or extramedullary plasmacytoma. Cases with immature-appearing morphology tend to express both cIg and sIg. Testing for heavy chains is helpful to distinguish this group of disorders from lymphoplasmacytoid neoplasms. IgM is characteristic of lymphoplasmacytoid neoplasms, whereas IgG is typical of multiple myeloma and plasmacytoma. IgA can be found in either group, however.
- Lymphoplasmacytoid lymphoma-leukemia/Waldenstrom's macroglobulinemia (see Section 27.5.5).
- High-grade lymphoma with plasmacytoid differentiation (also referred to as immunoblastic lymphoma). The dividing line between immunoblastic lymphoma and anaplastic plasmacytoma is not always clear.

The final diagnosis rests upon the correlation of the FCM results with other clinical and laboratory findings, such as serum and urine protein electrophoresis, a skeletal survey and the morphologic findings in the bone marrow or extramedullary sites.

Nonspecific pattern

The FCM pattern is considered nonspecific when the data are insufficient to establish either the maturity of a B-cell or T-cell population, or the critical cells express only monocytic markers.

30.1 Nonspecific B cell or T cell (maturity undetermined)

Based on the FCM studies contributed to the authors from multiple institutions in several countries, an inability to establish the maturity of a lymphoid population occurs more frequently than expected. Below are common examples of FCM data inadequate for assessment of the maturity of the lymphoid cells.

**Professor Fidelio
Case 52**

1. Positive B-cell antigens, and:

   - immature markers (TdT and CD34) and surface light chains (sIg) not tested; **or**
   - immature markers not done and both sIg negative; **or**
   - one immature marker negative, one not done, and sIg not tested.
2. Positive T-lineage associated antigens, but TdT and CD34 not done (or CD34 negative and TdT not done). Often only CD2, CD5, and CD7 were studied (i.e. CD3, CD4, and CD8 were omitted from the analysis).

Based on the above data, it is only possible to conclude that the cell population is of B-cell or T-cell lineage. In such situations, morphologic features become, by default, the final arbitrator of maturity (i.e. blasts vs. lymphoma cells). When analyzing blood or bone marrow, it is preferable to avoid relying on morphology, particularly when the neoplastic cells are medium to large without specific features, or when the term 'blast' is used to designate any large nucleolated cell. In lymph nodes or spleen, histological features such as the pattern of involvement may offer morphologic clues to distinguish an immature from a mature lymphoid neoplasm.

As shown in the following examples, FCM data interpretation should take morphologic findings into account, unless there is gross discordance between the immunologic data and the morphologic information.

1. CD19$^+$, CD20$^+$, T-cell and myeloid markers negative, TdT, CD34 and sIg not done, and the cells of interest reported as 70% blasts. Based on this information, the only plausible interpretation is precursor-B ALL, if the morphologic information was correct.

2. Identical FCM data to that of the above example but blasts are not present. This implies a mature B-cell population of undetermined clonality.
3. CD19$^+$, CD20$^+$, T-cell and myeloid markers negative, both TdT and CD34 negative, sIg not performed, and the cells of interest reported as 50% blasts. In this example, the lack of both TdT and CD34 (assuming that the negative results were not technical artifacts) indicates that the cells of interest are not immature cells. This, however, conflicts with the morphologic report of 'blasts'. It is possible that the 'blasts' seen in this example correspond to Burkitt's cells (ALL-L3), in which case the morphologic information should be more specific and testing for light chains should be carried out. The conflicting immunologic and morphologic data preclude any conclusion about the maturity of the malignant cells. Without more information, the interpretation can only be 'nonspecific B cell, maturity undetermined'.

30.2 Monocytic markers only

On rare occasions, the FCM data demonstrate positive CD14 (along with HLA-DR), but no other B-cell, T-cell or myeloid surface antigens. Since CD14 is a relatively nonspecific marker (present not only on myeloid proliferations but also in CLL, related LPDs, and plasma cell dyscrasias), it cannot be relied upon for lineage determination. Hence, the FCM pattern is considered 'nonspecific (monocytic marker positive)'. In the context of appropriate morphologic information, a more specific interpretation can be provided, as shown in the following examples.

1. CD2$^-$, CD3$^-$, CD13$^-$, CD14$^+$ (moderate to strong), CD19$^-$, CD33$^-$, HLA-DR^{strong}, myeloperoxidase cytochemistry negative, other markers not tested, and the cells of interest reported as 70% blasts. These data are most suggestive of AML-M5. The diagnosis needs to be confirmed with an NSE stain (ANBE).
2. A phenotype similar to the one above, but also with strongly expressed CD56 and negative CD16. Such cases should not be interpreted as 'blastic natural killer cell tumors'. This phenotype is another unusual manifestation of AML-M5 (Figure 30.1). Again, the diagnosis can be confirmed by ANBE cytochemistry.

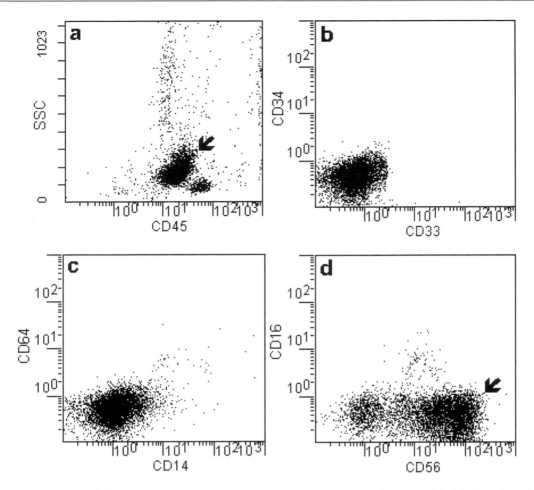

Figure 30.1 AML-M5. (a) Blast population (arrow) in the 'monocyte' region. (b)–(d) Gated on the blast population: the blasts are negative for CD34, CD33 and CD13 (not shown). The blasts express weak CD14 and strong CD56. The tumor cells also react strongly with ANBE (not shown)

Professor Fidelio
Case 53

Professor Fidelio
Case 54

In a small number of cases, FCM analysis may not yield any positive results, despite the application of an extensive panel to include immature markers, B-cell, T-cell and myeloid-associated antigens, surface and cytoplasmic immuno-globulins and several activation markers (e.g. CD38, CD30, CD71). The two most common scenarios include:

1. CD45$^-$, some activation markers present. The differential includes non-hematopoietic neoplasms that can be further characterized by immuno-stains on fixed tissue, and a small subgroup of LCLs, usually with plasmacytoid differentiation. Most of these should have monoclonal cIg, however.
2. CD45$^+$, variable expression of some activation markers. This is usually associated with large cell size and a high S-phase. The data indicate a high-grade NHL.

Either of the above scenarios can be seen in CD30$^+$ LCL. Because the activation marker CD30 is nonspecific, the category of CD30$^+$ lymphomas is hetero-geneous and poorly defined. Further testing with anti-ALK-1 (anaplastic large cell kinase), which identifies the protein encoded by the (2;5) translocation, is helpful to classify the tumor as anaplastic large cell lymphoma (see Section 40.7.2).

Bone
Marrow

Approach to the bone marrow

Bone marrow examination is an integral step in the diagnostic work-up and follow-up of patients with hematological malignancies, suspected metastatic disease and widespread systemic infections. For proper interpretation, sufficient bone marrow material should be obtained for all studies that may need to be performed. In addition, the quality of the sample dictates the conclusions that can be drawn from studying the marrow.

In hematopoietic malignancies, a bone marrow procedure is not just for morphologic evaluation. Representative fresh material is frequently needed for FCM immunophenotyping, cytogenetics and molecular studies. The bone marrow procedure causes some degree of anxiety and discomfort to the patient even in skillful hands. Therefore, to ensure that appropriate fresh material is collected and the procedure does not need to be repeated, it is important to think about the ancillary tests before obtaining the specimen.

The key element in the technique described below is to aspirate a large amount of marrow that is quickly anticoagulated and subsequently concentrated. Psychological coaching, in addition to a generous amount of local anesthetic to the periosteum, helps to allay the patient's anxiety and discomfort. In the rare patients allergic to local anesthetic agents, it is possible (in the authors' experience) to perform the bone marrow procedure based solely on good psychological coaching.

32.1 Equipment

A disposable bone marrow tray is convenient since it is sterile and provides sterile drapes, a scalpel and bone marrow needles. The following additional equipment is necessary, however:

- Sterile surgical gloves of the appropriate size.
- An additional bottle of local anesthetic. Often, the amount provided in the disposable bone marrow tray is insufficient.
- A large sterile syringe (at least 20 ml, preferably 50 ml). The syringe packaged in the disposable tray is usually a 10 ml syringe. With a larger syringe, a stronger suction force can be created and more marrow can be aspirated. Although a high-suction vacuum may cause more discomfort, trying to be 'gentle' to the patient by using a small aspiration syringe usually backfires since an inadequate specimen may be collected, which in turn would necessitate a repeat procedure.

- A bottle of heparin of the lowest concentration. The heparin is used for coating the bone marrow needles and the syringe.
- An appropriate fixative for the bone marrow core biopsy. The usual fixative provided in the tray is a small container of 10% buffered formalin. Formalin is not optimal for the morphologic evaluation of hematopoietic specimens. It is more appropriate to use a fixative with a heavy metal component to achieve good fixation and sharp cytologic detail. A commercially available fixative containing barium chloride is a good choice. Barium chloride is considered preferable to the mercury chloride in the B5 fixative for environmental reasons. Heavy metal fixatives also yield better and more consistent immunohistochemical stains.
- EDTA tubes and preservative-free heparin tubes for collecting the aspirate.
- If necessary, anaerobic culture media.
- One extra set of sterile bone marrow needles.

One of the advantages of the disposable bone marrow tray is the certainty that the bone marrow needles are sharp. If a disposable tray is not available, then it is necessary to organize a tray containing all of the necessary items. If reusable bone marrow needles are employed, it is important to ensure that they are still sharp.

There are several types of bone marrow needles. They can be divided into two groups: short needles (e.g. Illinois needle) for aspiration, and long needles (e.g. Jamshidi needle) for obtaining a bone marrow core biopsy.

It is also possible to use the long needle for aspiration. This is especially true when the patient has a thick layer of subcutaneous tissue.

32.2 Preparation for the bone marrow procedure

Proper evaluation of the bone marrow should take into account the peripheral blood findings, relevant clinical information and laboratory results. Before performing a bone marrow procedure, the responsible physician needs to check that a recent peripheral blood specimen (preferably within 7 days) is available. In case of doubt, it is always judicious to draw a fresh blood specimen at the time of the bone marrow procedure. If a sufficient number of circulating malignant cells is present, the peripheral blood is the specimen of choice for FCM immunophenotyping. Cytogenetics and molecular studies can also be performed on the blood.

Before the bone marrow procedure is performed, several key pieces of clinical information should be available. Good communication between clinical departments and laboratory services is necessary for optimal patient care. The more complete the clinical information, the better the service the laboratory can give back in return. In real life, clinical information is too often missing or erroneous. To circumvent this problem, the authors have routinely reviewed the patient's chart (if available), obtained a brief clinical history, and performed a quick hematologically oriented physical examination to detect the signs of anemia, thrombocytopenia and the presence of lymphadenopathy and/or splenomegaly, prior to the actual bone marrow procedure.

It is important to obtain the following clinical information before performing a bone marrow procedure:

- Exposure to any toxic substances (including smoking and alcohol), previous therapeutic regimens and current medications including growth factors (e.g. G-CSF).
- Previous major surgery on visceral organs (e.g. splenectomy, gastrectomy).
- A history of documented malignancies. In the case of hematological malignancies, it is most helpful to know the exact subtype (e.g. 'mantle cell lymphoma' instead of just the general category of 'NHL'). Preferably, the diagnostic material should be reviewed before the procedure is performed.
- Any history of infections, autoimmune disorders, and immune status (e.g. HIV infection).
- Constitutional symptoms, i.e. fever, night sweats and unexplained weight loss of > 10% of body weight.
- Any history of congenital/hereditary disease, especially when the bone marrow procedure is on a young patient.

Review of the clinical information, peripheral blood findings and key laboratory tests (e.g. serum protein immunoelectrophoresis if Waldenstrom's macroglobulinemia is in the differential diagnosis) is also useful to assess whether the bone marrow procedure is actually indicated. Examples of situations in which the procedure may not be required include:

1. Isolated neutropenia in childhood, unless there is a history of recurrent bacterial infections. In children, viral infections are frequent and can result in transient neutropenia. Therefore, it is preferable to follow the patient with peripheral blood studies for evidence of neutrophil recovery.
2. Isolated thrombocytopenia, especially in childhood. A bone marrow examination may be indicated if the patient has not responded to therapy for immune thrombocytopenia.
3. Isolated anemia. The underlying etiologies for anemia are multiple and should be narrowed down using noninvasive laboratory tests to exclude nutritional deficiencies, renal or liver impairment, and chronic inflammatory disorders prior to requesting a bone marrow. A bone marrow procedure is not indicated for microcytic anemia unless congenital sideroblastic anemia is suspected.
4. Erythrocytosis or thrombocytosis. A bone marrow procedure should be performed only if polycythemia or thrombocytosis have been persistent or progressive with no apparent etiology.
5. Reactive neutrophilia. A bone marrow procedure should be performed only if a metastatic malignancy is suspected.
6. A marked absolute lymphocytosis which has already been documented as CLL by FCM immunophenotyping. Since the tumor content in the blood reflects the extent of bone marrow infiltration, a bone marrow examination is often not necessary unless the patient has anemia and/or thrombocytopenia. Similarly, in patients with documented NHL presenting with apparent 'lymphocytosis', it is preferable to perform FCM immunophenotyping on

the blood. If the results indicate NHL in leukemic phase, a bone marrow procedure may not be necessary.

The bone marrow procedure should be deferred if the patient has taken aspirin within the preceding 48 hours. A bone marrow aspirate/biopsy can be performed in patients with coagulation factor deficiencies once adequate factor transfusions have been given to achieve at least 50% of normal levels. Platelet transfusions are usually not required for patients with thrombocytopenia. If necessary, an appropriate agent, e.g. des-aminoarginine vasopressin (DDAVP) can be administered to stimulate platelet function.

32.3 Performing the bone marrow procedure

The prospect of a bone marrow procedure usually renders the patient anxious and fearful. Much of the anxiety comes from not knowing what is taking place. Therefore, it is important to explain to the patient, in clear layman's terms, the 'why and how' of the procedure. Not only does this allay fear, it also allows the patient to cooperate better. For medical-legal reasons, the patient should sign a consent form prior to the procedure. It is advisable to perform the procedure with the help of an assistant or nurse.

32.3.1 Choosing a site

The preferred site for a bone marrow procedure is the posterior superior iliac crest (PSIC), which in nonobese patients should be easily visible as a dimple on the lower back. Other sites are employed only if attempts on the PSIC have been unsuccessful or the patient has had extensive pelvic irradiation. The anterior iliac crest is not a routine site since the cortical bone is much thicker in that location. In infants and neonates, the tibia can be chosen for marrow aspiration as the PSIC is incompletely ossified. Although a sternal bone marrow is quick and easy to perform, the sternum is not a preferred site for specific reasons:

- Only an aspirate can be obtained and often the amount of the aspirate is insufficient for necessary adjunctive tests.
- There is a potential risk of damaging mediastinal organs and causing a hemothorax.

32.3.2 The bone marrow procedure

The adequacy of the bone marrow specimen, crucial for subsequent analyses and interpretation, is dependent on how well the procedure is performed. In many institutions, only an aspiration is performed in suspected or known acute leukemias, myelodysplastic syndromes or MPDs. It is preferable, however, that a biopsy (along with touch imprints) be performed routinely.

The procedure described below is for both an aspirate and a biopsy, with the aspirate obtained first. Irrespective of whether the biopsy is done before or after the aspirate, it is important to use a different entry site on the bone (i.e. not to follow the same needle track) for each step. If the biopsy is done after the aspirate and the same track is used, the sample is invariably hemorrhagic and therefore unsuitable for evaluation. If the aspiration follows the biopsy (which can activate the coagulation cascade), it is important to perform the anticoagulation measures described below to prevent the aspirate from clotting.

Because of the coagulation cascade, the time-window for making an adequate number of good quality bone marrow spreads and allocating the marrow to appropriate tubes for adjunctive studies is limited. The authors advocate anti-coagulating the aspirate to provide adequate time to prepare good quality smears.

The recommended way to perform the bone marrow procedure is as follows:

1. Have the patient lay on their side with bent knees drawn up toward the chest. Palpate the PSIC and mark the site with a waterproof felt-tip marker. Cleanse the skin with iodine solution. The area to be cleansed must be larger than the window in the disposable sterile drape.

2. Once the disposable bone marrow tray is opened, the procedure must be performed in an aseptic manner wearing sterile surgical gloves. Ensure that the bone marrow needle and its obturator can lock and unlock properly. Apply the sterile drapes, leaving a small window over the marked area. Anesthetize the skin overlying the iliac crest by creating a subepidermal weal. Then, inject anesthetic into the subcutaneous tissue as the needle is pushed toward the periosteum. A generous amount of anesthetic should be given to a sizable area of the periosteum in multiple directions by changing the angle of the needle. It is best not to rush, but allow about 5–10 minutes for the anesthetic to take effect. Massaging the area improves the anesthetic's distribution, and has the added psychological effect of reducing the patient's anxiety.

3. Draw about 2 ml of heparin into a 20 ml syringe. Attach the bone marrow needle to the syringe and pull the plunger back and forth several times to coat the inner wall of the syringe and needle with heparin. Discard most of the heparin, leaving a minimal amount (less than 0.25 ml) in the syringe. This coating process is designed to counteract the coagulation cascade, which starts as soon as the aspirated marrow contacts a foreign surface. In addition, the resulting thin film of heparin facilitates pulling back the plunger smoothly during aspiration. This procedure does not result in heparin artifacts if the following precautions are taken: (a) the heparin is the lowest commercially available concentration; (b) a large amount of marrow is aspirated; and (c) the aspirated specimen is injected into an EDTA tube. The last two steps essentially eliminate the effects of heparin.

4. Make a small incision (about 0.5–0.8 cm) at the previously marked site. Insert the bone marrow needle with its obturator in a locked position until it touches the periosteum. At this point, it is important to coach the patient through deep breathing (a technique similar to that used in childbirth) since this technique reduces pain and anxiety. Rotate and advance the needle through the cortical bone. A feeling of 'yield' is usually experienced once the needle is through the cortical bone. Rotate and advance the needle by an additional 0.2–0.3 cm to ensure that the beveled tip of the needle is well

within the marrow cavity and the needle is well anchored. Unlock and remove the obturator. Attach the large aspiration syringe.

5. The quantity of marrow aspirated depends on the degree of vacuum created during the aspiration procedure, which in turn is proportional to the size of the syringe and the speed of pulling the plunger. The most intense pain is felt during the aspiration step as a vacuum suction force is applied to the marrow space. Therefore, the patient should be coached to perform quick deep breathing during this step, and the aspiration should be performed swiftly. Apply the maximum suction force by pulling the plunger of the syringe quickly and steadily, to draw about 10–15 ml of marrow and admixed blood. Although there is a relatively large amount of admixed blood, the number of marrow particles aspirated is actually higher than that obtained when only 1–2 ml are aspirated with a 5 ml syringe. In cases with a markedly hypocellular marrow, aspirating a large amount of marrow improves the possibility of harvesting the few spicules present. When the marrow is not hypocellular, it is the authors' experience that this one single aspirate pull yields a more than adequate specimen for a comprehensive evaluation, including special studies. If additional aspirates are needed, then it is best to repeat the procedure at a different entry site on the bone.

Mix and transfer the aspirated specimen to an EDTA tube and a preservative-free heparin tube. Ensure that the EDTA tube is well filled to maintain an optimal 'specimen to EDTA' ratio (this is one of the reasons why a large amount of marrow and admixed blood is drawn), thus avoiding EDTA artifacts. In general, most of the specimen should be allocated to the EDTA tube since the marrow from this tube is used for multiple studies including morphology, FCM analysis and molecular biology. The heparin tube is mainly for cytogenetics. Let the tubes stand upright in a tube holder to allow the marrow spicules to rise to the top, which usually occurs after about 30 minutes. With this procedure, the spreading of bone marrow smears can be done properly and in a 'leisurely' manner in the laboratory instead of racing against the coagulation cascade at the bedside.

6. To perform a biopsy, stretch the skin and subcutaneous tissue to overlay an adjacent but different site on the PSIC. Insert the biopsy needle with the obturator in a locked position. Ensure that a different needle track is made and a different site on the bone is entered. The biopsy procedure should not create any sharp pain, only a sensation of dull pressure. A sharp pain, which requires repositioning of the needle, occurs when the cortical bone and periosteum are tangentially sheared and lifted off. In performing a biopsy, rotation instead of pushing while advancing the needle will cut the core specimen without causing crushing artifacts.

Rotate and advance the needle through the cortical bone until a 'yield' is felt and the needle is well anchored. Remove the obturator. Continue to advance the needle with a rotating motion for about 2.5 cm. To release the marrow core from the surrounding marrow, vigorously rotate the needle in full circles in both directions several times. Remove the needle gently. Insert the stylet into the tip of the needle to push out the core specimen.

Before removing the needle, do not reinsert the obturator in an attempt to estimate the length of the biopsy since this may accidentally push the core out. Applying suction in an attempt to extract the biopsy is not recommended since this causes distortion artifacts in the biopsy.

It is possible to visually distinguish a good marrow core from cartilage, tendon and cortical bone. If the core specimen is marrow, the appearance is tan-pink with flecks of bone. In contrast, a homogeneous pale appearance is seen with cortical bone, connective tissue and cartilage (cartilage also has a glistening surface). In the following situations it is judicious to repeat the biopsy procedure, using a new biopsy needle if necessary:

- The core specimen is not bone marrow or the marrow core is too short for evaluation. Ideally, the core should be around 2 cm in length (Figure 32.1).
- The aspirate is a 'dry tap' in a patient in whom adjunctive studies are indicated. In such instances, it is necessary to obtain two additional cores (2–2.5 cm each) for cell suspensions.
- The patient has Hodgkin's disease. Because Hodgkin's disease disseminates in a 'metastatic-like' fashion, marrow involvement is often focal. A bilateral biopsy is usually indicated to increase the sensitivity of detection. For the same reasons, a bilateral procedure is often performed on patients with large cell lymphoma.

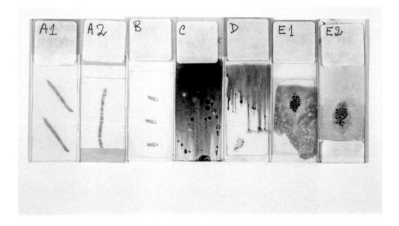

Figure 32.1 Examples of bone marrow core biopsies and aspirate preparations. (A1) An adequate biopsy specimen, 2.1 cm long (after fixation and processing). (A2) A 3.5 cm long bone marrow core from cortex to cortex. The procedure did not result in any complication, however. (B) A short and inadequate biopsy specimen, 0.4 cm long. (C) and (D) Bone marrow aspirate smears prepared at the bedside using the 'push' technique. Film C is unacceptable, with excessive admixed blood and the few particles located at the far third of the slide, hampering proper microscopic evaluation of the specimen. Smear D is acceptable with the scattered particles located in the middle third of the slide. There is still a considerable amount of blood associated with the particles, however. (E1) A better aspirate smear prepared at the bedside using the 'pull' technique. The particles are concentrated in one area. There is less blood associated with the particles. Most of the contaminated blood is distributed peripherally. (E2) An optimal bone marrow smear prepared from the concentrated particles collected in EDTA (see text). The smear is virtually free of blood contamination

32.3.3 Care of the patient after the procedure

Firm pressure should be applied to the wound until the bleeding stops. Then, apply appropriate bandages to the area. Cleanse the skin with alcohol to take off the iodine stain. Have the patient lay on their back with pressure on the marrow site for about 20–30 minutes. Explain to the patient when the results of the procedure can be expected. Complications after a bone marrow procedure, such as infection and hemorrhage, are extremely rare.

32.4 Handling routine bone marrow biopsy specimens

Before dropping any biopsy into fixative, ensure that it is not needed for imprints or adjunctive studies that require fresh tissue.

32.4.1 Imprints

It is preferable to make bone marrow imprints from core biopsies routinely. Good imprints should be free of excess blood and serum since excess fluid leads to slow drying and shrinkage artifacts (Figure 32.2). The procedure is as follows:

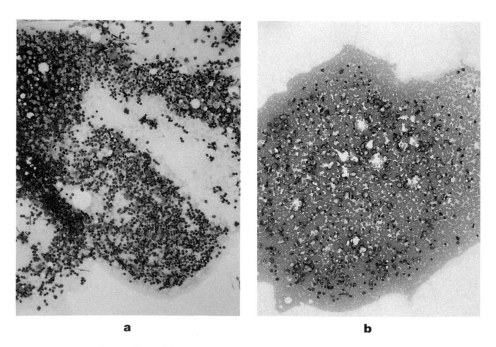

a   b

Figure 32.2 Examples of bone marrow imprints. (a) A good imprint with abundant hematopoietic elements and no excess RBCs and plasma. (b) An unacceptable imprint with excess blood. The nucleated cells are shrunken

1. Dab off the excess blood from the surfaces of the biopsy on blotting paper or a piece of non-shredded gauze.
2. Pick up the core with small forceps and place it on a glass slide.
3. Gently press (do not crush) the biopsy with gloved fingers against the slide. Repeat this about four times along the length of the slide. If the excess blood is well dabbed off, the core will actually stick to the gloved fingers and can be transported to the next spot on the slide for subsequent imprints. Repeat the process on several slides. A higher number of imprint slides should be prepared in cases that may need special stains.

32.4.2 Preparing cell suspensions from fresh biopsies

The material required for preparing cell suspensions includes tissue culture media, a Petri dish, forceps, a scalpel and pipettes. Immerse the cores in the culture media. Mince the core as finely as possible. The culture media becomes cloudy as cells get released. Transfer everything to a sterile specimen tube when finished. The cell suspension can be sent for FCM immunophenotyping, cytogenetics and molecular studies.

32.4.3 Fixing the biopsy

The preferred fixative for hematopoietic tissues is one that contains a heavy metal element such as barium or mercury chloride (B5). This allows better cytologic detail on H&E sections (Figure 32.3). Post-fixation with B5 can also be used to 'rescue' a biopsy that has been accidentally fixed in formalin. If a heavy metal fixative is used, the biopsy is fixed for about 3–4 hours, then transferred to a decalcifying solution for 2–3 hours. Ensure that the specimen is not over-decalcified which can result in artifacts. Rinse the specimen before putting it in a cassette to be loaded on the automated tissue processor.

32.4.4 Special stains on biopsy sections

At the time of initial sectioning, several unstained slides should be prepared from paraffin-embedded biopsies in case special stains or extra H&E slides are needed. Preparing extra sections at the time the block is first sectioned reduces the risk of cutting through the block when additional slides are needed.

In most institutions, the reticulin stain is performed routinely to evaluate the stromal reticulin network. In patients with suspected widespread infection (e.g. HIV-positive patients), stains for acid-fast and fungal organisms should be done routinely, even if no obvious granulomata are present. An iron stain on biopsy sections is of limited value, since fixation and decalcification can result in false-negative results.

Immunohistochemical staining, which employs either peroxidase- or alkaline phosphatase-conjugated antibodies can be applied to biopsy sections. The technique is useful mainly for confirming the identity of a nonhematopoietic infiltrate, e.g. carcinoma or melanoma. It is also helpful for identifying Reed-Sternberg cells to document bone marrow involvement by Hodgkin's disease. The ability of

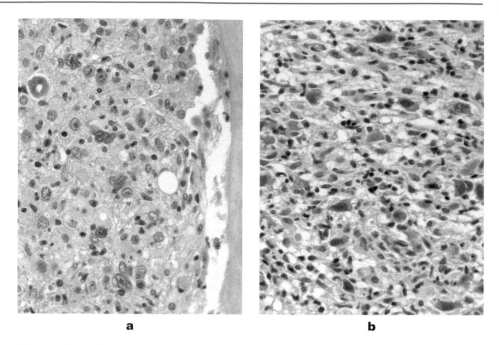

a   b

Figure 32.3 Bone marrow biopsies (with involvement by Hodgkin's disease) fixed in different fixatives. (a) Sharp cytologic details obtained with a fixative containing barium chloride. (b) Suboptimal morphology when fixed in formalin

immunohistochemistry to characterize involvement by sarcomas (a rare occurrence) is less satisfactory because of the limited number of available reagents. With proper FCM immunophenotyping on peripheral blood, bone marrow aspirates, or cell suspensions prepared from fresh core biopsies, the need for immunohistochemistry on biopsy sections should rarely arise in the work-up of leukemias and lymphomas. Immunostaining on glass slides (smears and tissue sections) is popular as a routine technique in institutions where FCM is not available. Immunohistochemistry on paraffin-embedded sections for leukemia and lymphoma is called for when adequate fresh marrow is unavailable (e.g. referral material or a suboptimal bone marrow procedure). The limitations of immunohistochemistry on paraffin-embedded sections are mentioned in Section 20.1.2.

32.5 Handling the anticoagulated bone marrow aspirates

The specimen collected in EDTA can be used for preparing aspirate smears, as well as FCM immunophenotyping and molecular studies. The specimen in preservative-free heparin can be sent for cytogenetics, FCM immunophenotyping, molecular studies and microbiological cultures.

32.5.1 The advantages of the bone marrow buffy coat

To prepare bone marrow smears, the EDTA tube is left in an upright position to allow the spicules to rise to the surface. There is no need to subject the specimen to centrifugation, which often causes nuclear irregularities that may be misidentified as a feature of malignancy. Marrow smears must be prepared soon after the spicules rise to the top of the tube to avoid EDTA/storage artifacts.

Bone marrow smears prepared from this concentrated top layer (buffy coat) are essentially devoid of excess blood. In contrast, aspirate smears prepared at the bedside are invariably contaminated with blood, which has several disadvantages:

- Excess blood on the slide can cause poor spreading and shrinkage artifacts that obscure nuclear and cytoplasmic details. When using the 'push' technique for smear preparation (described below), the excess blood can result in a marrow film too long for adequate examination (Figure 32.1), with the tail of the smear located at the gap on the microscope stage.
- Excess blood decreases the accuracy of the bone marrow differential because of contamination with peripheral leukocytes. For example, the percentage of lymphocytes can easily be artificially elevated, with a concomitant falsely reduced percentage of blasts or lymphoma cells. This is a frequent phenomenon seen on 'push' marrow films prepared at the bedside, particularly when there are few spicules on the slides.

Use a small pipette to draw spicules from the top layer of the EDTA specimen. The number of films to be made depends on the need for cytochemistries and/or immunocytochemistry to detect cytoplasmic antigens. Usually, three Romanovsky-stained smears should be adequate. In the work-up for metastatic disease, a higher number of smears should be stained to improve detection when only a few metastatic clusters are present.

There are two ways to spread bone marrow aspirates, the 'push' and 'pull' techniques. Irrespective of the method used, ensure that the following steps are performed properly:

1. The specimen drop applied to the slide should not have excessive fluid (pipette off the excess if necessary).
2. The smear should be quickly fan-dried (or dried vigorously by arm and hand motion) to prevent slow-drying artifacts.

32.5.2 Bone marrow spreading techniques

The 'push' technique for preparing bone marrow smears is similar to that used for making a blood film. A small drop of marrow fluid containing spicules is applied to the end near the frosted portion of the glass slide. The spreader (e.g. a hematocytometer coverslip attached to an alligator clip) is applied at an appropriate angle in front of the drop, and pulled back to it. As soon as the specimen has run along the edge of the spreader, the spreader is pushed forward in a smooth and steady manner.

Using the 'push' technique, the quality of the slide depends on the size of the drop (a small drop is preferred), the spreader angle applied, and both the speed and steadiness in pushing the spreader.

The 'pull' technique has been misnamed a 'squash (or crush) preparation'. After a drop of marrow fluid containing spicules is applied near the frosted portion of the glass slide, a second slide is put on top perpendicular to the first one. Allow the marrow fluid to spread out between the two slides and gently pull the top slide across the bottom slide. There is no need to put pressure on the slides, one against the other, since a 'heavy handed' approach results in cellular disruption and naked nuclei. If well prepared, i.e. without crushing the cells, 'pull' preparations offer several advantages over 'push' preparations, including:

1. The spicules are concentrated in one area (Figure 32.1), thus facilitating morphologic evaluation and the bone marrow differential.
2. A more accurate semiquantitative assessment of megakaryocytes is possible than in the 'push' preparation. In a 'push' preparation, large cells are preferentially distributed to the lateral edges, and are detectable only if the lateral edges of the film are narrower than the sides of the slides. Large cells may be lost when the lateral edges of the smear encroach on the sides of the slide. This is the most likely reason why the number of megakaryocytes in 'push' marrow smears appears lower than in 'pull' smears.

32.5.3 Fixing and staining aspirate smears

Once dried, the marrow films should be fixed as soon as possible in methanol. It is better to overfix since underfixation causes dissolution of nuclear chromatin. Ensure that the methanol is not contaminated with water, especially if the ambient humidity is high. The quality of staining can be altered if the smears are left unfixed for more than 24–48 hours with resulting breakdown of plasma proteins.

Current staining procedures are variations of the Romanovsky stain, using a combination of basic and acid dyes. For optimal results, free of deposits, ensure that the stain has been filtered and the pH of the staining buffer is correct.

Since bone marrow films contain a much higher density of nucleated cells than peripheral blood films, the exposure time to the staining mixture must be lengthened accordingly. For this reason, the staining process is usually done manually. If the marrow smears are stained with May-Grünwald-Giemsa they can be loaded on an automatic 'dipping' stainer used for staining blood films. A 'flat bed' stainer should be avoided, since the smears are not well immersed in the staining baths, and the exposure time to the staining mixture is inadequate. With the Wright stain the nuclei often stain too pink. Therefore, it is preferable to use either the May-Grünwald-Giemsa or Wright-Giemsa stains.

32.5.4 To fix marrow particles

In the 'traditional' bone marrow procedure, the clotted aspirate is either discarded or put into fixative to yield a clot preparation, which can be cut into

H&E sections. The excess blood in a clot preparation can interfere with cutting thin sections, however. In the procedure described above, the aspirate is collected anticoagulated. If desired, any 'left-over' particles may be filtered through fine filter paper (e.g. lens paper) for fixation and processing. H&E sections from either fixed marrow particles or clot preparations provide little additional information to that already obtained from the biopsy, however. Therefore, it is preferable to use the 'left-over' anticoagulated aspirate either as controls (e.g. for special stains or molecular studies) or to make extra smears for teaching purposes.

32.5.5 Special stains on air-dried preparations

Air-dried preparations (aspirates/imprint smears) are the material of choice for the iron stain (Prussian blue reaction). In most institutions, an iron stain is routinely performed for evaluating iron stores in macrophages and iron incorporation in RBCs.

In the work-up of acute leukemia, the two most important cytochemical stains are MPO to establish a myeloid lineage and the NSE stain to confirm monocytic differentiation. Myeloperoxidase is the most reliable marker for myeloid cells, since the reaction detects the activity of the MPO enzyme. Reaction with diaminobenzidine yields the most sensitive MPO results, despite its overpublicized carcinogenic potential. Enzymatic activity decreases with time. Therefore, an MPO stain on a smear that is several weeks old can be falsely negative. In such instances, Sudan black B (SBB), a lipophilic dye, can be used as an alternative. Although SBB reactivity in most cases correlates with the presence of MPO granules, it does not detect the activity of the MPO enzyme *per se*. Sudan black can be positive in ALL, with the reactivity seen as a few scattered coarse globular granules (Figure 32.4). The reaction with SBB is often accompanied by stain deposits, which can interfere with microscopic evaluation and lead to misinterpretation. The enzyme chloroacetate esterase (CAE) appears relatively late in

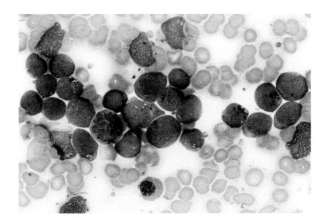

Figure 32.4 Sudan black B positive ALL

myeloid maturation, and is therefore less useful than MPO. If only fixed, paraffin-embedded material is available, then staining for CAE may be included as part of the work-up for a mononuclear cell infiltrate composed of large cells.

The substrate employed can affect the quality of cytochemical stains, especially the NSE stain. The ANBE procedure is preferred since myeloid precursors do not give a positive reaction with the butyrate substrate. Dot positivity for ANBE is normally seen in T-helper lymphocytes, a feature that is useful as an internal control. The use of the butyrate substrate obviates the need for the fluoride inhibition step. Although ANAE may be somewhat more sensitive, the reactivity can be present in nonmonocytic cells, including some cases of ALL. The combined esterase procedure to detect NSE and CAE is not recommended, as reaction with CAE can inhibit reaction with NSE.

Other cytochemistries, such as the PAS reaction (which detects cytoplasmic glycogen) and the acid phosphatase stain, can be omitted in view of their low sensitivity and specificity as compared to FCM immunophenotyping.

The TRAP stain, performed on trephine imprints, remains a useful test for hairy cell leukemia, especially when no specimen has been allocated for FCM studies.

Immunostaining can be performed on air-dried preparations by the alkaline phosphatase technique, primarily to detect cytoplasmic antigens, such as cCD3 and cCD22, myeloperoxidase antigen and cytoplasmic light chains. Detection of the nuclear enzyme TdT can also be performed on smears that have been quickly frozen to preserve the enzyme activity. Plasma immunoglobulins present on the smears and a variable degree of cellular disruption during smear preparation can easily cause background staining, however. It is preferable to perform these tests by FCM, since multicolor FCM immunophenotyping allows simultaneous detection of surface, nuclear and cytoplasmic antigens.

Air-dried preparations can also be used for FISH to detect chromosomal abnormalities if the appropriate molecular probes are available. Ensure that the air-dried preparation is a monolayer to avoid false-positive results.

32.6 Special studies

In suspected hematopoietic malignancies, an adequate amount of representative marrow (aspirate or cell suspensions from fresh biopsies) should be allocated for potential FCM immunophenotyping, cytogenetics and molecular analysis. These studies provide valuable diagnostic and/or prognostic information, and add to the understanding of the biology of the disorder in question.

In contrast to FCM immunophenotyping, the results of cytogenetics are often not necessary for diagnosis although they can be of prognostic value. The availability of molecular probes and the FISH technique have overcome some of the technical limitations inherent to standard cytogenetics (e.g. the need for adequate metaphase spreads). In addition to FISH, other molecular techniques such as PCR can be applied to detect:

1. Cellular oncogenes or suppressor genes, resulting from: (a) chromosomal translocations, such as c-*myc* associated with the (8;14) translocation in

Burkitt's lymphoma-leukemia; (b) point mutations (e.g. *ras* mutations in some acute myeloid leukemias); or (c) deletions (e.g. loss of the *p53* gene from chromosome 17).
2. Infectious agents, e.g. HTLV-I involved in the pathogenesis of ATLL.
3. Minimal residual disease (MRD), especially in acute leukemias.
4. B-cell and T-cell rearrangements. For diagnostic purposes, these studies are only needed if clonality has not been established after extensive FCM immunophenotyping.

In general, molecular analyses rarely provide diagnostic information beyond that already obtained by a properly performed multiparameter FCM study. Furthermore, clonal rearrangements may be present in benign lymphoid aggregates.

Since the majority of acute leukemias demonstrate one or more immunophenotypic aberrancies, such as cross-lineage expression, asynchronous expression, overexpression, or aberrant light scatter, MRD detection can also be performed by multiparameter FCM.

Because of its high sensitivity, the PCR technique has been applied to MRD detection if the DNA motif of the given acute leukemia is known. The RT-PCR assay is based on the presence of an abnormal fusion mRNA transcript resulting from a particular chromosomal translocation, e.g. the AML1/ETO fusion resulting from the (8;21) translocation. With technological advances, the sensitivity of RT-PCR assays has improved from 10^{-3}–10^{-4} to 10^{-5}–10^{-6}. At this level of sensitivity, persistence of abnormal transcripts has been found in patients with long-term remission, however. For this reason, an important issue to consider in PCR detection of MRD is the threshold at which positive PCR results are clinically significant to predict relapse.

An additional difficulty in judging the clinical significance of positive PCR results is the fact that some molecular abnormalities, such as *bcl*-2 and *bcr-abl,* can be present at low levels in normal individuals. Similarly, recent studies have found the t(4;11) fusion transcripts in normal hematopoietic cells. Such findings suggest that these molecular rearrangements are just one of the initial steps in the development of hematopoietic malignancies, and additional events are necessary for progression to clinical malignancy. For these reasons, data from molecular analyses should be interpreted cautiously and always in the context of other clinical and laboratory findings.

32.7 Storage of bone marrow slides

After the bone marrow slides and the corresponding blood film have been examined, the entire set should be stored for at least the lifetime of the patient. The marrow and blood smears should be coverslipped to facilitate examination and avoid scratches.

32.8 Bone marrow evaluation and reporting

The repertoire of observable qualitative and quantitative changes in hemato-poietic precursors is limited. Similar abnormalities can occur in unrelated disorders. For instance, the same qualitative erythroid abnormalities (also referred to as dysplastic features or dyserythropoiesis) can be seen in MDS, HIV infections and following multiagent chemotherapy. Therefore, a thorough bone marrow evaluation must take into account the relevant clinical information, peripheral blood data and laboratory findings. In leukemias and lymphomas, the results of FCM immunophenotyping are critical to the final bone marrow interpretation. The morphologic assessment of the bone marrow and peripheral blood can be seriously hampered if the specimens are of suboptimal quality.

32.8.1 Bone marrow artifacts

A number of common artifacts in bone marrow specimens can lead to erroneous interpretation if they are not recognized. These artifacts can result from faulty technique during the bone marrow procedure and suboptimal staining, as well as problems with decalcification and processing of the biopsy.

32.8.1.1 Procedure-related artifacts

Artifacts secondary to faulty technique on aspirate smears include:

- An inadequate aspirate (i.e. few or no spicules) when there is no evidence of reticulin fibrosis or severe hypocellularity on the biopsy. This is seen when the bone marrow needle has not been inserted deep enough into the marrow space (i.e. the beveled tip is just barely through the cortical bone) or a small syringe is used for aspiration.
- Storage (EDTA) artifacts occurring when preparation of the aspirate smears from an EDTA specimen was delayed, or the EDTA tube was only partially filled. Examples include cytoplasmic vacuoles and nuclear irregularities, which may be misinterpreted as dysplastic or malignant features.
- Crush artifacts, resulting in naked nuclei or nuclear streaking caused by too much pressure during the 'pull' preparation of the bone marrow smear.
- Slow drying, resulting in various degrees of cell shrinkage (Figures 1.7 and 1.8). The artifacts here manifest as villi, hairs and blebs, encountered mainly in lymphoid cells (especially plasmacytoid lymphocytes) and any large agranular mononuclear cells such as blasts or large lymphoma cells. Shrinkage causes the nuclear chromatin to appear coarse and nucleoli to become indistinct.

Poor bone marrow core biopsy technique can lead to:

- An inadequate biopsy composed mostly of cartilage and/or cortical bone. Subcortical marrow is hypocellular and therefore not a representative specimen for evaluation (Figure 32.5). Note that the subcortical marrow becomes more prominent in older individuals.

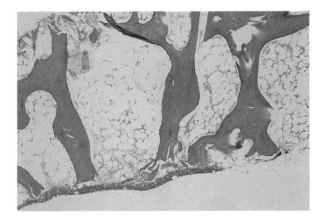

Figure 32.5   Subcortical hypocellular marrow in a 70-year-old male. The deeper marrow is actually normocellular

- A biopsy with 'negative pressure' effects, which occur when a suction force has been applied during the removal of the biopsy specimen from the surrounding tissue. The sections demonstrate empty marrow spaces and distorted, displaced or fragmented bony trabeculae (Figure 32.6a).
- Crush artifacts. These occur in the biopsy when too much pushing force has been applied to advance the biopsy needle.

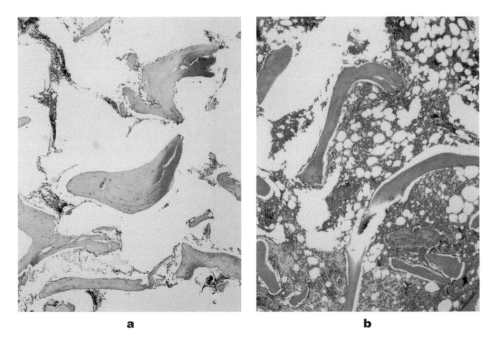

a   b

Figure 32.6   Unacceptable bone marrow core specimens with no marrow tissue and disorganized bony trabeculae (a) or excessive hemorrhage (b)

• A hemorrhagic biopsy. This is the result of the biopsy having been taken too close to the area of aspiration (Figure 32.6b).

32.8.1.2 Processing and staining artifacts

Staining artifacts (see Section 1.3) are mainly seen on the aspirate smears. The quality of the staining can be gauged by the color of the (few) RBCs present on the slide. With optimal staining, the RBCs should be tan. Delayed fixation of the aspirate smears or an excess of heparin anticoagulant are some of the causes of poor staining.

Excessive decalcification of the biopsy results in the nuclei of erythroid precursors having a glassy appearance. Normally, erythroid precursors appear dark and homogeneous (reminiscent of an 'ink dot'). Pigments mimicking hemosiderin granules can appear when the biopsy has been inadequately rinsed of the fixative. Suboptimal preparation of H&E sections results in sections that are too thick or of uneven thickness. When the paraffin block is not properly faced and a superficial level is obtained, the resulting section can be discontinuous, and the critical areas (e.g. small foci of lymphomatous involvement) can be missed. For these reasons, it is important to obtain at least three H&E sections at different levels.

32.8.2 Morphologic examination

The standard sequence to morphologic review is:

1. Peripheral blood film
2. Bone marrow aspirate smears
3. Biopsy sections

Proper evaluation of the bone marrow requires correlation with peripheral blood data and clinical information. Too often, especially in the case of referral material, only the bone marrow specimen is received with no blood film and minimal, if any, clinical information.

The blood and bone marrow aspirate smears are ready the same day as the procedure. Therefore, a preliminary interpretation can be rendered within hours of the procedure.

Since the critical elements may be unevenly distributed on the slides, all available strips of the biopsy sections and all aspirate smears need to be scanned thoroughly at low power (20 × objective) before rushing to high power. Fields with many smudge cells and bare nuclei on the smears should be avoided. Areas where cytologic details are suboptimal because of shrinkage artifacts or cellular overcrowding should also be omitted.

32.8.2.1 Low-power assessment of the bone marrow

Features that can be evaluated at low power include cellularity, megakaryocytes, increased mast cells, and the presence of clusters of foreign cells. Clusters of metastatic cells are preferentially distributed at the periphery of the aspirate films prepared by the 'pull' technique. On 'push' preparations, they are mostly found at the feather-edge.

On the biopsy, low-power examination allows evaluation of: (1) the pattern and extent of neoplastic infiltration; (2) the presence of granulomata; and (3) abnormal processes affecting the bony trabeculae or stroma (serous fat atrophy, fibroblastic proliferations, osteoblasts and osteoclasts).

The bone marrow cellularity is defined as the relative proportion of cells to fat in the marrow. It is best to evaluate cellularity on a representative core biopsy. The cellularity can be relatively accurately assessed on aspirate smears (Figure 32.7), especially 'pull' preparations. The central part of the spicule is composed of stroma, where macrophages and mast cells (if present) accumulate. Most megakaryocytes are distributed in the vicinity of the spicules as well. In between the spicules are the hematopoietic elements, often arranged along the convexity of the rims of fat spaces. The relationship between the cellular components and the fat spaces gives an estimate of the cellularity.

On a 'push' preparation, the cellularity can also be assessed if the smears have been prepared from anticoagulated concentrated marrow as described above. With 'push' preparations performed at the bedside, accurate estimates of cellularity can be difficult, especially when adequate cell trails are not present. This may be true even when the spicules give an impression of being normocellular. In the authors' experience, there is a tendency to overestimate or underestimate the cellularity on 'push' smears prepared at the bedside.

A semiquantitative estimate of megakaryocytes (i.e. decreased, normal, increased) is best done on the biopsy sections and/or 'pull' marrow smears. Megakaryocytes may be underestimated on 'push' preparations. Qualitative changes in megakaryocytes are of limited diagnostic usefulness, mirroring the limited role of platelet morphology in peripheral blood interpretation. For example, hypolobulated, small megakaryocytes can be seen in MDS and CML, as well as in immune thrombocytopenia.

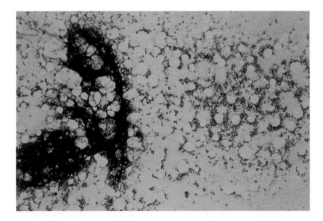

Figure 32.7 Normocellular marrow ('pull' preparation made from concentrated particles)

32.8.2.2 Bone marrow differential

The usual recommendation for bone marrow differentials is a 500-cell count, performed on air-dried preparations. In general, a 200–300 cell differential count is adequate after all the smears have been carefully screened. The differential does not include elements such as macrophages, mast cells or osteoblasts, which are related to the bone marrow stroma. To avoid skewed differential counts, ensure that the differential is performed from several noncontiguous areas of the slide, and that the areas are representative, with good cytologic detail.

On smears prepared at the bedside by the 'push' technique, the spicules are scattered from one lateral edge of the slide to the other. The differential should be concentrated on the cell trails closely adjacent to the spicules. If the individual cell trails are scanty, the differential should incorporate several cell trails. Areas on either side of a cell trail are to be avoided because of blood contamination. Enumerating cells in these areas can easily result in an erroneous marrow lymphocytosis, especially when the differential includes only 100–200 cells. The area of the cell trail far away from the spicule should also be avoided, since it is toward the thick end of the smear with a higher number of RBCs and more serum. In such areas, cellular details are less discernible due to shrinkage artifacts from slow drying, making the distinction between lymphocytes and polychromatophilic erythroid precursors unnecessarily difficult.

Because bone marrow differential counting is considered time-consuming, it is often replaced by visual estimates. It is good practice to do an actual differential count, however, when the relative proportion of blasts is estimated to be around established diagnostically important cut-off levels (e.g. 5%, 20% or 30%). Furthermore, a differential is necessarily accompanied by a thorough review of the smears, which allows experienced individuals to detect a low level of lymphomatous involvement (e.g. 3–5% large NHL cells). When individuals with insufficient experience review the smears without performing a differential, there is a high frequency of overestimating or underestimating both the quantitative and qualitative features in the marrow. The actual counting process can be replaced by an overall estimate of the differential (i.e. a scan marrow differential) when neoplastic cells overrun the marrow (e.g. acute leukemia with 95% blasts).

32.8.2.3 Assessment of cytology and qualitative features

The assessment of the qualitative features is performed on the aspirate smears or biopsy imprints. The range of cytologic features discernible on fixed sections (clot preparation, core biopsy) is limited.

Assessment of the erythroid and myeloid lineages includes their maturation, the relative percentage of erythroid and myeloid precursors, and the presence of qualitative abnormalities ('dysplastic' features). When air-dried preparations are not available, a rough estimate of the M:E ratio and the maturation within the myeloid and erythroid series can be made from the biopsy. On the biopsy, myeloid maturation is estimated by comparing the proportion of myeloid cells with round nuclei (which encompasses blasts, promyelocytes and myelocytes) to those with lobulated or segmented nuclei (metamyelocytes, bands and neutrophils).

Erythroid maturation is judged from the number of erythroid precursors with dense 'ink dot' nuclei (late precursors) relative to larger erythroid cells with sharp nuclear contours, amphophilic cytoplasm and fine nuclear chromatin (early precursors).

Other elements to be evaluated include:

1. **Lymphoid cells and plasma cells**. The cytology of lymphocytes and plasma cells is best appreciated on air-dried preparations. Neoplastic lymphocytes and plasmacytoid lymphocytes in disorders such as CLL/SLL, LPC lymphoma-leukemia and Waldenstrom's macroglobulinemia are morphologically similar to benign/reactive lymphocytes. Although the malignant nature of the lymphocytes and/or plasmacytoid lymphocytes can usually be inferred from the marked extent of the infiltrate, immunophenotyping is necessary to subclassify the disorder correctly. The pattern of the infiltrate can be assessed on the biopsy sections.
2. **Bony trabeculae, stroma and related elements**. The stroma and its associated elements include adipose cells, osteoblasts, osteoclasts, mast cells and macrophages. Osteoblasts, often seen in marrow aspirates from young children, may be misidentified as plasma cells. Features such as hemophagocytosis and increased mast cells are best appreciated on air-dried preparations.
3. **Routine special stains** on aspirate smears and biopsy sections. On the aspirate, iron in stromal macrophages manifests as coarse coalescent blue granules with the Prussian blue reaction. High power magnification (i.e. 50–100 × oil objective) is required to assess iron incorporation, which is seen as one to four small blue granules in RBCs and late erythroid precursors. Alterations in the stromal reticulin network can be semiquantitatively estimated on silver-impregnated sections (i.e. a reticulin stain).

32.8.3 Bone marrow reporting

The bone marrow report integrates the clinical information, peripheral blood and bone marrow findings, and other relevant laboratory results in order to communicate the diagnosis (and, if necessary, recommendations or requests) to the treating physicians. Optimally, the bone marrow report should be completed within 24–36 hours after the procedure. There may be an extra day of delay because of immunostaining on biopsy sections. When only an aspirate is performed, the report should be available the same day, unless cytochemistries or FCM immunophenotyping is needed. A succinct bone marrow report should include:

1. The CBC results and pertinent morphologic features on the blood film.
2. The bone marrow differential and qualitative (or semiquantitative) findings based on a combined assessment of the aspirate (and/or imprint) smears and biopsy sections.
3. The results of special stains.
4. In leukemias and lymphomas, a summary of the peripheral blood or bone marrow FCM immunophenotyping results.

5. A final diagnostic interpretation. The final interpretation is usually a specific diagnosis if the available data are complete. When a specific diagnosis cannot be reached, it is often appropriate to append a comment listing the differential diagnosis, along with recommendations for additional clinical information and/or laboratory tests to establish the diagnosis.

32.9 Terminology

Some of the confusion that has plagued the field of hematology/hematopathology has been caused by the inconsistent use of terminology, namely the same term applied to different entities, or one entity with multiple names. Concise terminology is important to improve communication.

Below are explanations for some of the terms employed or avoided in the subsequent chapters:

- **Blasts**. The term 'blast' should be reserved for phenotypically immature mononuclear cells, based on immunophenotyping evidence (e.g. lymphoblasts) or combined immunologic, cytochemical and morphologic evidence (e.g. blasts with myeloid or monocytic differentiation). Problems can arise if the term blast is employed for any transformed cell with a distinct nucleolus (see Section 20.5). While awaiting additional evidence, it is judicious to describe large cells as 'abnormal mononuclear cells' with a comment on the appropriate differential diagnosis. Exceptions to this are the terms 'immunoblast' and 'plasmablast', in which the prefixes 'immuno-' and 'plasma-' infer that the cells are mature.
- **Blast crisis, blastic transformation**. The term 'blast crisis' (e.g. CML in blast crisis) indicates the transformation of a pre-existing disorder into a leukemia composed of immature cells. 'Blast crisis' and 'blastic transformation' are synonymous. The term 'blastic transformation' has also been used, inappropriately, to designate the progression of a low-grade NHL to a high-grade NHL.
- **Atypical monocytes**. The morphology of monocytes is variable, with some degree of overlap between reactive monocytosis, CMMoL, and acute myeloid leukemia with monocytic differentiation. In neoplastic monocytosis, blasts are often present in the peripheral blood along with variable numbers of immature-appearing monocytes. It is preferable to designate these immature-appearing monocytes as promonocytes rather than 'atypical monocytes'. The term 'promonocyte' conveys a malignant process more explicitly.
- **Atypical lymphoid cells**. This is an abused term designating a range of mononuclear cells, both benign and malignant and of different lineages (see Section 5.11). Based on the clinical and laboratory data, the appropriate terminology should be employed instead of the ambiguous term 'atypical lymphocytes'.
- **Cell size**. The term 'cell size' in hematopathology actually refers to the size of the nucleus, especially when the assessment is performed on tissue sections where cytoplasmic borders are indistinct. Because most malignant cells

demonstrate an increased nuclear/cytoplasmic ratio, cell size and nuclear size are used interchangeably.

The terminology for NHL used in this book is derived from the revised European–American classification of lymphoid neoplasms (REAL) (Table 32.1). The REAL classification of lymphoid neoplasms represents an improvement over its predecessors in that it advocates the use of a multiparameter approach (immunologic, morphologic, genetic and clinical) in defining disease entities.

Table 32.1 The REAL classification of mature lymphoid neoplasms

Mature B-cell neoplasms
  B-cell CLL/SLL
  Prolymphocytic leukemia
  Lymphoplasmacytoid lymphoma
  Mantle cell lymphoma
  Follicular center cell lymphoma, grades I, II and III
  Plasmacytoma/multiple myeloma
  Hairy cell leukemia
  Marginal zone lymphoma (includes MALT lymphoma and monocytoid B-cell lymphoma)
  Diffuse large cell lymphoma (including the subgroup of large cell lymphoma with plasmacytoid differentiation)
  Primary mediastinal large B-cell lymphoma
  Burkitt's lymphoma
Mature T-cell neoplasms
  T-prolymphocytic leukemia
  Mycosis fungoides/Sezary syndrome
  Large granular leukemia, T-cell and NK types
  Adult T-cell lymphoma leukemia
  Anaplastic large cell lymphoma
  Peripheral T-cell lymphomas
  Angioimmunoblastic lymphoma
  Intestinal T-cell lymphoma (a $CD8^+$ lymphoma prevalent in areas with gluten-sensitive enteropathy)
  Angiocentric lymphoma (closely related to the aggressive LGL/NK leukemia)

Normocellular marrow pattern

The age of the patient is taken into account when estimating cellularity. In infants and young children, a cellularity in the range of 90–100% is still normocellular. The cellularity gradually decreases with age as fat cells increase in size and number. In adults, an overall cellularity of 30–70% is considered to be within the normal range. Even with advanced age the cellularity in healthy individuals remains in the low normal range (30–35%). The bone marrow may remain normocellular in both benign and malignant infiltrative processes (e.g. involvement by NHL, granulomata, infections and metastatic tumors), which are discussed in other chapters.

In the absence of obvious infiltration, a normocellular marrow may demonstrate:

1. Virtually no abnormalities, i.e. an essentially normal marrow, as seen in bone marrow donors, patients with underlying malignancies but negative staging marrows, or systemic disorders without specific hematological manifestations (e.g. anemia of chronic disease).
2. Variable degrees of qualitative and/or quantitative abnormalities. The conditions in this category include red cell aplasia, myeloid maturation arrest, metabolic bone disorders, Chediak-Higashi syndrome, AIDS, chemotherapy, viral infections and low-grade MDS.

The common qualitative and quantitative abnormalities are discussed in this chapter. These abnormalities can be present in hypocellular and hypercellular marrows in addition to normocellular marrows.

33.1 The essentially normal bone marrow

An essentially normal marrow is characterized mainly by negative findings:

1. The relative proportion of erythroid and myeloid precursors is not reversed. In most normal marrows, the M:E ratio ranges from 2:1 to 4:1. Disorders presenting with a normocellular marrow and increased erythroid elements are discussed in Chapter 35.
2. Megakaryocytes are adequate. Estimating the number of megakaryocytes is best done in conjunction with the platelet count. It is difficult to give an exact figure for the number of megakaryocytes per unit area in a normal marrow. However, marked deviations from normal are easily

appreciated. Disorders with increased megakaryocytes are discussed in Chapter 37.

3. The maturation of erythroid and myeloid precursors is not left-shifted. The morphologically recognizable stages of myeloid maturation are blasts, promyelocytes, myelocytes, metamyelocytes, bands and neutrophils. Promyelocytes, myelocytes and metamyelocytes are also known as intermediate myeloid precursors. The myeloid cell pool in the marrow is normally composed of more bands and neutrophils than myelocytes and metamyelocytes. Promyelocytes are infrequent.

The sequence of erythroid maturation includes proerythroblasts, basophilic erythroblasts, polychromatophilic erythroblasts and orthochromatic erythroblasts. The synthesis and accumulation of hemoglobin accounts for the gray cytoplasm of polychromatophilic erythroblasts. This process is accompanied by progressive condensation of the nuclear chromatin. In a normal marrow, the erythroid series is composed predominantly of late precursors (mostly polychromatophilic erythroblasts). Early erythroid precursors with basophilic cytoplasm normally account for about 10–15% of the erythroid elements.

4. Eosinophils or basophils are not present in excess. The top normal range of eosinophils is 7%. Basophils are normally rare, at most 1–2%.

5. No evidence of plasmacytosis or lymphocytosis. Plasma cells should comprise less than 10% of the marrow differential and no more than 20% lymphocytes should be present in adults. A higher proportion of lymphocytes is allowed in pediatric marrows. A few reactive lymphocytes (Downey cells) may be present, especially in children. Older individuals have a higher frequency of benign lymphoid aggregates. This age group also has a higher incidence of LPD/NHL, which can manifest as focal lymphoid infiltrates, however. Disorders with an increase in plasma cells or lymphocytes are discussed in Chapter 39.

6. No increase in the percentage of blasts (i.e. <5%). Disorders with increased blasts are discussed in Chapter 40.

7. No evidence of granulomata, infectious agents, hematological malignancies or metastatic tumors.

8. Cytologic abnormalities are virtually absent. If present, they are minimal and often represent long-term effects of intensive or cumulative chemotherapy. In such instances, the most common finding is mild nuclear/cytoplasmic asynchrony in erythroid precursors.

9. No overwhelming evidence of hemophagocytosis in macrophages.

10. The bone marrow framework is normal, i.e. without fibrosis or bony abnormalities.

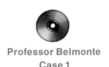

Professor Belmonte
Case 1

A routine iron stain on aspirate smears makes it feasible to identify disorders that would otherwise pass as essentially normal marrows. The evaluation is more accurate on aspirate smears stained with Prussian blue than on biopsy sections. In the normal marrow, iron storage is neither decreased/absent nor increased, and iron incorporation is not increased. RBCs may contain from one to four siderotic granules (best viewed with the 100× oil objective) but ring sideroblasts are not detectable.

33.1.1 Disorders with the morphology of an essentially normal marrow

The bone marrow in anemia of chronic disease (ACD) and most cases of iron deficiency has an essentially normal morphology, except for the abnormalities in iron storage and iron incorporation on Prussian blue stains. The presence of anemia alone rarely necessitates a bone marrow examination, unless the cause cannot be established from the clinical information and laboratory data or there is a suspicion of malignant disease. Anemia of chronic disease and iron deficiency are therefore 'incidental' diagnoses.

In iron deficiency, iron storage is markedly decreased or absent. RBCs with one to four siderotic granules are essentially nonexistent, indicating that iron incorporation is also markedly decreased. These features correspond to the patient's decreased serum and RBC ferritin.

While iron incorporation is also decreased in ACD, iron storage is increased. Excess iron is manifest as hemosiderin deposits (golden granules) on biopsy sections (Figure 33.1). The underlying etiologies of ACD are multiple, including AIDS, autoimmune disorders, chemotherapy, malignancies and metabolic disorders. The diagnosis is usually based on clinical information and other laboratory tests. The diagnosis of HIV infection can be inferred if opportunistic infectious agents are present in the bone marrow (see Chapter 42).

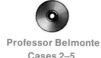

**Professor Belmonte
Cases 2–5**

The bone marrow in thalassemia minor can be essentially normal. Myeloproliferative disorders (CML, ET and PRV), either in their early stages or following treatment, can also exhibit a normal-appearing bone marrow.

33.2 Normocellular marrow with abnormalities of the stromal component

The nonhematopoietic component of the bone marrow includes the bony trabeculae, osteoblasts, osteoclasts, fat cells, fibroblasts, mast cells and histiocytes/

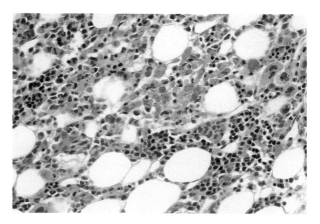

Figure 33.1 Abundant hemosiderin granules in the bone marrow of an HIV-positive patient. There is also a mild reactive plasmacytosis

macrophages. Apart from the bony trabeculae and fat cells, the other elements are inconspicuous under normal conditions.

Abnormalities of the stromal component include:

1. Occasional macrophages with erythrophagocytosis. The presence of widespread hemophagocytosis should raise the suspicion of an infection-associated hemophagocytic syndrome, however (see Chapter 42).
2. Alterations of the fatty tissue reflecting recent bone marrow injury secondary to chemotherapy (see Chapter 34).
3. A variable degree of reticulin fibrosis (Figure 33.2). Under normal conditions, reticulin fibers are nearly nonexistent except around blood vessels. Mild reticulin fibrosis, occurring as part of a transient repair process, is a common finding in patients exposed to chemotherapy and/or radiotherapy for systemic malignancies. More intense reticulin fibrosis occurs mainly in association with MPDs and NHL. The common non-neoplastic conditions with increased bone marrow reticulin include AIDS, Paget's disease and renal osteodystrophy.
4. Alterations in the thickness of the trabeculae. The bony trabeculae are often overlooked during bone marrow evaluation. In children, osteoblasts, osteoclasts and woven bone are easily identified, indicating active new bone formation, mineralization and remodeling. In contrast, very few osteoblasts and osteoclasts are found in adults and only pyknotic osteocytes are seen within the bone matrix. In the absence of malignancies which can induce osteosclerosis (e.g. mast cell infiltration, metastatic tumors and AMM)

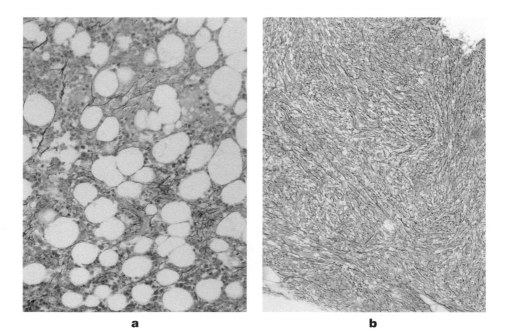

a   b

Figure 33.2 Increased reticulin: (a) mild; (b) severe

or osteoporosis (e.g. acute leukemia), the main causes of altered bone resorption and new bone formation include Paget's disease and renal osteodystrophy.

33.2.1 Metabolic bone disorders

Metabolic bone disorders are usually incidental findings in a bone marrow being evaluated for other reasons. It is preferable to confirm the diagnosis with laboratory/radiological data and clinical information.

Paget's disease is a rare disorder, more common in males than females. The pelvis is the most commonly affected bone. The abnormality consists of excessive bone resorption which is compensated by defective new bone formation (poorly mineralized osteoid matrix) and extensive fibrosis, resulting in enlargement and softening of the affected bones. The hematological manifestations are nonspecific, usually mild NCNC anemia. Bone marrow aspiration from the affected pelvis yields scanty material. Hematopoietic elements are decreased but appear normal. The biopsy demonstrates fibroblastic proliferation and thickened bony trabeculae with widened osteoid seams (increased woven bone). In addition, there is osteoblastic rimming along with osteoclasts scalloping the medullary surface of the trabeculae (Figure 33.3). A mosaic pattern of the trabeculae, which results from the haphazard bone resorption and new bone formation, is essentially pathognomonic of Paget's disease.

Chronic renal failure can result in secondary hyperparathyroidism, which in turn results in demineralization and progressive resorption of bones. This condition is known as renal osteodystrophy (Figure 33.4). The morphologic manifestations include thin bony trabeculae, increased osteoblastic and osteoclastic activity, and deposition of poorly mineralized osteoid at the periphery. Paratrabecular collagen fibrosis is common.

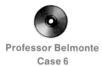

Professor Belmonte
Case 6

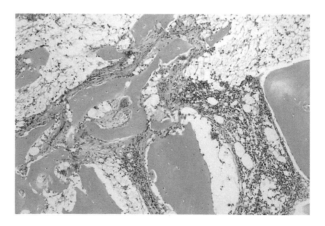

Figure 33.3 Paget's disease: thickened bony trabeculae rimmed by osteoblasts and osteoclasts. Loose fibroblastic proliferation adjacent to the trabeculae can also be seen

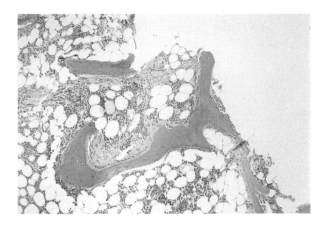

Figure 33.4 Renal osteodystrophy: thinned bony trabeculae with osteoblastic rimming and adjacent loose fibroblastic proliferation

33.2.2 Hemophagocytosis/erythrophagocytosis

Phagocytosis of hematopoietic elements can be seen in both benign and malignant disorders. The hemophagocytosis in reactive conditions occurs in benign-appearing macrophages (Figure 33.5). In malignant disorders, the phagocytosis is nearly always associated with the neoplastic cells. The process affects primarily erythroid cells, especially mature RBCs. Therefore, hemophagocytosis and erythrophagocytosis are essentially synonymous.

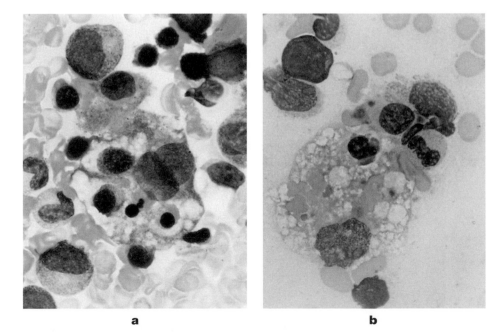

a   b

Figure 33.5 Erythrophagocytosis from two different patients. (a) HIV-positive patient. (b) Immunocompetent patient with infectious mononucleosis

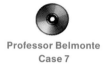

Professor Belmonte
Case 7

A variable degree of hemophagocytosis can be found in a host of conditions, such as immune hemolytic anemia (e.g. following transfusion), drug-induced immune neutropenia, and infections (most commonly viral). In immune neutropenia, the ingested elements consist mainly of granulocytes. The more severe the infection and the less immunocompetent the patient is, the more extensive the hemophagocytosis. The acute manifestation of severe infections in subjects with either congenital or acquired immunosuppression is known as infection-associated hemophagocytic syndrome (IAHS).

In addition to hemophagocytosis, the bone marrow in viral infections often demonstrates mild lymphocytosis or scattered large reactive lymphoid cells. These may simulate the morphology of large lymphoma cells.

33.3 Quantitative abnormalities in hematopoietic precursors

The main quantitative abnormalities consist of an altered relative proportion of erythroid and myeloid elements, and alterations in the number of megakaryocytes. The quantitative changes may be accompanied by cytologic abnormalities. The quantitative alterations include:

1. **Bone marrow eosinophilia**. A host of benign conditions can present with mild to moderate bone marrow eosinophilia, including skin disorders, allergens/medications, infectious/parasitic agents, chemotherapy and Hodgkin's disease without bone marrow involvement. Peripheral blood eosinophilia is often present. The hypereosinophilic syndrome is a diagnosis of exclusion (see Chapter 10 and Section 36.2.3).
2. **A reversed M:E ratio**. Several conditions share the picture of a normocellular marrow with erythroid preponderance. These include HIV infection (see Chapter 42), PNH, bone marrow recovery following chemotherapy/bone marrow transplantation, MDS, and neutropenia of various causes. Some of these disorders also share peripheral blood manifestations, e.g. cytopenias and macrocytosis. The erythroid predominance may be accompanied by a variable degree of qualitative abnormalities.
3. **Marked hypoplasia of the erythroid series**. Pure red cell aplasia (RCA), which can be either congenital or acquired, characteristically presents as a normocellular marrow with erythroid hypoplasia. A decrease in erythroid precursors may also be a feature of stem cell disorders (e.g. 5q– syndrome) secondary to the marked proliferation of abnormal myeloid precursors.
4. **Increased or decreased megakaryocytes**. In most instances, quantitative changes in megakaryocytes occur in association with abnormalities of the myeloid and/or erythroid series as part of a stem cell disorder (e.g. aplastic anemia, MPD, MDS), multilineage injury (e.g. chemotherapy/drug effect) or bone marrow infiltration. An isolated increase or decrease in megakaryocytes is more suggestive of a reactive process than a stem cell malignancy. Disorders with increased megakaryocytes are discussed in Chapters 37 and 38.

33.3.1 Congenital red cell aplasia (Diamond-Blackfan anemia)

Congenital RCA manifests within the first year of life as a severe macrocytic anemia in which the RBCs retain high levels of Hgb F and expression of the i antigen. The WBC and platelet counts are within normal limits. The bone marrow cellularity is normal for age (i.e. packed) with abundant hematogones but a marked decrease in erythroid precursors, composed mostly of early forms, some with cytoplasmic vacuoles. This bone marrow morphology is indistinguishable from acquired RCA occurring in young children. Serum erythropoietin is increased and skeletal abnormalities may be present.

It is important to differentiate congenital RCA from Fanconi's anemia, which in its initial stage may manifest as RCA. Sequential blood counts or bone marrow studies, and especially a chromosomal breakage study (positive in Fanconi's anemia) are helpful in making this distinction. Current therapeutic strategies for congenital RCA include corticosteroids, growth factors and bone marrow transplantation.

33.3.2 Acquired red cell aplasia

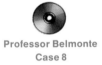

**Professor Belmonte
Case 8**

The pathogenesis and duration of acquired RCA (Figure 33.6) differs between children and adults. In adults, the disorder is chronic and associated with a variety of underlying processes. Immune mechanisms are presumably involved in the pathogenesis. The diagnostic work-up should focus on the search for a cause, such as thymoma, drugs, HIV infection (see Chapter 42), underlying malignancies, and autoimmune disorders (with or without an associated proliferation of LGLs).

In childhood, acquired RCA is a self-limited disorder, frequently associated with a recent viral infection. One manifestation, the disorder known as 'transient erythroblastopenia of childhood', occurs in children without underlying RBC abnormalities. It is possible that parvovirus B19 is involved in this form of RCA. However, in the few cases investigated, the serologic and viral studies have been negative. During an acute episode, the morphologic manifestations in the bone marrow and peripheral blood are similar to those of congenital RCA. A spontaneous recovery occurs within a month with a marked reticulocytosis and rebound erythroid hyperplasia in the bone marrow.

RCA superimposed on a pre-existing hemolytic anemia can be secondary to either parvovirus infection or folate deficiency, manifesting as a sudden exacerbation or a gradual worsening of the anemia, respectively.

33.3.2.1 Parvovirus-associated RCA

The viral infection responsible for acquired RCA in pre-existing severe chronic hemolytic anemia (e.g. sickle cell disease, hereditary spherocytosis) or ineffective erythropoiesis (e.g. thalassemia, CDA) is caused by parvovirus B19 (Figure 33.6). Infection with parvovirus B19 is common, especially in late winter or early spring. The virus has selective tropism for erythroid progenitors and repli-

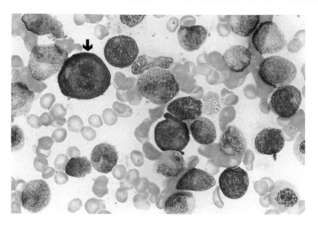

Figure 33.6 Acquired red cell aplasia associated with parvovirus infection in a 7-year-old male. One of the four early erythroid precursors in this field is enlarged (arrow) with visible intranuclear viral inclusions

cates while the infected cells are in S-phase. Synthesis of nonstructural viral proteins impairs the survival of host cells. The number of erythroid precursors in S-phase is increased in patients with either stressed or ineffective erythropoiesis. Therefore, these patients are more susceptible to parvovirus infection.

The selective affinity for erythroid cells appears to be related to the P blood group antigen, which functions as a cellular receptor for parvovirus B19. The clinical manifestations of parvovirus infection reflect the balance between viral suppression of erythropoiesis and the status of both the host's immune system and erythropoietic activity. In normal subjects, the infection is biphasic, with an initial phase of viremia and suppression of erythropoiesis. This results in a transient reticulocytopenia and a slight decrease in hemoglobin. This phase lasts for 1–2 weeks, followed by the appearance of IgM and IgG antibodies against the virus. The second phase is accompanied by a rash and arthralgia. These symptoms are presumably secondary to immune complex formation.

Because of the long lifespan of RBCs in normal individuals, a brief suppression of erythropoiesis usually does not cause clinical manifestations. In contrast, in individuals with an underlying hemolytic anemia or impaired erythropoiesis, any transient interruption in erythropoiesis can lead to a profound drop in hemoglobin. Therefore, in the predisposed patient, parvovirus-induced RCA can be suspected clinically by a sudden exacerbation of the existing anemia.

Parvovirus-induced RCA can also occur in immunocompromised patients (e.g. chemotherapy, SLE, HIV infection) without underlying hemolytic anemia. Because of the lack of an effective antibody response to the virus, the infection can persist, resulting in a profound chronic anemia. A rash and arthralgia are not present initially. They may appear, however, as the patient recovers immunologically or during high-dose intravenous immunoglobulin therapy. Relapse is common if the immunodeficiency persists. The situation may require indefinite immunoglobulin therapy.

In parvovirus-induced RCA, intranuclear viral inclusions may be present in erythroid precursors. Identification of the inclusions can be facilitated by appropriate immunostaining. The diagnosis can be further confirmed by the detection of IgM and IgG antibodies in the patient's serum. Testing for viral DNA in the blood or bone marrow is the method of choice if the patient is immunocompromised, however.

33.3.3 Megakaryocytic hypoplasia

Isolated megakaryocytic hypoplasia, either congenital or acquired, is an uncommon condition. The congenital megakaryocytic hypoplasias are a heterogeneous group of rare disorders with various modes of inheritance, characterized by congenital cardiac and/or skeletal anomalies (e.g. absent radii), neonatal thrombocytopenia, and markedly decreased to absent megakaryocytes in an otherwise normal marrow. Because of coexisting skeletal abnormalities, the main differential to consider is Fanconi's anemia (see Chapter 34).

In addition to immune mechanisms, some drugs and infectious agents can sporadically cause selective suppression of megakaryopoiesis. One of the offending agents is alcohol. Alcohol-induced thrombocytopenia is multifactorial, involving both peripheral destruction and inadequate compensatory megakaryocytic proliferation. The effects of alcohol are usually also evident in the erythroid lineage.

Acquired megakaryocytic hypoplasia may be secondary to viral infections, such as measles, varicella, EBV, CMV, hepatitis and HIV. Direct viral invasion in megakaryocytes may result in nonspecific cytologic abnormalities such as cytoplasmic vacuoles. Viral infections can also induce destruction of platelets via an immune mechanism. The latter is the most common pathogenesis of thrombocytopenia in HIV patients.

Rarely, pure megakaryocytic hypoplasia can develop in patients with underlying disseminated SLE.

33.4 Qualitative abnormalities in hematopoietic precursors

Qualitative abnormalities in hematopoietic precursors have been termed 'dysplastic' changes because they have been extensively described in myelodysplastic syndromes. It should be noted, however, that such abnormalities are seen frequently in benign/reactive conditions, such as B_{12}/folate deficiency, HIV infection, hemolytic anemias, administration of growth factors and chemotherapy. Furthermore, the peripheral blood manifestations of some of these disorders often overlap with those of MDS. Therefore, the presence of 'dysplastic' features is not synonymous with MDS.

Note that the abnormalities described below are not restricted to normocellular marrows. They can occur against a background of a hypocellular or hypercellular marrow.

33.4.1 Abnormalities in the erythroid precursors

Under normal conditions, most of the erythroid cells are polychromatophilic erythroblasts. Early erythroid precursors account for about 10–15% of the erythroid elements. It is unusual for early erythroid precursors to outnumber late precursors even in left-shifted maturation. In general, erythroid maturation can be considered left-shifted when the early precursors represent approximately one-third of the total erythroid cells. This abnormality is usually present in association with erythroid preponderance or erythroid hyperplasia (see Chapter 35), and accompanied by one or more qualitative changes. Very few of these 'dyserythropoietic' features are specific for any given disease, however. Among the following abnormalities, some (e.g. nuclear/cytoplasmic asynchrony and nuclear lobulation) are more 'ubiquitous' than others:

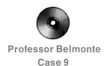

Professor Belmonte
Case 9

1. Nuclear/cytoplasmic asynchrony (Figure 33.7), i.e. the nuclear maturation lags behind that of the cytoplasm. As a result, the chromatin remains 'open' with a speckled appearance, instead of becoming condensed in the late erythroid stage. This is the most ubiquitous abnormality, seen in stressed erythropoiesis as well as ineffective erythropoiesis. Because the affected cells are also slightly enlarged, this feature has been referred to as 'megaloblastoid' maturation.

2. Giant precursors, i.e. erythroid or myeloid cells that demonstrate an overt increase in cell size. Giant precursors with nuclear/cytoplasmic asynchrony represent megaloblastic maturation (Figure 33.8). The morphology is best appreciated in late erythroid cells. Megaloblastic maturation is striking in

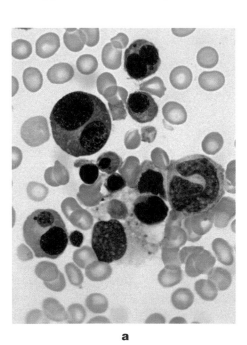
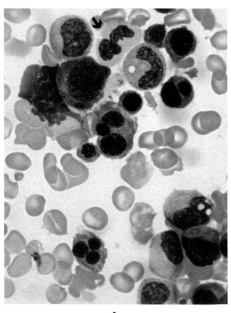

a

b

Figure 33.7 Bone marrow aspirate from a 6-year-old male in the recovery phase following induction chemotherapy for ALL. (a) Erythroid precursors with nuclear/cytoplasmic asynchrony, binucleation and karyorrhexis. Note the giant myeloid precursor. (b) Binucleated and multinucleated erythroid precursors. One of the granulocytes is also hypogranulated (arrow). The features are identical to those seen in myelodysplastic syndromes

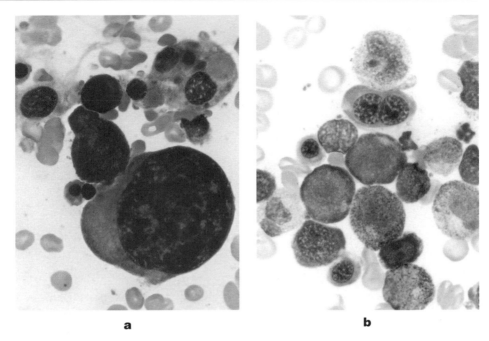

a   b

Figure 33.8 (a) An enormous erythroid precursor in a myelodysplastic syndrome. The appearance of the nuclear chromatin is in concordance with that of the cytoplasm, however. (b) Increased erythroid precursors with megaloblastic maturation resulting from a case of B_{12} deficiency. Note the giant myeloid precursor

B_{12}/folate deficiency, unless there is coexisting iron deficiency. A similar picture can also be seen in erythroleukemia (AML-M6). In other conditions, such as chemotherapy, MDS, and HIV infection, small numbers of megaloblastic erythroid precursors can be present.

3. Cytoplasmic vacuolization, primarily in early erythroid precursors, is a feature associated with AML-M6, exposure to toxic agents (benzene, chemotherapy), alcohol abuse, malnutrition and antibiotics (especially chloramphenicol). Other abnormalities include basophilic stippling, karyorrhexis, nuclear lobulation, binucleation (Figure 33.7) and multinucleation. These abnormalities are seen mainly among late erythroid precursors and can occur in both stressed and ineffective erythropoiesis.

4. Increased iron incorporation indicates either iron overload (e.g. repeated transfusions) or impaired iron metabolism due to ineffective erythropoiesis. The siderotic granules in RBCs are increased (more than four granules) and coarser than normal. In ring sideroblasts, the accumulation of siderotic granules takes place in mitochondria, resulting in a ring (or partial ring) around the nucleus. The diagnosis of sideroblastic anemia, either acquired or congenital, rests on the presence of abundant ring sideroblasts (see Chapter 35) on Prussian blue stained aspirate smears (Figure 33.9).

5. Late erythroid precursors with unevenly stained cytoplasm indicating poor hemoglobinization (Figure 33.10). This feature can result from advanced iron deficiency as well as ineffective erythropoiesis secondary to hemoglobin

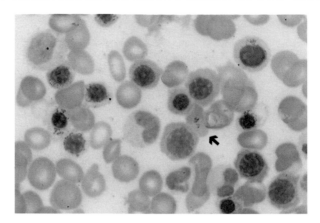

Figure 33.9 Ring sideroblasts and increased iron incorporation (arrow) from a case of RARS

synthesis defects or altered DNA synthesis (thalassemias, congenital or acquired sideroblastic anemia). Another finding in iron deficiency is erythroid cells with ragged cytoplasmic contours.

33.4.2 Abnormalities in myeloid maturation

Left-shifted myeloid maturation is present when intermediate myeloid precursors outnumber mature granulocytes in the bone marrow. The causes include altered proliferation of myeloid elements, drug-induced myelosuppression, excessive intramedullary cell death and early release of mature precursors into the peripheral blood. A severe left shift results in a maturation arrest picture with a preponderance of myelocytes and a lesser number of promyelocytes (Figure 33.11). Table 33.1 lists the morphologic criteria that distinguish myelocytes from promyelocytes.

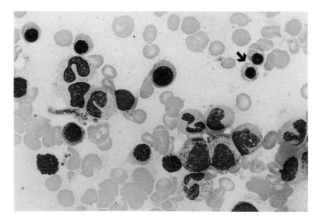

Figure 33.10 Iron deficiency: a few late erythroid precursors with defective hemoglobinization (arrow)

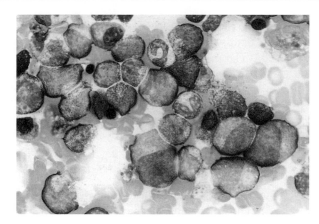

Figure 33.11 Severe left-shifted myeloid maturation secondary to sepsis in an immunosuppressed patient

Table 33.1 Features that allow the distinction between myelocytes and promyelocytes

Promyelocytes
Promyelocytes have a higher nuclear/cytoplasmic ratio and less condensed chromatin. The cytoplasm is basophilic with abundant azurophilic primary granules. A prominent Golgi hof is frequent.
Myelocytes
The appearance of secondary granules confers a pale orange hue (initially focal, then diffuse as the number of secondary granules increases) to the cytoplasm of myelocytes. Early myelocytes still contain ample primary granules. In myelocytes, the nucleus is often eccentrically located, and one side of the nucleus can appear flattened.

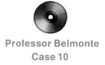

Professor Belmonte
Case 10

A marked preponderance of promyelocytes in excess of myelocytes is unusual in maturation arrest. Even when promyelocytes are abundant, the proportion rarely exceeds 30%. Acute promyelocytic leukemia (AML-M3) is in the differential diagnosis when promyelocytes reach 30% of the bone marrow differential count. Normal promyelocytes can be distinguished from the heavily granulated neoplastic cells in AML-M3 by their Golgi hof and the lack of nuclear irregularities.

A variable degree of left-shifted myeloid maturation can be observed in many conditions including infections, AIDS (see Chapter 42), MDS, MPD, G-CSF administration (see Chapter 36), chemotherapy (see Chapter 34) and congenital/acquired neutropenias (see Chapter 13). Kostmann's disease, chronic benign granulocytopenia of infancy and childhood and cyclic neutropenia are the main constitutional neutropenias.

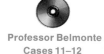

Professor Belmonte
Cases 11–12

In the evaluation of neutropenia, a bone marrow examination (to exclude an infiltrative process) is more commonly performed in adults than in children. The diagnosis of the various types of non-neoplastic neutropenia, whether constitutional or acquired, rests primarily on the clinical picture and family studies (if indicated), since these disorders share similar blood and bone marrow pictures.

The bone marrow in non-neoplastic neutropenia is normocellular in the great majority of cases. The M:E ratio can be normal or reversed (erythroid preponderance). The myeloid population is composed primarily of myelocytes and a lesser number of promyelocytes and metamyelocytes. The mature elements (neutrophils and bands) are few, often accounting for no more than 10% of the total myeloid cells. The proportion of blasts remains below 5%. In affected children, the bone marrow contains an increased number of hematogones (Figure 33.12) which can be easily misidentified as blasts. The bone marrow in adult patients may demonstrate a relative increase in LGLs with or without a mild lymphocytosis. An occasional benign lymphoid aggregate may be present.

33.4.3 Cytologic abnormalities in myeloid precursors

Qualitative abnormalities in myeloid cells reflect impaired hematopoiesis with different underlying mechanisms such as an altered bone marrow microenvironment and altered DNA synthesis (drug therapy, stem cell disorders). Cytologic abnormalities in myeloid precursors (i.e. 'dysgranulopoietic' features) include:

1. Nuclear/cytoplasmic asynchrony and giant precursors (Figure 33.13a). In most cases, these two features coexist and indicate megaloblastic maturation. Indeed, nuclear/cytoplasmic asynchrony in myeloid cells can be difficult to recognize if the cells are not enlarged. These features are best appreciated in metamyelocytes and bands. Impaired DNA synthesis also manifests as excessive contortions of the nuclei at the band stage.

   Megaloblastic maturation is most striking in B_{12}/folate deficiency (see Chapter 35) where hypersegmented neutrophils are usually present in both the bone marrow and peripheral blood. A small number of myeloid

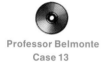

Professor Belmonte
Case 13

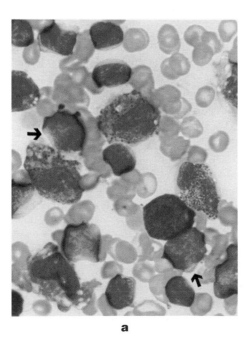

a

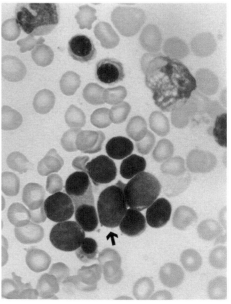

b

Figure 33.12 Increased hematogones (arrow) in two different children with congenital neutropenia (a) and neuroblastoma (b)

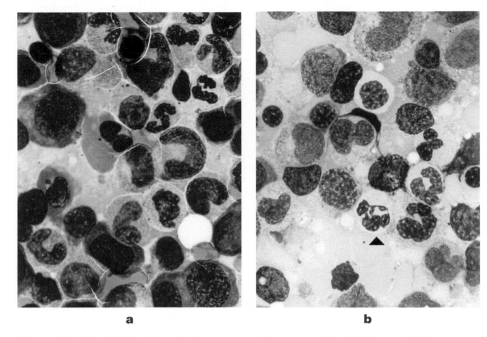

a   b

Figure 33.13   (a) Giant myeloid precursors in a case of B$_{12}$ deficiency. (b) Hypogranulated myeloid precursors (arrowhead) in a myelodysplastic syndrome

precursors with megaloblastic changes can be observed in other conditions, such as hydroxyurea therapy, AIDS and MDS. G-CSF therapy also induces large cells but this feature is overshadowed by the prominent hypergranulation.

2. Hypogranulation (Figure 33.13b). Hypogranulated myeloid precursors are a frequent feature in MDS, AIDS and MPD. When assessing this feature, one should be careful to exclude hypogranulation caused by suboptimal staining (alkaline pH of the staining buffer). In MDS and AIDS, the hypogranulated granulocytes are also hyposegmented. Hypogranulation can be so extreme as to yield a negative peroxidase reaction.

3. Hyposegmentation (Figure 15.5). Frequent hyposegmented neutrophils indicate either congenital Pelger-Huët anomaly or pseudo-Pelger-Huët anomaly. Pseudo-Pelger-Huët anomaly is a common manifestation in MDS, AML and HIV infection. Rarely, it may also represent a residual effect of previous myeloablative chemotherapy or bone marrow transplantation in patients without evidence of therapy-related MDS.

4. Binucleation, nuclear fragments, and neutrophils with ring nuclei (Figure 33.14). Binucleated myeloid precursors may be seen in AIDS, MDS and G-CSF therapy. Nuclear fragments (Figure 12.5) are indicative of recent exposure to intensive chemotherapy or toxic substances. Neutrophils with ring nuclei have been described frequently in MDS. This feature is also present in other conditions, however.

5. Abnormal granulation. The presence of large abnormal orange-pink cytoplasmic granules in the peripheral blood and bone marrow leukocytes of a

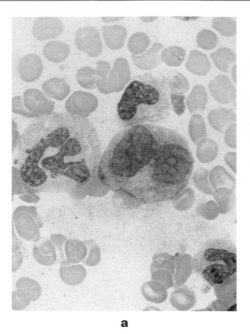
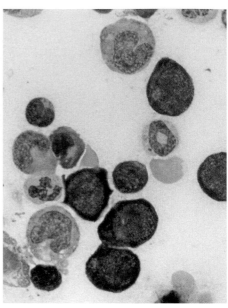

a   b

Figure 33.14 (a) Two binucleated myeloid precursors in an immunosuppressed patient (HIV-negative). (b) One neutrophil with a ring-shaped nucleus and a nuclear fragment in B_{12} deficiency (note the giant myeloid precursors)

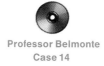

Professor Belmonte
Case 14

child should elicit the suspicion of Chediak-Higashi syndrome (Figure 33.15). This rare fatal disorder, characterized by defective granule formation in leukocytes and melanocytes, is readily diagnosable in the peripheral blood (see Section 12.3).

33.4.4 Cytologic abnormalities in megakaryocytes

Megakaryocytes are the most easily recognizable hematopoietic elements in the bone marrow because of their large cell size and multilobulated nuclei. The cytoplasm is normally deep purple-blue and granular on aspirate smears. The less mature-appearing megakaryocytes are hypolobulated or mononuclear. They can be easily overlooked because of their smaller size, especially on biopsy sections.

Qualitative abnormalities in megakaryocytes are most commonly observed in association with abnormalities of the other lineages. The abnormal cytology is manifest primarily as small megakaryocytes, either monolobed or bilobed. Such cells are referred to as micromegakaryocytes or dwarf megakaryocytes. The cytoplasm is usually ample and hypogranular, possibly with prominent cytoplasmic vacuoles.

Abnormal megakaryocytes have been emphasized in MDS and AML as part of the trilineage dysplasia. Several other conditions, such as regenerative bone marrows, AIDS, chemotherapy, CML and ITP can exhibit similar features, however.

Monolobed megakaryocytes with cytoplasmic vacuoles (Figure 33.16a) may be seen in ITP, as well as stem cell disorders. The mononuclear megakaryocytes in CML are virtually indistinguishable from those seen in MDS. In the proper

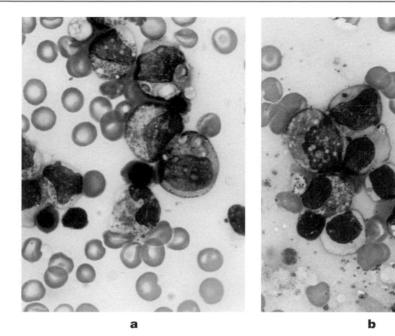

a   b

Figure 33.15   Chediak-Higashi syndrome in a 5-year-old male, exhibiting prominent azurophilic granules in intermediate myeloid precursors (a) and reactive lymphoid cells (b). In eosinophils (b), the granules appear gray

clinical context, however, megakaryocytic abnormalities can be a useful morphological adjunct in identifying a specific entity such as the 5q– syndrome (see Section 37.2.2.1).

Megakaryocytes with disconnected nuclear lobes are less frequently observed (Figure 33.16b). This appearance, that of a multinucleated giant cell, simulates the morphology of cells such as osteoclasts and Langhan's giant cells. Helpful clues to differentiate megakaryocytes with disconnected nuclear lobes from other cell types are listed in Table 33.2.

Table 33.2 Clues to help differentiate megakaryocytes with disconnected nuclei from other giant cells

- Osteoclasts and multinucleated giant cells are rarely aspiratable.
- Osteoblasts are typically located along the rim of bony trabeculae on biopsy sections.
- Multinucleated giant cells occur in association with granulomata.
- Megakaryocytes with disconnected nuclei occur in MDS and megaloblastic anemias where obvious abnormalities in erythroid and myeloid precursors are also evident.

33.5 The diagnosis of MDS in a normocellular marrow

The term MDS implies a clonal stem cell disorder. The subtypes (as defined by the FAB group) can be separated into high-grade and low-grade MDS. The

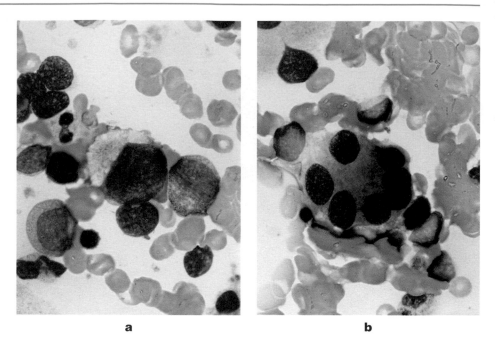

a   b

Figure 33.16 (a) A monolobed megakaryocyte with prominent cytoplasmic vacuoles in a myelodysplastic syndrome. (b) A megakaryocyte with disconnected nuclear lobes from the same case

majority of high-grade MDSs demonstrate a hypercellular marrow with an increased number of blasts. These disorders are discussed in Section 36.1.2.

Low-grade MDS consists of refractory anemia and refractory anemia with ring sideroblasts (RARS). While the diagnostic criteria for RARS have been well established (see Section 35.2.3.1), the diagnosis of refractory anemia can be problematic unless there are overwhelming qualitative abnormalities.

A mild to severe anemia can be the sole peripheral blood abnormality in refractory anemia. Although the anemia is usually macrocytic, it can also be normocytic. The bone marrow has been described as either normocellular or hypercellular with variable degrees of dyserythropoiesis, with or without abnormalities in the myeloid and megakaryocytic series. Iron stores are normal or increased. The relative proportion of erythroid elements can be increased, normal or decreased. These same findings can be seen in patients with a variety of disorders including RCA, AIDS, alcohol abuse, and patients exposed to multiple chemotherapy regimens over a long period (Figure 33.17). In these patients, the morphologic abnormalities are usually transient and nonprogressive. Caution should be taken not to over-interpret these changes as therapy-related MDS unless cytogenetic abnormalities are also present.

An iron stain on aspirate smears can be helpful to identify refractory anemia. While the iron stores are normal or increased, similar to ACD, increased iron incorporation in the absence of repeated transfusions points to the diagnosis of refractory anemia. The granules are usually coarse and there may be a few ring sideroblasts (albeit fewer than those seen in RARS). These features are not always present, however.

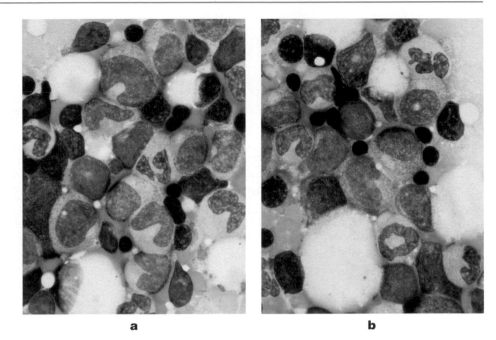

a   b

Figure 33.17 Bone marrow aspirate from a patient with long-standing low-grade lymphoma exposed to multiple chemotherapy regimens. Frequent hypogranulated myeloid cells are visible with an occasional giant form (a) and one myeloid cell with a ring-shaped nucleus (b). There were no cytogenetic abnormalities and the patient has remained clinically stable for several years

The definitive diagnosis of refractory anemia is therefore a challenging one, especially in a normocellular marrow. To make this diagnosis requires ample clinical information and laboratory data at the time of the bone marrow and peripheral blood evaluation. For practical purposes, it is often preferable to render a descriptive diagnosis (e.g. 'normocellular marrow with erythroid preponderance and dyserythropoietic features') along with a comment to include the diagnostic possibilities, rather than basing the diagnosis of a clonal stem cell disorder on morphology alone.

CHAPTER 21

Hypocellular marrow pattern

Since an aspicular/hemodilute aspirate can reflect either a markedly hypocellular marrow or a suboptimal bone marrow procedure, the assessment of a hypocellular bone marrow is best made on a representative biopsy. A biopsy of adequate length is critical since the cellularity of the marrow may not be homogeneous. Bone marrow smears made at the bedside have a higher probability of being aspicular/hemodilute. The technique of concentrating spicules described in Section 32.5 is useful to ensure the best morphology in hypocellular marrows, especially when evaluating hypocellular MDS, hypocellular acute leukemia, and residual disease (Figure 34.1). Since a hypocellular marrow may exhibit increased reticulin, especially in HIV patients, touch imprints of the biopsy should be made routinely.

34.1 Differential diagnosis of a hypocellular marrow

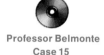

**Professor Belmonte
Case 15**

It is generally accepted that a marrow cellularity of less than 30% indicates hypocellularity. The differential includes neoplastic and non-neoplastic diseases (Table 34.1).

34.1.1 Hypocellular leukemia and hypocellular MDS

About 10% of AMLs present with a hypocellular bone marrow. Similarly, reported cases of hypoplastic MDS account for about 10% of all MDSs. Hypocellular acute leukemia and hypoplastic MDS are relatively more common in the elderly. Rare cases of ALL in children may also present initially with a hypocellular marrow. The criteria for the diagnosis of hypocellular leukemia and hypocellular high-grade MDS (Figure 34.1) are no different than those applied to these entities when they present with hypercellular marrows (see Chapters 36 and 40). Therefore, good smear preparations are essential to assess

---

Table 34.1 Differential diagnosis of a hypocellular marrow

- Chronic debilitating disorders such as HIV infection, malnutrition, anorexia nervosa.
- Aplastic anemia, paroxysmal nocturnal hemoglobinuria.
- Hypocellular acute leukemia and hypoplastic myelodysplastic syndromes.
- Following myeloablative high-dose multiagent chemotherapy or bone marrow transplantation with or without residual disease. Therapy-induced bone marrow suppression accounts for the majority of hypocellular marrows in most hematology laboratories.

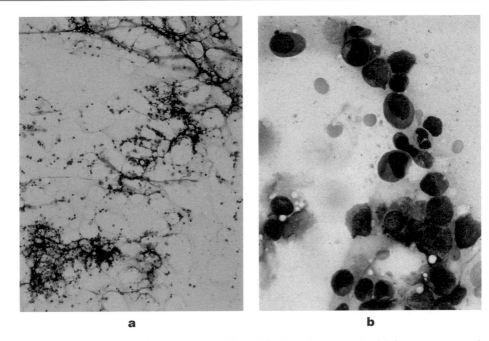

a   b

Figure 34.1 Hypocellular marrow with residual acute leukemia. (a) Smear prepared from the bone marrow collected in EDTA, using the technique of concentrating spicules. In this case, the bone marrow smears prepared at the bedside were all aspicular and hemodilute. (b) Residual blasts admixed with immature myeloid precursors

the proportion of blasts. On biopsy sections, clusters of abnormally located immature myeloid precursors (so-called ALIP) are usually present in these disorders.

The diagnosis of hypocellular low-grade MDS (i.e. without excess blasts) is to be made with caution in the absence of typical cytogenetic abnormalities, since the morphologic features can overlap with those of aplastic anemia or HIV infection. A variable degree of cytologic abnormalities, the sparse number of cells available for evaluation and the subjective grading of qualitative abnormalities are some of the factors to account for the diagnostic difficulty. The great majority of hypocellular MDSs are therapy-related and are invariably associated with cytogenetic aberrations, especially those of chromosomes 5 and 7. Therefore, hypocellular low-grade MDS is more reliably diagnosed based on chromosomal abnormalities or sequential bone marrow studies. Sequential bone marrow examinations usually reveal a progression from hypocellular to hypercellular MDS. Following this progression, a substantial number of cases evolve into overt acute (hypercellular) leukemia.

34.2 Morphologic features in hypocellular marrows

The degree of hypocellularity reflects the severity of the decreased hematopoiesis. As a result, lymphocytes and plasma cells appear relatively more prominent, even though their absolute numbers remain essentially unchanged from those in normal bone marrow. In general, the decreased hematopoiesis is most pronounced in the myeloid and megakaryocytic lineages. Hypocellular marrows usually contain scattered islands of hematopoiesis, composed mostly of erythroid precursors (Figure 34.2). This morphology is not specific to aplastic anemia or PNH. Early regenerative bone marrows and AIDS-related hypocellular marrows can display an identical appearance. Iron stores are invariably increased. In addition to this relative erythroid preponderance, hypocellular marrows may demonstrate some of the following features:

- **Increased mast cells**. Mast cells adhere to the stromal particles and are best appreciated on aspirate smears. In the context of a hypocellular marrow, an increased number of mast cells is a feature supportive of aplastic anemia.
- **Stromal injury**. This feature suggests that the hypocellularity is secondary to toxic agents such as chemotherapy. The authors use the term 'chemotherapy effects' (Figure 34.3a) to designate the various morphological features of stromal damage seen in post-chemotherapy bone marrows, including fibrinoid necrosis, edema and fat necrosis. Fibrinoid necrosis can be distinguished from true bone marrow necrosis. In bone marrow necrosis secondary to either a rapidly growing neoplasm that outstrips its blood supply or ischemic vascular occlusion from sickle cells or tumor emboli, the outline of the bone marrow architectural framework and the shadow of cells can still be recognized.

Other features indicating injury to the bone marrow stroma include serous atrophy (also known as gelatinous transformation) and increased reticulin. The background in serous atrophy (Figure 34.3b) appears amorphous and glassy, admixed with small adipocytes. Serous atrophy is prominent in patients with severe malnutrition or chronic debilitating illness. Increased reticulin fibrosis is a common feature in AIDS-associated hypocellular marrows. Chemotherapy can also induce a transient increase in reticulin.

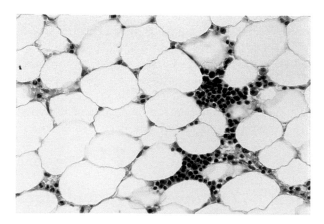

Figure 34.2 Hypocellular marrow with small islands of erythropoiesis in a regenerative marrow following chemotherapy

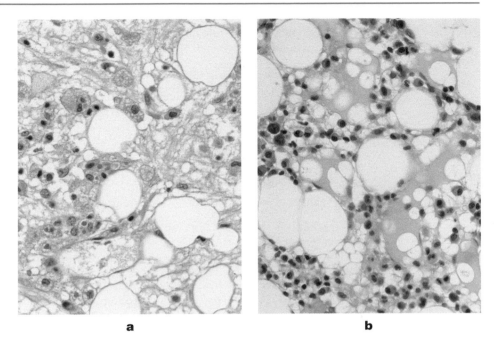

Figure 34.3 (a) Chemotherapy effects with damage to the fatty stroma. Histiocytes, plasma cells and fibroblasts constitute the main residual cellular elements. (b) Serous fat atrophy in an HIV-positive patient

- **Lymphoid aggregates**. Benign lymphoid aggregates are uncommon in a hypocellular marrow. Lymphoid aggregates more often represent residual or relapsed disease (e.g. low-grade LPD/NHL) after chemotherapy. The nature of the lymphoid infiltrate can be established by FCM immunophenotyping.
- **Qualitative abnormalities in hematopoietic precursors**. Erythroid precursors, and less frequently myeloid precursors, may display nuclear/cytoplasmic asynchrony and nuclear lobulation. Florid cytologic abnormalities are unusual in aplastic anemia, but common in other conditions such as postchemotherapy, HIV infection, and hypocellular therapy-related MDS.

34.3 Aplastic anemia

Once conditions such as HIV infection and high-dose chemotherapy can be excluded, the combination of peripheral pancytopenia and a hypocellular marrow is consistent with a diagnosis of aplastic anemia. Aplastic anemia can be congenital or acquired. Most cases are acquired.

34.3.1 Acquired aplastic anemia

Most acquired aplastic anemias are considered idiopathic. The underlying pathogenesis appears to be multifactorial, including stem cell defects, immune suppression of hematopoiesis, and stromal abnormalities.

In aplastic anemia, an etiologic agent can be identified in only a small number of cases, such as:

- Medications, including certain analgesics, anticonvulsants and antibiotics. Chloramphenicol is responsible for nearly half of all drug-induced aplastic anemia. The onset of aplasia is sudden and unrelated to the dosage. The aplasia may or may not be reversible.
- Toxins, such as chronic excessive exposure to benzene.
- Massive ionizing radiation.
- Hepatitis C virus, causing a severe and irreversible bone marrow aplasia 1–2 months after the acute infection.
- Pregnancy, which can induce a self-limited aplasia.

The mechanisms proposed for the pathogenesis of idiopathic aplastic anemia include:

1. Defects in the bone marrow microenvironment. However, much of the evidence indicates that the stroma in aplastic anemia is functionally normal. Normal CD34-positive cells can proliferate on the stroma from aplastic anemia patients. Clinically, this is reflected in the high efficacy of engraftment in patients receiving allogeneic bone marrow transplantation.
2. A reduced stem cell pool secondary to increased apoptosis.
3. Immune suppression of hematopoiesis. The majority of patients with aplastic anemia respond to immunosuppressive therapy (usually a combination of antithymocyte globulin and cyclosporin). The blood and bone marrow of affected patients contain increased numbers of activated cytotoxic T cells ($CD8^+$ cells with expression of activation markers HLA-DR and/or CD25) associated with abnormal production of γ-interferon. Furthermore, γ-interferon can induce increased apoptosis.

Patients with aplastic anemia have normal cytogenetic studies. However, clonal stem cell abnormalities, including PNH and acute leukemia, develop in a substantial number of patients, especially following immunosuppressive therapy. The emergence of clonal hematopoiesis in aplastic anemia most likely follows somatic mutations producing a stem cell clone lacking recognition sites for cytotoxic cells. In a marrow under immune attack, this defect confers a survival advantage to the mutated clone. The close relationship between aplastic anemia and PNH supports this hypothesis.

34.3.2 Congenital aplastic anemia

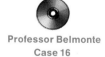

Professor Belmonte
Case 16

In children, aplastic anemia is associated with congenital disorders characterized by chromosomal instability and a defective ability to repair DNA damage. The best known example is Fanconi's anemia (FA).

Most patients with FA present with cutaneous hyperpigmentation and/or a hypoplastic thumb or radius. Because of the variability in the clinical manifestations, the diagnosis of FA currently rests on the demonstration of increased chromosomal breakage in peripheral blood lymphocytes incubated with DNA cross-linking agents such as diepoxybutane or mitomycin C. Diepoxybutane testing can be used to diagnose FA before the development of overt aplasia, including at the prenatal stage.

In FA, the increased chromosomal instability and accumulation of unrepaired DNA damage leads to delayed transit through the cell cycle, arrest in the G2-phase, and ultimately cell death. The genomic defects predispose to the development of solid and hematopoietic malignancies.

The diverse clinical manifestations of FA and the different sensitivities to DNA cross-linking agents observed among different patients reflect the underlying genetic heterogeneity. Recently, complementation studies on somatic cell hybrids have identified multiple different FA genes as defined by the different complementation groups (named in alphabetical order, thus far from A to H). The chromosomal locations for some of these genes have been recently identified, e.g. the *FA-C* gene on chromosome 9q22.3, the *FA-A* gene on 16q24.3 and the *FA-D* gene on 3p22-26. Some of these genes may be involved in the correction of DNA cross-link damage.

34.4 Post-chemotherapy/transplantation bone marrows

Systemic chemotherapeutic agents target both benign and malignant cells indiscriminately. The appearance of the bone marrow reflects the intensity of the regimen administered to the patient. The effects on normal hematopoiesis depend on the potency of the particular regimen, as well host factors.

Single agent chemotherapy usually produces mild changes manifesting primarily as qualitative abnormalities in the erythroid series (e.g. nuclear/cytoplasmic asynchrony). Severe myelosuppresion occasionally occurs, especially with nucleoside analogs.

Administration of intensive multiagent chemotherapy, such as the protocols employed in the induction phase of acute leukemia, invariably result in marked bone marrow suppression. Bone marrow transplantation, which in most instances involves myeloablative preparatory regimens, produces similar affects in the early post-transplantation period.

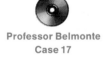

The bone marrow after intensive chemotherapy or bone marrow transplantation demonstrates features of both cellular damage and hematopoietic regeneration.

Sequential bone marrow studies following high-dose chemotherapy are performed for evaluating disease clearance. In bone marrow transplant recipients, the sequential marrow examinations allow the evaluation of engraftment, rejection, superimposed infection and any subsequent secondary malignancies.

34.4.1 Hematopoietic regeneration

Following chemotherapy or bone marrow transplantation, hematopoietic regeneration progresses through four overlapping stages: (1) nadir; (2) early recovery (mainly erythroid); (3) progressive recovery; and (4) essentially normal marrow.

In bone marrow samples taken during the first week after chemotherapy or bone marrow transplantation, marked hypocellularity and widespread chemotherapy effects predominate. Foamy macrophages containing cellular debris may be prominent. Erythroid and myeloid precursors become evident in bone marrow samples around the second to third week, appearing as clusters of a single lineage, with a preponderance of erythroid clusters.

Erythroid regeneration usually manifests as solid aggregates in the middle of the medullary space, whereas myeloid proliferation occurs interstitially (around fat cells), sometimes forming paratrabecular foci. The regenerative process is accompanied by conspicuous cytologic abnormalities ('dysplastic features'), especially among erythroid precursors (Figure 33.7). Since these recovery-associated changes are reactive and transient, it is better not to stress the term 'dysplastic features' in the bone marrow report. The regenerative erythropoiesis is reflected peripherally by an increased proportion of early reticulocytes (with high fluorescence detectable by FCM analysis).

The early phase of myeloid recovery is accompanied by left-shifted maturation. Because of the difficulty in distinguishing promyelocytes from blasts on biopsy sections, small foci of markedly left-shifted myeloid cells may be misinterpreted as residual foci of blasts. This pitfall can be overcome by examining good quality imprints and smears prepared from concentrated spicules. Another potential pitfall, especially in children, is the abundance of hematogones in post-treatment bone marrows. It is important to avoid misinterpreting hematogones as residual leukemia (see Section 25.4 and Chapter 40). High numbers of hematogones can persist for up to a year in some children.

Bone marrow samples obtained at 4–8 weeks after treatment show further recovery with less evidence of bone marrow damage, less erythroid preponderance and fewer cytologic abnormalities. The regenerative foci are larger, with a mixed lineage composition and a higher content of more mature elements. Mild bone marrow eosinophilia is common (Figure 34.4). The continuing recovery in the marrow is reflected by a progressive increase in the peripheral counts, with the absolute neutrophil count reaching $1 \times 10^9/l$ around 5–6 weeks. Megakaryocytes are the last elements to recover. Between the eighth and twelfth weeks,

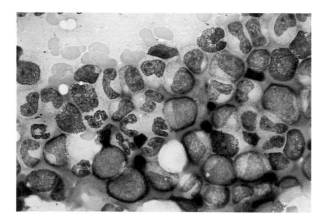

Figure 34.4 Bone marrow eosinophilia in the late phase of bone marrow recovery. There is myeloid preponderance. The intermediate myeloid precursors are still in excess of the mature precursors

the bone marrow appears essentially normal (i.e. normocellular with a normal M:E ratio). Mild to moderate cytologic abnormalities, mainly in erythroid precursors, may persist. Development of pseudo-Pelger-Huët anomaly has also been reported in some patients. For these reasons, any subsequent diagnosis of therapy-related MDS based solely on qualitative features (i.e. without excess blasts, ring sideroblasts or cytogenetic abnormalities) should be rendered with caution.

In post-transplantation bone marrow specimens, persistence of hypocellularity at day 28 is an ominous sign indicating failure of engraftment. The long-term follow-up after engraftment can be done via periodic blood counts. A bone marrow sample is only deemed necessary if the peripheral counts drop, as in graft rejection. There are no specific features in the marrow to diagnose this condition, however, apart for the progressive hypocellularity.

In recent years, G-CSF has been used to enhance recovery following myelosuppressive therapy. Studies have shown that G-CSF shortens the time for the recovery of the neutrophil count by 1 week, with a resulting decrease in neutropenic febrile episodes, infections and hospitalization. When G-CSF is used at the end of intensive induction chemotherapy, the bone marrow morphology follows a recovery sequence similar to that described above, with a shorter time span, however. If G-CSF is integrated into the induction regimen, the sequential morphologic changes in the post-induction bone marrows can differ. At day 8, the marrow may not be markedly hypoplastic. Under the influence of G-CSF, it remains normocellular or hypercellular with a marked myeloid preponderance, left-shifted myeloid maturation and the telltale hypergranularity in myeloid precursors. These features can hamper the morphologic assessment of residual acute leukemia, especially when the initial diagnosis is AML. Often, by the fourth to eighth week, however, the myeloid hyperplasia subsides and the marrow appears less cellular, with a relative erythroid preponderance. By the tenth to twelfth week, the marrow is usually normocellular with no significant quantitative or qualitative changes.

34.4.2 Assessment of residual disease following transplantation or induction chemotherapy

After chemotherapy or bone marrow transplantation, adjunctive techniques, such as FCM immunophenotyping, DNA ploidy analysis and molecular biology, are particularly useful for assessing residual hematological malignancy. If appropriate probes are available, PCR techniques can be applied. The validity of positive PCR results is questionable in the early post-therapy stage, however, since RNA/DNA from nonviable residual tumor cells may be detected.

34.4.2.1 Acute leukemia

The morphologic criteria for residual acute leukemia are straightforward, i.e. at least 5% blasts in the bone marrow. However, there are two potential pitfalls to avoid: (1) abundant hematogones in pediatric marrows, which may be

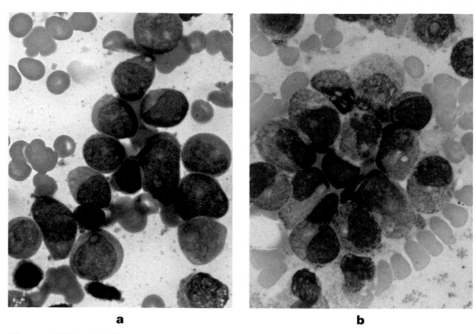

Figure 34.5 (a) Bone marrow at diagnosis in a case of AML-M1. (b) Four weeks after induction chemotherapy which included G-CSF: hypercellular marrow with similar appearing hypergranular myeloid cells which did not express HLA-DR (note the excess of granules in the background derived from ruptured cells). Residual leukemia was more easily identified by FCM immunophenotyping, which revealed 10% CD34[+] myeloblasts

misinterpreted as residual ALL; and (2) synchronous maturation of large numbers of heavily granulated cells, which may be confused with AML-M3 (Figure 34.5), espccially when G-CSF is administered as part of the induction regimen. Since the synchronous maturation associated with G-CSF can result in a transient absence of HLA-DR expression, even the phenotype can mimic that of AML-M3.

The following situations can pose diagnostic dilemmas:

1. The bone marrow differential reveals less than 5% blasts but the biopsy contains a focus or small foci of 'blasts'. In such instances, it would be helpful to have optimally prepared touch imprints of the core biopsy to determine whether the mononuclear cells are blasts or promyelocytes/myelocytes. Immunostaining for CD34 can also be helpful. A preponderance of CD34[+] cells in such foci is strongly suspicious of residual acute leukemia and overt disease usually becomes evident in the peripheral blood or bone marrow within 1–2 weeks.

2. The bone marrow aspirate and biopsy are negative for excess blasts, but 3–5% blasts are detectable in the peripheral blood. This phenomenon is often transient, but appears to correlate with a subsequent late relapse. Transient circulating blasts are also observed with G-CSF therapy.

34.4.2.2 Other hematological malignancies

Unlike acute leukemia, morphologic criteria have not been proposed for residual involvement by LPD/NHL and multiple myeloma. The morphologic detection of residual LPD/NHL can be difficult since the neoplastic cells may be indistinguishable from benign lymphocytes and the disease can manifest only as one or two small lymphoid aggregates.

Unless small aggregates are composed of mostly transformed cells, it is difficult to distinguish them from benign lymphoid aggregates. In most instances, the presence of lymphoid aggregate(s) in the post-treatment bone marrow of a patient with previous marrow involvement is indicative of residual LPD/NHL. It is judicious to obtain confirmatory evidence by FCM immunophenotyping, however. Residual low-grade NHL can be identified with confidence if a substantial number of the small lymphoid cells exhibit nuclear abnormalities or the pattern of infiltration on the biopsy is paratrabecular.

The morphologic identification of residual multiple myeloma and high-grade NHL is relatively easier since the large cell size of immature-appearing plasma cells or large lymphoma cells facilitates their detection on aspirate smears, even when present in low numbers. Sequential serum/urine immunoelectrophoresis (or immunofixation) remains the preferred method to follow-up a patient with multiple myeloma, however.

CHAPTER 35

Erythroid preponderance/hyperplasia pattern

Professor Belmonte
Case 11

The mechanisms that can lead to an increased number of erythroid elements with a bone marrow M:E ratio of less than 1:1 are listed in Table 35.1. The erythroid series can also appear relatively increased if myeloid proliferation is suppressed. In such instances, there is invariably left-shifted myeloid maturation with a myeloid maturation arrest picture and peripheral neutropenia (see Section 33.4.2).

In erythroid preponderance, the bone marrow can be hypocellular or normocellular, whereas the term erythroid hyperplasia infers a hypercellular marrow with a reversed M:E ratio. To distinguish the various underlying processes, it is crucial to take into account the peripheral blood data and pertinent clinical information when evaluating the bone marrow. An increase in erythroid precursors is often accompanied by a variable degree of the cytologic abnormalities ('dyserythropoietic' features) described in Section 33.4.1. Left-shifted erythroid maturation may also be present, as well as abnormalities in the myeloid and/or megakaryocytic lineages.

The common conditions that can manifest with erythroid preponderance or erythroid hyperplasia are listed in Table 35.2. A bone marrow aspirate/biopsy is not necessary in the work-up of some of these diseases, including most hemolytic anemias, thalassemias and nutritional deficiencies. These entities can usually be diagnosed based on peripheral blood examination (including an absolute reticulocyte count, which is increased in stressed erythropoiesis) and/or other appropriate laboratory tests (Coombs test, enzyme studies, or hemoglobin electrophoresis and ferritin levels).

In AIDS and alcohol abuse, the increase in erythroid precursors results from a combination of peripheral RBC destruction, ineffective erythropoiesis and myelosuppression. Similarly, in thalassemia, production defects and decreased RBC survival coexist. A characteristic of ineffective erythropoiesis, especially if associated with DNA synthesis abnormalities, is the low absolute reticulocyte count despite bone marrow erythroid hyperplasia.

Table 35.1 Mechanisms leading to erythroid preponderance/hyperplasia

- An excessive proliferation of erythroid precursors, either autonomous or secondary to increased erythropoietin production.
- Ineffective erythropoiesis (increased spontaneous intramedullary cell death among the erythroid precursors).
- Compensatory or regenerative erythropoiesis (e.g. in response to the peripheral destruction of RBCs).

Table 35.2 Diseases with erythroid preponderance/hyperplasia

- Erythrocytosis, either secondary or primary (i.e. PRV).
- Hemolytic anemias, either hereditary (e.g. hemoglobinopathies, RBC membrane disorders or enzyme deficiencies) or acquired (e.g. immune hemolytic anemia, paroxysmal cold hemoglobinuria, PNH).
- AIDS.
- Alcohol abuse.
- Disorders with ineffective erythropoiesis:
  (1) Hemoglobin synthesis disorders, i.e. thalassemias and congenital sideroblastic anemia.
  (2) DNA synthesis defects, i.e. B_{12}/folate deficiency, CDA, MDS, drugs interfering with nucleic acid synthesis.

35.1 Erythroid preponderance/hyperplasia and peripheral erythrocytosis

In general, the diagnostic work-up for erythrocytosis does not require bone marrow evaluation. A thorough clinical investigation should be sufficient to elucidate the underlying etiologies of secondary erythrocytoses, which include primarily physiological causes such as hypoxia (heavy smoking, chronic pulmonary diseases), hemoglobinopathies with high oxygen affinity, and inappropriate production of erythropoietin secondary to renal disease or various neoplasms. When a peripheral basophilia is present, along with splenomegaly, pruritus and symptoms secondary to an increased RBC mass (e.g. thrombosis), the findings are suggestive of PRV.

The diagnostic criteria for PRV and the work-up to distinguish PRV from reactive erythrocytosis are presented in Chapter 6. Bone marrow morphologic changes are not part of the diagnostic criteria for PRV as proposed by the Polycythemia Vera Study Group. The bone marrow in most cases of PRV is hypercellular with an increased number of megakaryocytes resulting in either bihyperplasia (erythroid/megakaryocytic) or panhyperplasia (see Chapter 38). There are no specific bone marrow features that are diagnostic for PRV. Furthermore, the bone marrow in the early stages of the disease may appear deceptively normal.

35.2 Erythroid preponderance/hyperplasia and peripheral cytopenia(s)

A bone marrow aspirate/biopsy is often necessary for unexplained or persistent cytopenia(s), namely macrocytic anemia, NCNC anemia, neutropenia, bicytopenia or pancytopenia. Since the differential diagnosis of these cytopenias includes numerous disorders, both benign and malignant, it is important that a thorough clinical and laboratory work-up (e.g. an absolute reticulocyte count, B_{12}/folate levels, HIV status, immunoelectrophoresis) precedes the request for a bone marrow investigation. Conditions with erythroid preponderance, cytopenias and a hypocellular marrow, such as aplastic anemia and a regenerative marrow, are discussed in Chapter 34.

The combination of erythroid preponderance/hyperplasia and macrocytic anemia, bicytopenia or pancytopenia suggests ineffective erythropoiesis. The most common disorders with ineffective erythropoiesis include low-grade MDS, B_{12}/folate deficiency (and less common causes of megaloblastic anemia), alcohol abuse, HIV infection (discussed in Chapter 42), and some cases of PNH. Depending on the predominant clinical manifestations (bone marrow failure vs. hemolysis), the bone marrow findings in PNH can range from a markedly hypocellular marrow to erythroid hyperplasia. The diagnosis of PNH is discussed in Section 12.2.

In the other disorders with ineffective erythropoiesis, the bone marrow is hypercellular in the majority of cases. Certain constellations of qualitative abnormalities in erythroid and myeloid precursors can offer clues to identify the disorder.

35.2.1 Megaloblastic maturation

The term 'megaloblastic' refers to erythroid and/or myeloid precursors that uniformly exhibit large cell size (giant precursors) and asynchronous nuclear/cytoplasmic maturation. Megaloblastic morphology is best appreciated in late erythroid precursors on aspirate smears (Figure 33.8b). In these cells, hemoglobin production (i.e. cytoplasmic maturation) proceeds normally while nuclear maturation is delayed. The nuclear chromatin remains 'open', resulting in a sieve-like, speckled appearance. Note that the terms 'megaloblastic' and 'megaloblastoid' are not synonyms of each other. In megaloblastoid morphology, nuclear/cytoplasmic asynchrony is present, but the cells are not markedly enlarged. In the myeloid series, megaloblastic changes manifest as abundant giant metamyelocytes and giant bands (Figure 33.13a).

Professor Belmonte
Case 18

With megaloblastic maturation, other abnormalities, including karyorrhexis, nuclear lobulation and occasional binucleated or multinucleated erythroid precursors, may be present, as well as hypersegmented neutrophils. Megakaryocytes with disconnected nuclear lobes, simulating multinucleated giant cells, may also be detectable. The constellation of widespread megaloblastic abnormalities among erythroid and myeloid elements, erythroid hyperplasia, and a peripheral macrocytic anemia essentially defines megaloblastic anemia, the most common cause of which is B_{12}/folate deficiency (see Section 15.5). In a hypercellular biopsy, the morphology may be mistaken for a malignant process since the sheets of megaloblastic erythroid precursors simulate the appearance of leukemic blasts (Figure 35.1).

The diagnosis of B_{12}/folate deficiency can be confirmed by appropriate assays for serum B_{12} and RBC folate, with additional investigations, if necessary, to determine the causes of the deficiency. If the B_{12}/folate levels are normal, other less common causes of megaloblastic anemia need to be considered, including drug-induced alterations of DNA synthesis and rare congenital disorders such as CDA or deficiency of transcobalamin II.

The presence of coexisting iron deficiency can mask several features of B_{12}/folate deficiency. Megaloblastic changes among the erythroid precursors are less

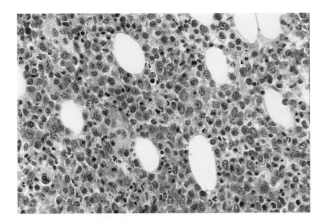

Figure 35.1 Erythroid hyperplasia with a preponderance of early erythroid precursors in pernicious anemia (B$_{12}$ deficiency). On the biopsy section, the sheets of early erythroid precursors simulate the appearance of acute leukemia or high-grade lymphoma

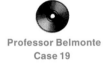

Professor Belmonte
Case 19

obvious, and the peripheral blood MCV can fall within the normal range. The bone marrow may not demonstrate erythroid hyperplasia. The picture may be that of a hypercellular marrow with myeloid preponderance (Figure 35.2), usually associated with megakaryocytic hyperplasia.

35.2.2 Abundant binucleation and/or multinucleation

Scattered binucleated or multinucleated erythroid precursors are not unusual in the bone marrows of patients with either ineffective erythropoiesis or stressed erythropoiesis secondary to peripheral RBC destruction. Erythroid hyperplasia with abundant binucleation or multinucleation, together with a low absolute reticulocyte level, and no laboratory evidence of known RBC disorders, should raise the suspicion of CDA. Pronounced multinucleation in giant late erythroid precursors, also referred to as multinucleated gigantoblasts, is essentially pathognomonic for CDA type III (Figure 35.3), whereas binucleation is more prominent in CDA types I and II.

The congenital dyserythropoietic anemias are rare familial disorders which have been classified based on blood and bone marrow morphology and the results of an acidified serum test. The most common subtype is CDA II. It is characterized by mild to moderate NCNC anemia and abundant binucleated late erythroid precursors. Erythroid maturation is otherwise normal. Mature RBCs exhibit increased sensitivity to acid hemolysis (hence the name HEMPAS, hereditary erythroblast multinuclearity with positive acidified serum test), but the sugarwater test is negative.

Binucleation is also frequent in CDA I. The anemia is macrocytic and the erythroid precursors are megaloblastic in CDA I, however. Other common features described in CDA I include internuclear bridges between erythroid precursors, karyorrhexis and nuclear lobulation.

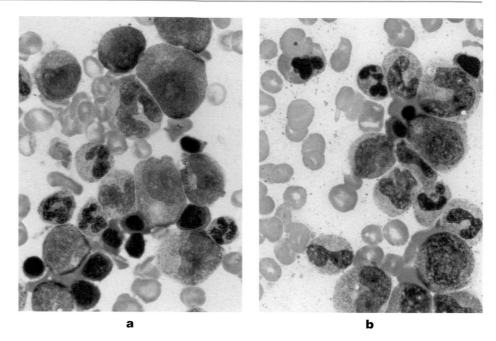

a   b

Figure 35.2   (a), (b) Coexisting B_{12} and iron deficiencies. Myeloid precursors predominate, with abundant giant forms. The erythroid precursors do not appear to be megaloblastic. A rare abnormal erythroid precursor with nuclear lobulation and karyorrhexis is present (b)

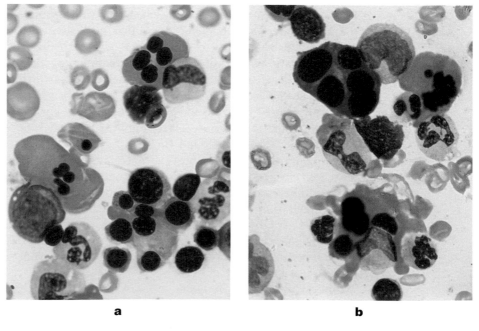

a   b

Figure 35.3   (a), (b) Frequent multinucleated gigantoblasts in both fields in CDA III

35.2.3 Other dyserythropoietic features

Dyserythropoietic features are manifestations of either a high proliferative rate (stressed erythropoiesis) or ineffective erythropoiesis resulting from either hemoglobin synthesis defects or altered DNA synthesis. In general, alterations in DNA synthesis also produce abnormalities in the other cell lineages, i.e. dysmyelopoietic and/or dysmegakaryopoietic features. In the absence of widespread megaloblastic changes or striking binucleation/multinucleation, which facilitate the identification of megaloblastic anemia and CDA respectively, a broader differential (e.g. MDS, AIDS or chemotherapy) needs to be considered.

Most low-grade MDSs (i.e. MDSs without excess blasts) demonstrate erythroid hyperplasia and cytologic abnormalities in one or more cell lineages. Since the presence of 'dysplastic' features does not necessarily imply myelodysplasia and the clinical manifestations in MDS are rather nonspecific, conditions which can simulate low-grade MDS should be excluded (Table 35.3).

The FAB classification divides MDS into five subtypes (refractory anemia, RARS, RAEB, RAEB-T and CMMoL) based on the peripheral blood and bone marrow morphology. The key features in the differential diagnosis are the percentage of blasts, the percentage of ring sideroblasts in the bone marrow, and the proportion of monocytes. Refractory anemia with excess blasts, RAEB-T and CMMoL are usually accompanied by myeloid hyperplasia and are therefore discussed in Chapter 36.

Although RAEB can occur with erythroid hyperplasia, the percentage of blasts would necessarily be on the low side of the 5–20% range proposed by the FAB group. This is true because the FAB definition of AML-M6 is met when the percentage of blasts reaches 30% of nonerythroid cells (NEC) and the M:E ratio is less than 1:1. In cases with marked erythroid proliferation, (e.g. an M:E ratio of 1:4), a slight change in the blast count (from 4% blasts to 6% blasts) can shift the diagnosis from MDS to AML-M6 according to the FAB definitions. Such instances are fortunately infrequent. Including a much larger number of cells in the bone marrow differential (> 500 cells) may help to resolve a borderline situation.

35.2.3.1 Low-grade myelodysplastic syndromes

Refractory anemia and RARS are considered together to be low-grade MDSs (Figure 35.4). Both entities present with anemia, macrocytosis, a low absolute reticulocyte count and variable qualitative abnormalities in hematopoietic precursors. The bone marrow is usually hypercellular with an M:E ratio of less than 1:1. The following criteria apply to both refractory anemia and RARS:

Table 35.3 Work-up to exclude conditions simulating low-grade MDS

1. Measurements of serum B_{12} and RBC folate levels to exclude the vitamin deficiencies.
2. Laboratory studies to exlude PNH and HIV infection irrespective of the age group.
3. Drug history, including chemotherapy or toxic substances which can induce sideroblastic changes.
4. History of autoimmune disorders or liver disease.
5. Family history to exclude CDA in young patients.
6. Karyotyping analysis. The presence of certain cytogenetic abnormalities is supportive of MDS.

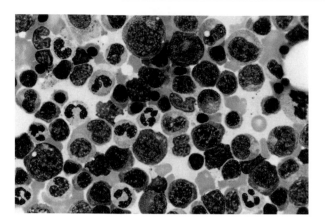

Figure 35.4 Erythroid hyperplasia in a case of RARS. There is preponderance of early erythroid precursors. Nuclear/cytoplasmic asynchrony is present

- Blasts, if present in the peripheral blood, do not exceed 1%.
- Bone marrow blasts account for less than 5% of all nucleated cells and less than 30% of NEC.
- There is no evidence of a peripheral monocytosis.

The proportion of ring sideroblasts on a bone marrow iron stain (aspirate or touch imprint) is used to separate refractory anemia from RARS. In RARS, ring sideroblasts account for more than 15% of the erythroid precursors. Abnormalities in the other cell lineages may or may not be present. Dysplastic features in the myeloid series may not be easily detectable because of the abundance of erythroid precursors.

Note that the presence of ring sideroblasts is not synonymous with RARS. In particular, alcohol abuse can simulate the morphology of RARS. Ring sideroblasts can also be present in occasional MPDs (Figures 35.5 and 35.6). However, these cases can be distinguished from RARS by their CML-like peripheral blood picture.

In its original description, the FAB group claimed that in low-grade MDSs, 'the granulocytic and megakaryocytic series almost always appear normal'. For this reason, many institutions consider that MDS with abnormalities in all three lineages but without excess blasts should be considered 'unclassifiable MDS' or 'MDS with trilineage dysplasia'. The majority of such cases are therapy-related MDSs. The multiple underlying cytogenetic abnormalities, rather than the presence of the trilineage dysplasia *per se*, confer a relatively poor prognosis on this group of patients. For communicating with clinical colleagues, these secondary MDSs can be assigned to the categories of refractory anemia or RARS if excess blasts are not present.

The diagnosis of refractory anemia is less straightforward, especially when qualitative abnormalities in the bone marrow are few. A helpful diagnostic clue is increased iron incorporation (see Section 33.5). HIV infection is one of the most common conditions that can manifest with a blood and bone marrow picture closely similar to refractory anemia. The trilineage dysplasia in AIDS patients

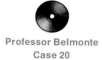

Professor Belmonte
Case 20

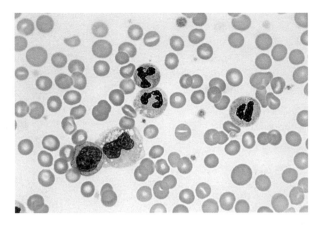

Figure 35.5 A CML-like myeloproliferative disorder in a 76-year-old female with moderate anemia (Hgb 8 g/dl), a normal platelet count (250×10^9/l) and a slowly rising WBC count (from 30×10^9/l to 50×10^9/l over 4 years). The bone marrow has an increased number of ring sideroblasts (see Figure 35.6)

does not imply a clonal disorder, but rather reflects the combined effect of infections, altered immune status and various drug therapies.

One low-grade MDS not included in the FAB classification that can manifest with erythroid hyperplasia is the 5q– syndrome. The number of megakaryocytes is normal or increased. Although the presence of hypolobulated megakaryocytes is a consistent finding in all reported cases of the 5q– syndrome, the same feature is present in other MDS subtypes, including those without cytogenetic abnormalities. This syndrome is described in more detail in Section 37.2.2.1.

35.2.4 Erythroid hyperplasia in stressed hematopoiesis

A bone marrow aspirate/biopsy is not necessary for the work-up of hemolytic anemias, thalassemias and hemoglobinopathies. In some patients, however, a

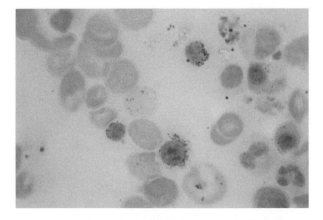

Figure 35.6 Prussian blue stain on a bone marrow aspirate from the patient shown in Figure 35.5, showing ring sideroblasts and increased iron incorporation

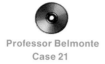

Professor Belmonte
Case 21

bone marrow examination is performed because marked splenomegaly raises the suspicion of a possible malignancy. The bone marrow in severe hemolytic anemia invariably demonstrates erythroid hyperplasia, and variable degrees of 'dyserythropoietic' abnormalities (e.g. karyorrhexis, binucleation or multinucleation).

35.2.5 Erythroid preponderance/hyperplasia and microcytic anemia

The work-up of microcytic anemia rarely calls for bone marrow evaluation since other appropriate laboratory tests (serum and RBC ferritin, hemoglobin electrophoresis) confirm the diagnosis of iron deficiency or thalassemia in the great majority of patients. In a patient with moderate to severe microcytic anemia, a negative hemoglobin electrophoresis and increased ferritin (indicative of iron overload), a bone marrow aspirate/biopsy may be necessary to establish the diagnosis of congenital sideroblastic anemia.

Congenital sideroblastic anemia is clinically and genetically heterogeneous, with variable severity and a variable response to pyridoxine therapy. The majority of reported cases demonstrate an X-linked inheritance, whereby the female carriers exhibit a dimorphic blood picture without evidence of anemia. Dimorphism in the female carrier may not be evident, however, in subjects with skewed lyo-

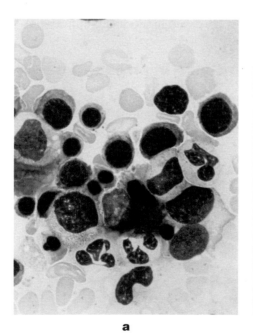

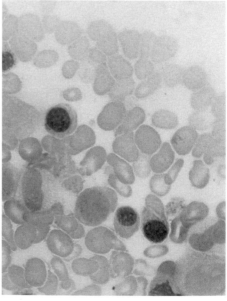

a   b

Figure 35.7 Congenital sideroblastic anemia. (a) Erythroid preponderance (the bone marrow is normocellular). (b) Prussian blue stained smear, showing ring sideroblasts and increased iron incorporation

Professor Belmonte
Case 22

nization in favor of the normal X chromosome. The ineffective erythropoiesis in congenital sideroblastic anemia reflects the impaired activity of the enzyme 5-aminolevulinic acid synthetase 2, a mitochondrial enzyme involved in the rate-limiting step of heme synthesis. Several mutations of the gene involved have been identified on chromosome Xp11.21 to account for the enzyme defects. The affected patients have moderate to severe microcytic anemia with a dimorphic blood picture (Figure 14.1) and evidence of iron overload (including hepatosplenomegaly). The bone marrow demonstrates erythroid preponderance/hyperplasia with increased iron incorporation and ring sideroblasts (Figure 35.7).

Hypercellular marrow, myeloid preponderance/hyperplasia pattern

In a normal marrow, there is myeloid preponderance with an M:E ratio in the range of 2:1 to 4:1. The myeloid preponderance can be maintained in a hypercellular marrow if there is a proportional increase in both myeloid and erythroid precursors. Myeloid hyperplasia, in contrast, represents an excessive increase of myeloid elements in a hypercellular marrow. A hypercellular marrow with a normal M:E ratio can be encountered in both reactive conditions and clonal stem cell disorders. Myeloid hyperplasia occurs primarily in MPDs, e.g. CML.

The increased myeloid proliferation can result from:

1. Endogenous production of growth factors and/or cytokines. This mechanism of increased myelopoiesis, which often results in peripheral leukocytosis, operates in infectious processes, tissue damage/necrosis and underlying neoplasms with or without bone marrow involvement (e.g. solid tumors, Hodgkin's disease). Similarly, increased myelopoiesis can be induced by exogenous administration of G-CSF. In G-CSF therapy, the WBC count can vary widely, depending on the bone marrow reserve and underlying condition.
2. DNA abnormalities and cytogenetic aberrations at the stem cell level, giving rise to an autonomous proliferation or survival advantage of myeloid cells. Alterations at the DNA level occur in MPD, MDS and B_{12}/folate deficiency. In MPD, granulopoiesis is effective, resulting in a peripheral leukocytosis. In contrast, because of the ineffective hematopoiesis in MDS, the peripheral counts are not elevated.

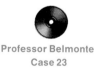

Professor Belmonte
Case 23

Increased myeloid proliferation, whether benign or neoplastic, can be accompanied by left-shifted maturation and variable qualitative abnormalities. Therefore, the bone marrow evaluation should always include the peripheral blood findings and adequate clinical information.

36.1 Hypercellular marrow with myeloid preponderance/ hyperplasia and peripheral cytopenia(s)

Isolated neutropenia in adults may not require a bone marrow procedure if the work-up uncovers an etiology such as a drug reaction or an underlying immune disorder (often associated with an indolent proliferation of LGLs). When an unexplained persistent or progressive leukopenia is associated with anemia and/

or thrombocytopenia, however, evaluation of the bone marrow is often indicated.

The combination of increased myeloid proliferation and peripheral cytopenias is seen mainly in MDS, HIV infection (see Chapter 42), and B_{12}/folate deficiency with coexisting iron deficiency (see Section 35.2.1), and as a transient phenomenon in association with the use of growth factors.

36.1.1 The effect of growth factors and cytokines

Growth factors (referred to together as G-CSF in this section) have been widely used for the following purposes:

- To facilitate the mobilization of progenitors in preparation for autologous peripheral blood stem cell transplantation.
- To prevent febrile neutropenia, especially in oncology patients following high-dose chemotherapy or allogeneic bone marrow transplantation.
- To treat acquired and congenital neutropenia.

**Professor Belmonte
Cases 13 and 24**

In the peripheral blood, the quantitative and morphologic changes of G-CSF therapy vary depending on the WBC count prior to the start of therapy and the ability of the patient's bone marrow to respond. Patients with repeated exposure to chemotherapy have a decreased bone marrow regenerative capacity and a blunted response to G-CSF. Therefore, in the context of G-CSF therapy, the WBC can vary from low to increased. Occasionally, the WBC count climbs into the leukemoid range ($> 50 \times 10^9$/l). Circulating intermediate myeloid precursors are common, along with a small number of NRBCs resulting in a leukoerythroblastic picture. Usually, there are fewer than 5% circulating NRBCs. In individuals with good bone marrow reserve, the brisk response to G-CSF can release a small number of circulating blasts. In rare cases, the peripheral blast count may be as high as 10%. In such instances, the blood picture may be indistinguishable from that of CML, although without basophilia. The phenomenon is transient, however, lasting for about a week.

In patients with acute leukemia receiving G-CSF as an adjunct to high-dose chemotherapy, the presence of circulating blasts raises the concern of persistent leukemia. Peripheral blood follow-up over a 1–2 week period should resolve the dilemma. If the blasts persist and the peripheral counts do not normalize after discontinuation of G-CSF, a bone marrow evaluation is warranted to determine the status of the leukemic process.

The bone marrow morphology varies depending on the patient's marrow reserve (cellularity, proliferative activity) prior to G-CSF therapy and the time of the bone marrow examination. In patients with prior bone marrow damage (from intense or repeated chemotherapy), or an inadequate stem cell pool (e.g. severe aplastic anemia), the response to G-CSF can be absent or blunted. Therefore, the bone marrow cellularity can vary from low (in minimal responders) to increased (in good responders). The most dramatic changes seen in the early phase of G-CSF therapy include:

- An increased M:E ratio. The myeloid hyperplasia is not as marked as that seen in CML, however (i.e. < 10:1).
- Markedly left-shifted myeloid maturation, primarily myelocytes but with a moderate number (< 30%) of promyelocytes. Blasts are not increased. The myeloid precursors are mildly enlarged. Nuclear/cytoplasmic asynchrony and occasional binucleated forms can be found.
- Hypergranulation in myeloid cells (Figure 36.1). The increased azurophilic granulation probably results from the shortened maturation time in the bone marrow and therefore represents cytoplasmic immaturity in granulocytes. Myelocytes are frequently misidentified as promyelocytes because of the heavy granulation. The granulocytes are usually enlarged and Döhle bodies may be present.
- Nuclear abnormalities, including hyposegmentation (pseudo-Pelger-Huët anomaly), hypersegmentation, and occasional ring nuclei. Rare granulocytes may be binucleated.
- Eosinophilia may be present. This is more commonly associated with GM-CSF.

Because the hypergranulation is not discernible on biopsy sections, the G-CSF-induced myeloid hyperplasia with left-shifted maturation can simulate the appearance of an MPD or MDS. After the growth factor has been discontinued, the M:E ratio, myeloid maturation and cellularity progressively return to normal.

Whereas G-CSF and GM-CSF stimulate committed progenitors, IL-3 acts on pluripotent hematopoietic stem cells. This may account for the delayed effects in the peripheral blood. The effects of IL-3 on the blood and bone marrow are less striking than those induced by growth factors. The changes reported in IL-3 therapy include improved leukocyte counts, a variable increase in reticulocytes and platelets, left-shifted maturation of all three cell lines, bone marrow eosinophilia and mild reticulin fibrosis.

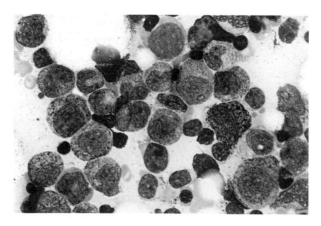

Figure 36.1 Effects of G-CSF therapy in the bone marrow in a case of Felty's syndrome. Left-shifted myeloid maturation and hypergranulated myeloid precursors are apparent

36.1.2 High-grade myelodysplastic syndromes

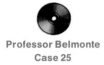

A key characteristic of most cases of MDS is the contrasting picture between the peripheral cytopenia and the bone marrow hypercellularity. A hypocellular marrow is unusual and is associated primarily with therapy-related MDS (see section 34.1.1). Most cases of low-grade MDS present with erythroid preponderance/hyperplasia (see Section 35.2.3.1). The occasional case of RARS with myeloid hyperplasia can be identified by the presence of greater than 15% ring sideroblasts.

Most high-grade MDSs present with myeloid preponderance/hyperplasia. The peripheral blood demonstrates bicytopenia or pancytopenia with a decreased or low normal WBC count. In the bone marrow, myeloid maturation is left-shifted and dysplastic features are common, including hypogranulated myeloid precursors, hyposegmented neutrophils, small hypolobulated megakaryocytes and dyserythropoiesis. The diagnosis does not rest on these cytologic abnormalities but on the percentage of blasts in the peripheral blood and bone marrow. The higher the number of cells included in the bone marrow differential, the higher the 95% confidence limit for the accuracy of the enumeration. This is most important in situations where the bone marrow blast count is close to 5%.

High-grade MDSs can develop *de novo* or secondary to alkylating agents, toxic substances (e.g. benzene) or intense radiation. Secondary MDS usually occurs 4–6 years after exposure to the injurious agent. The frequent occurrence of severe reticulin fibrosis in therapy-related MDS and AML results in aspicular aspirates and causes difficulty in diagnosis and classification. Well-prepared touch imprints, which should be a routine component of the bone marrow procedure, are crucial in such instances to reduce the number of cases of 'unclassifiable MDS'.

Myelodysplastic syndromes are less common in children than in adults. In children, high-grade MDS is often associated with cytogenetic abnormalities including monosomy 7. There is also a high frequency of underlying constitutional disorders such as DNA repair defects (e.g. Fanconi's anemia) or congenital immune disorders.

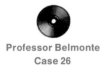

The FAB group classified high-grade MDS into RAEB and RAEB in transformation (RAEB-T). The FAB criteria for RAEB are shown in Table 36.1. Ring sideroblasts may be present. This suggests that the high-grade MDS has been preceded by RARS as part of the natural progression from MDS to AML. Irrespective of the proportion of ring sideroblasts, the presence of increased blasts takes precedence in the diagnosis of RAEB (Figure 36.2).

According to the FAB criteria, RAEB-T is defined by any of the following: (1) 5% or more blasts in the peripheral blood; (2) blasts with Auer rods in the blood

---

Table 36.1 FAB criteria for refractory anemia with excess blasts

1. Less than 5% blasts in the peripheral blood AND
2. No absolute monocytosis in the peripheral blood (i.e. monocytes $< 1 \times 10^9$/l) AND
3. Bone marrow blasts account for 5–20% of all the nucleated cells.

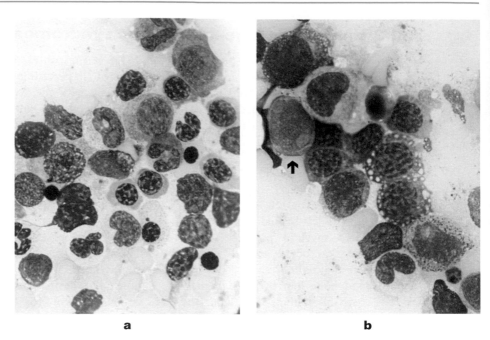

a   b

Figure 36.2 High-grade MDS. (a) Myeloid cells with hypogranulation and a ring-shaped nucleus. Nuclear/cytoplasmic asynchrony is evident in erythroid precursors, and one with karyorrhexis. (b) One blast (arrow) and vacuolated erythroid precursors. In this case, blasts account for 10% of all nucleated cells

or bone marrow (with less than 30% blasts in the marrow); or (3) 21–29% bone marrow blasts.

Recent evidence has raised questions concerning the relevance of RAEB-T, however. Patients diagnosed as RAEB-T based solely on the presence of Auer rods follow a clinical course similar to that of RAEB, whereas those classified according to the blast percentage criteria behave similar to AML. Furthermore, there exist cases of RAEB-T in which the karyotypic abnormalities, e.g. t(8;21), inv(16) or del(16), are those associated with a good prognostic group of AML. In cases with typical cytogenetic abnormalities, the bone marrow morphology is similar to that of the corresponding AML (e.g. abnormal eosinophils in AML-M4E) except for the blast percentage falling slightly short of the established 30% requirement. The clinical behavior and therapeutic response in these cases also correspond to AML.

In view of these findings, the arbitrary 30% bone marrow blast threshold for AML may need to be re-evaluated. In addition, patients presenting with at least 30% blasts in the peripheral blood but fewer than 30% blasts in the marrow behave as AML and are currently diagnosed as AML (see Chapter 40). A recent therapeutic trend has been to administer intensive chemotherapy (i.e. an AML regimen) to patients labeled RAEB-T, especially those in the pediatric or young adult age group, suggesting that these cases should be diagnosed as AML.

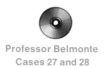

Professor Belmonte
Cases 27 and 28

36.1.2.1 Common cytogenetic abnormalities in MDS

About 90% of cases of secondary MDS and 30–50% of *de novo* MDS demonstrate chromosomal aberrations. Many of the same cytogenetic abnormalities are also found in AML and some MPDs. The predominance of partial chromosomal deletions and loss of chromosomes is characteristic of MDS, however. The most frequent chromosomal gain is trisomy 8.

In both *de novo* and secondary MDS (including the 5q– syndrome), the most frequent partial chromosomal deletion is del(5q), with 5q12–14 and 5q31–33 being the most common proximal and distal breakpoints, respectively. In secondary MDS, partial deletion of 5q can also result from unbalanced translocations such as t(5;7) and t(5;17). Monosomy 5 occurs less frequently than del(5q) and is associated mainly with secondary MDS.

In comparison to *de novo* MDS, secondary MDS has a much higher incidence of chromosome 7 abnormalities. The most common, in about 50% of cases, is monosomy 7 (either as the sole abnormality or as part of a complex karyotype) followed by del(7q) in 5–10% of cases. The del(7q) is a short interstitial deletion with the proximal breakpoint at q22 and the distal breakpoint between q32 and q36. In a small number of cases, the partial deletion of 7q results from an unbalanced translocation such as t(1;7), t(5;7) or t(7;17).

Less common rearrangements include chromosome 17p deletion and abnormalities of chromosome 3, found in approximately 6% and 2% of cases of MDS, respectively. The rearrangements of 17p appear to be associated with pronounced pseudo-Pelger-Huët changes and small vacuoles in neutrophils. Chromosome 3 abnormalities consist mainly of inv(3), t(3;5) and t(3;3). Patients with these rearrangements present with normal or increased platelet counts and abundant small megakaryocytes; features that simulate those of the 5q– syndrome (see Section 37.2.2.1).

36.2 Myeloid hyperplasia and peripheral leukocytosis

A marked increase in both peripheral blood leukocytes and bone marrow myeloid elements is the characteristic manifestation of MPDs, particularly CML and CMMoL. The entity referred to as 'juvenile CML' has morphologic features more akin to CMMoL than CML and, as suggested by the International Myelomonocytic Leukemia Working Group, should be renamed juvenile CMMoL. Myeloproliferative disorders not diagnostic of CML but presenting with a CML-like picture (referred to in the literature as 'atypical CML') are less frequent. Chronic neutrophilic leukemia and neoplastic hypereosinophilic syndromes are rare and are essentially diagnosed by exclusion. The diagnosis and classification of these disorders are best made in the peripheral blood (see Chapters 10, 11 and 18) since the bone marrow features often overlap between one MPD and another.

The differential diagnosis between CML and the CML-like MPDs is most reliably resolved at the cytogenetics and molecular level. Molecular studies can be performed on the peripheral blood whereas the bone marrow is usually a better choice for standard karyotyping analysis.

36.2.1 Chronic myeloid leukemia

CML and, less commonly, CML-like MPDs are the two main groups of disorders presenting with a leukemoid pattern in the blood. The peripheral blood manifestations of CML reflect the stage of the disease at the time of diagnosis. The typical peripheral blood findings in CML are discussed in Section 18.1.

36.2.1.1 Morphology of CML

The bone marrow findings in CML (Figures 36.3, 36.4 and 36.5) are often less diagnostic than the peripheral blood picture. In CML, the bone marrow is hypercellular with an increased M:E ratio, often in the range of 10:1. Myeloid maturation can be normal or moderately left-shifted with a preponderance of myelocytes and metamyelocytes. On the biopsy, the immature myeloid precur-

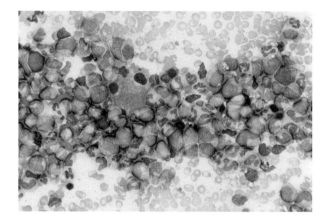

Figure 36.3 Myeloid hyperplasia in CML. Myeloid maturation is normal. There are occasional giant myeloid precursors

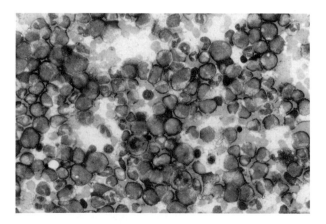

Figure 36.4 Myeloid hyperplasia with left-shifted myeloid maturation and hypergranulated myeloid precursors in CML

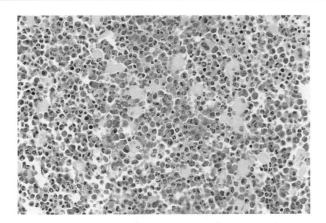

Figure 36.5   Abundant monolobated megakaryocytes in CML. The bone marrow demonstrates hyperplasia in the myeloid and megakaryocytic series

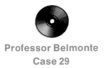

Professor Belmonte
Case 29

sors can be found away from the bony trabeculae, similar to the pattern seen in high-grade MDS (abnormal localization of immature precursors, ALIP). The blast proportion does not exceed 10% in the chronic phase. Basophilia and/or eosinophilia, including abnormal eosinophils with basophilic granules, can also be present.

Nuclear/cytoplasmic asynchrony, hypersegmentation and hypogranulation can occur. These 'dysplastic' features become more obvious with advanced disease or in association with therapy.

Megakaryocytes are predominantly small and hypolobulated (i.e. dwarf mega-karyocytes) in most, but not all, cases. When megakaryocytes are markedly increased, large, and hyperlobulated, the bone marrow picture may be mistaken for ET if the peripheral blood data are not taken into account. Karyotyping and/or molecular genetic studies should establish the diagnosis of CML. Such cases should not be diagnosed as Philadelphia chromosome-positive ET.

Reticulin may be increased on the biopsy sections in CML. The combination of severe reticulin fibrosis, myeloid hyperplasia and increased megakaryocytes results in a bone marrow morphology similar to that of AMM in cellular phase (see Section 38.2.2). In such instances, the differential diagnosis relies heavily on the peripheral blood findings (see Section 4.2). Marked reticulin fibrosis is often associated with an increase in circulating blasts and splenomegaly, two features that can adversely affect prognosis. The presence of increased reticulin *per se* does not imply transformation into the accelerated phase, however, since some patients with reticulin fibrosis have a prolonged survival.

A common nonspecific finding, more easily appreciated on the aspirate than the biopsy sections, is the presence of sea-blue histiocytes and pseudo-Gaucher cells filled with cellular membrane debris secondary to the increased cell turnover in CML (Figure 36.6).

36.2.1.2 Molecular pathogenesis of CML

The pathognomonic molecular abnormality in CML is *bcr-abl* rearrangement. The different molecular breakpoints are discussed in Section 18.4.

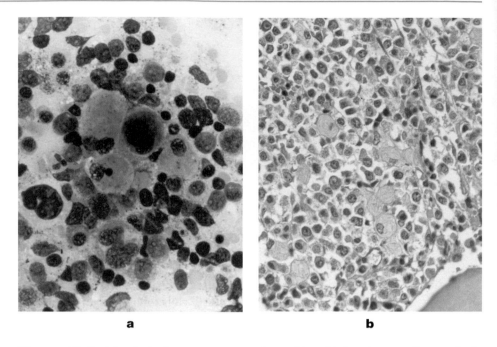

a   b

Figure 36.6 Morphologic appearance of sea-blue histiocytes on the aspirate smear (a) and biopsy section (b)

The growth advantage of CML over normal hematopoietic cells is most likely related to the *bcr-abl* rearrangement. Neoplastic stem cells in CML have been shown to have normal responses to colony-stimulating factors and negative feedback mechanisms, and to be actually less proliferative than their normal counterparts. This suggests that the massive accumulation of neoplastic cells is secondary to increased cell survival, i.e. that the fusion bcr-abl protein may function to suppress apoptosis. Another possible mechanism is that the fusion bcr-abl protein reduces adhesion of progenitor cells to the stroma. The stroma normally plays a role in the regulation of hematopoiesis. Consequently, the normal proliferation/maturation sequence is altered in CML with more cells remaining in the late proliferative phase before differentiation. The decreased stromal adhesion may also explain the premature release of neoplastic granulocytes into the peripheral blood.

36.2.1.3 Disease course in CML

CML is considered to be a triphasic disorder with a long chronic phase progressing to an accelerated phase and terminating in an acute blast crisis. The duration of the chronic phase (about 3-7 years) appears to depend in part on the aggressiveness of the disease in a given patient. Currently, many more patients are diagnosed early in the chronic phase, with less splenomegaly and fewer circulating blasts, and therefore with a 'longer' chronic phase. This partially accounts for the observed improvement in the survival in CML over the past two to three decades.

The term, 'accelerated phase' refers to patients under therapy who develop evidence of disease progression, but who do not meet the criteria for a blast crisis. The time to progression to the blastic phase is not uniform among patients in the accelerated phase, however, partly because the definition of 'accelerated phase' has been vague in the literature. In the authors' experience, the accelerated phase can be suspected based on the peripheral blood findings (see Section 18.2). The most reliable evidence of an accelerated phase is the presence of additional cytogenetic abnormalities, however. These commonly involve a gain of chromosome 8, or abnormalities of chromosome 17. Chromosome 17 abnormalities are associated with a pseudo-Pelger-Huët appearance.

The blastic phase of CML is discussed in Chapter 40. There is, however, a lack of consistency in the literature for the definition of a blast crisis. Whereas the threshold of 20% blasts has been accepted for lymphoid blast crisis, the level of 30% blasts has been applied for a myeloid blast crisis in line with the blast cut-off established for AML. In view of the issues surrounding the 30% blast threshold in RAEB-T (Section 36.1.2), it would seem logical to adopt the International CML Prognostic Study Group's criteria defining blast crisis as 20% or more blasts in either the peripheral blood or bone marrow.

The terminology 'second chronic stage of CML' is actually a misnomer. This stage is better designated as a remission of the blastic phase following high-dose chemotherapy. The remission is invariably of short duration.

36.2.2 Chronic myelomonocytic leukemia (CMMoL)

The typical peripheral manifestation of CMMoL is a leukocytosis with increased monocytes and promonocytes. Although CMMoL is included in the FAB classification of MDS, the hematological picture and clinical manifestations more closely resemble the features of an MPD. Although dysplastic features are often present in CMMoL, they are not important as diagnostic criteria. The differential diagnosis between RAEB and CMMoL is rarely a problem, whereas diagnostic difficulty may arise between CMMoL, CML and a CML-like MPD. Cases with a high percentage of blasts and promonocytes meet the criteria for the 'mononuclear cell infiltration' pattern (Chapter 40) and need to be distinguished from AML with monocytic differentiation.

The FAB criteria for CMMoL are listed in Table 36.2. Whereas monocytes and promonocytes are prominent in the peripheral blood in CMMoL (Section 11.1.1), the monocytic component in bone marrow aspirates can appear deceptively insignificant for the following reasons:

1. The circulating monocytic elements are composed mostly of the mature forms, whereas in the bone marrow promonocytes predominate over monocytes. A similar picture may be seen in AML-M5b.

Table 36.2 FAB criteria for chronic myelomonocytic leukemia

1. Absolute monocytosis ($> 1 \times 10^9$/l) in the peripheral blood AND
2. Peripheral blasts less than 5% AND
3. Bone marrow blasts up to 20%.

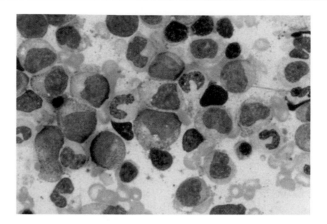

Figure 36.7   CMMoL: many of the round mononuclear precursors are actually pro-monocytes

2. Because of their round/ovoid nuclei, promonocytes in the bone marrow can be easily mistaken for hypogranulated myeloid precursors (Figure 36.7). This difficulty in cell identification is further accentuated in areas with shrinkage artifacts or cellular crowding on the aspirate smears. It is therefore important to perform the ANBE stain to avoid this problem (Figure 36.8). On biopsy sections, staining for lysozyme or immunostaining using antibodies against monocytic epitopes facilitates the identification of the monocytic elements. In CMMoL, the monocytic component accounts for at least 20% of bone marrow cells.

Similar to CML, the bone marrow in CMMoL typically demonstrates marked hypercellularity, an increased M:E ratio, a low proportion of blasts and mild cytologic abnormalities. With disease progression, the percentage of blasts increases. The term 'CMMoL in transformation' has been used to designate patients with more than 20% blasts. Some institutions diagnose these cases as AML with monocytic differentiation.

Patients with either low-grade MDS or RAEB can have a transient monocytosis in excess of 1×10^9/l. Based on FAB criteria, it is not possible to distinguish this group of 'MDS with peripheral monocytosis' from CMMoL. One difference is that the peripheral blood in CMMoL often has a granulocytosis in addition to the monocytosis, whereas neutropenia is the rule in MDS. The transient absolute monocytosis in some patients with MDS is reminiscent of the compensatory monocytosis associated with non-neoplastic neutropenia.

36.2.2.1 Juvenile CMMoL (or juvenile CML)

Juvenile CMMoL (JCMMoL) constitutes the majority of childhood myeloid disorders. The clinical and hematological features are essentially the same as those observed in adult CMMoL. Because the disease occurs in early childhood, bone marrow hypercellularity may be difficult to appreciate. As in

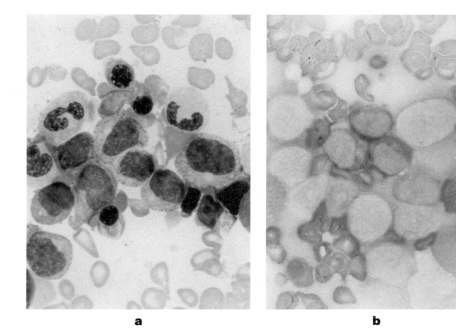

Figure 36.8 CMMoL. (a) Promonocytes with round and regular nuclear contours. Because of this appearance, the promonocytes in this case were initially misidentified as hypogranulated intermediate myeloid precursors. (b) The monocytic differentiation of these cells is confirmed by the ANBE stain. A positive reaction was seen in 30% of the cells

CMMoL, an ANBE stain on the aspirate smears or a lysozyme stain in bone marrow sections and biopsies of involved tissues (skin, lymph nodes) facilitates the identification of the neoplastic monocytic component. As in adults, the myeloproliferative features are more pronounced than the dysplastic changes.

In the literature, JCMMoL has not always been well separated from the 'monosomy 7 syndrome', since both conditions commonly present with anemia, thrombocytopenia and splenomegaly and occur predominantly in young males, and both are associated with a poor prognosis. Only 6–25% of cases of JCMMoL have monosomy 7, however. Furthermore, monosomy 7 has been reported in other pediatric myeloid malignancies and certain constitutional disorders including Fanconi's anemia, Kostmann's syndrome, familial monosomy 7 and neurofibromatosis type I.

In JCMMoL, Hgb H may be increased. This feature, previously considered the hallmark of JCMMoL, appears to be present only in cases without monosomy 7.

Cell culture studies are becoming an important adjunctive test to confirm the diagnosis of JCMMoL. The hematopoietic progenitors in JCMMoL proliferate normally in the presence of G-CSF or IL-3, but exhibit a selective hypersensitivity to GM-CSF. This results in the spontaneous growth of colonies which can be blocked by either antibodies to GM-CSF or removal of monocytes from the cell culture. The exact molecular abnormality underlying the hypersensitivity to GM-CSF remains to be elucidated.

36.2.3 Marked neutrophilia or persistent severe eosinophilia

A marked peripheral neutrophilia and a severe persistent eosinophilia raise the diagnostic possibilities of chronic neutrophilic leukemia and chronic eosinophilic leukemia, respectively. Both entities are uncommon and difficult to diagnose. In the literature, chronic eosinophilic leukemia has usually been discussed together with the idiopathic hypereosinophilic syndrome (HES). Chronic eosinophilic leukemia can be considered a subset of HES with bone marrow and cytogenetic abnormalities.

The diagnostic difficulties stem primarily in distinguishing these disorders from reactive conditions. Both a marked peripheral eosinophilia and a neutrophilic

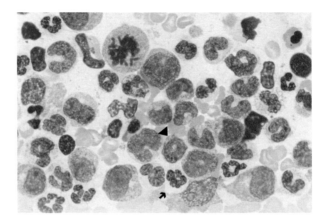

Figure 36.9 Chronic neutrophilic leukemia in a 70-year-old male: abundant mature myeloid precursors are apparent with occasional giant forms. Some precursors are hypogranulated (arrow). A rare cell has a ring-shaped nucleus (arrowhead). Cytogenetic studies revealed trisomy 8

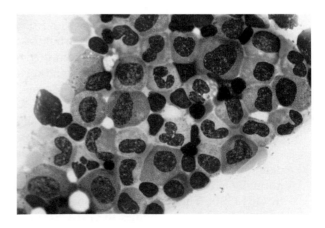

Figure 36.10 Chronic eosinophilic leukemia with a hypercellular marrow and 60% eosinophilic precursors. The CBC revealed an absolute eosinophilia of 40×10^9/l

leukemoid blood picture can be induced by underlying solid tumors via production of cytokines or growth factors. Basophilia, a helpful clue in identifying an MPD, is not present in either instance. Production of IL-3 by some lymphoid malignancies, e.g. ALL with t(5;14), can also result in a sustained reactive eosinophilia. In rare cases of CML or PRV, a marked eosinophilia may mask other features of the disease.

Chronic neutrophilic leukemia and chronic eosinophilic leukemia can be suspected when the respective peripheral manifestations (Figures 18.2 and 10.1) are accompanied by hepatosplenomegaly and a packed marrow with a markedly increased M:E ratio. In chronic neutrophilic leukemia, the myeloid hyperplasia is composed mostly of mature granulocytes (Figure 36.9). Cytologic abnormalities such as hypersegmentation and hypogranulation may be present. In chronic eosinophilic leukemia, the myeloid hyperplasia is accompanied by a marked preponderance of eosinophilic precursors, accounting for 33–50% of the bone marrow cells (Figure 36.10). Abnormal eosinophils with basophilic granules, and hypogranulated, hypersegmented eosinophils can also be found. The definitive diagnosis rests on the presence of clonal cytogenetic abnormalities to confirm the neoplastic nature of the process.

Megakaryocytic hyperplasia pattern

The proliferation and maturation of megakaryocytes is regulated by the interaction of several cytokines such as GM-CSF, interleukins, erythropoietin and thrombopoietin. Cells in the very early stages of megakaryocytic differentiation are not recognizable under normal circumstances, as they are rare and lack distinguishing morphologic features. FCM immunophenotyping (see Chapter 24) or platelet peroxidase ultracytochemistry can identify proliferations of these immature forms.

The maturation of megakaryocytes is an endomitotic process (i.e. nuclear division without cytoplasmic division) which results in large cells with multilobulated nuclei. Immature megakaryocytes are smaller with hypolobulated nuclei. Despite the great variation in nuclear lobulation and cell size (ranging from 15 to 80 μm), megakaryocytes can be recognized by their typical purple-blue granular cytoplasm.

Megakaryocytic hyperplasia can be either an isolated finding, or it can coexist with hyperplasia of erythroid and/or myeloid precursors (see Chapter 38). The quantitative and qualitative megakaryocytic abnormalities in hematological malignancies overlap with those in reactive conditions. Therefore, to reliably separate reactive from malignant processes, the evaluation of megakaryocytic hyperplasia must include peripheral blood data and ample clinical information.

37.1 Megakaryocytic hyperplasia and peripheral thrombocytopenia

Peripheral thrombocytopenia and megakaryocytic hyperplasia are the characteristic findings in ITP. The pathogenesis and clinical course of ITP, which are different between children and adults, are discussed in Section 9.2.

A bone marrow aspirate/biopsy is not usually performed in children with ITP unless the clinical course raises the suspicion of a more serious process. The procedure is more frequently performed in adults with isolated thrombocytopenia, however, because the early stages of an LPD or multiple myeloma can masquerade as ITP.

The bone marrow in ITP is normocellular for age with compensatory megakaryocytic hyperplasia. Many of the megakaryocytes are small with hypolobulated nuclei but there are no other significant abnormalities (Figure 37.1). Megakaryocytes may contain large cytoplasmic vacuoles. Late megakaryoblasts may also be recognizable morphologically by their deep basophilia, round nuclear contour, coarse chromatin, and larger size than erythroid precursors.

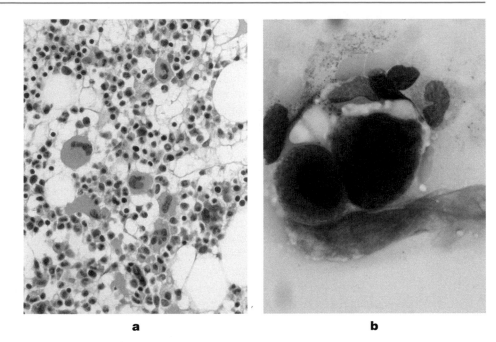

a   b

Figure 37.1 ITP. (a) Normocellular marrow with increased megakaryocytes. (b) Many of the megakaryocytes on the aspirate smears are small and monolobed with darkly stained cytoplasm

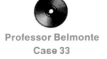

Professor Belmonte
Case 33

Hematogones, which may simulate ALL blasts morphologically, are often prominent in the bone marrows of children with ITP. In HIV patients with the clinical manifestations of ITP, the bone marrow does not necessarily demonstrate a compensatory increase in megakaryocytes.

Increased megakaryocytes and peripheral thrombocytopenia can also be a manifestation of some cases of MDS. Additional cytopenias, macrocytosis and hyposegmented/hypogranulated neutrophils are common findings. Confusion with ITP is unlikely. In such cases, the main diagnostic difficulty lies between AIDS and an MDS with increased megakaryocytes.

37.2 Increased megakaryocytes and peripheral thrombocytosis

Essential thrombocythemia is a diagnosis of exclusion since the disease has no distinctive diagnostic features. The diagnostic criteria are presented in Chapter 7. As discussed below, the combination of megakaryocytic hyperplasia and peripheral thrombocytosis should not lead to a 'reflex' interpretation of ET.

37.2.1 Reactive versus neoplastic megakaryocytic hyperplasia

Chronic inflammatory disorders, brisk bone marrow regeneration and underlying solid tumors can simulate the blood and bone marrow picture of ET. In nonhematopoietic malignancies, with or without bone marrow metastases, the reactive megakaryocytosis and thrombocytosis are presumably due to the release of thrombopoietin-like substances by the tumor cells. Most reactive processes have a platelet count lower than $1000 \times 10^9/l$ and a normocellular marrow. Some cases present with a more severe thrombocytosis and a hypercellular bone marrow, closely simulating an MPD.

Peripheral basophilia, a leukoerythroblastic peripheral blood pattern, bone marrow fibrosis in the absence of detectable bone marrow metastases, and a packed bone marrow (i.e. 90% + cellularity) are all features which favor a neoplastic megakaryocytic hyperplasia. Although not always present, enlarged hyperlobulated megakaryocytes, in the context of thrombocytosis and megakaryocytic hyperplasia, are supportive evidence of ET as opposed to another form of MPD. The diagnosis of ET is based primarily on the appropriate clinical manifestations, i.e. symptoms related to thrombosis or hemorrhage. Basophilia and bone marrow fibrosis are not typical features of ET.

In vitro cultures of hematopoietic precursors are useful for separating ET from reactive thrombocytosis. Approximately 75% of patients with ET demonstrate megakaryocyte and/or erythroid spontaneous colony formation without added growth factors or erythropoietin. Spontaneous growth is practically never seen in reactive thrombocytosis. Furthermore, it has been shown that patients with spontaneous megakaryocyte growth have a higher risk of thromboembolic complications.

37.2.2 Megakaryocytic hyperplasia in other MPDs and MDS

Megakaryocytic hyperplasia and thrombocytosis also feature in other subtypes of MPD. In particular, the distinction between ET and PRV can be difficult because of overlapping hemoglobin levels, platelet counts and bone marrow morphology (see Chapter 38).

Essential thrombocythemia is typically associated with a normal hemoglobin level and a normal to minimally elevated WBC count. However, the hemoglobin can vary widely from moderate anemia to erythrocytosis (6.4–18.8 g/dl) and the WBC count from normal to moderate leukocytosis (6–41.1 $\times$ 10^9/l). The low hemoglobin and normal WBC count overlap with that seen in low-grade MDS. Therefore, ET with anemia and leukopenia may be difficult to distinguish from the few cases of MDS with thrombocytosis and megakaryocytic hyperplasia. The distinction depends on the clinical behavior of the patient.

The main subgroups of MDS with thrombocytosis and megakaryocytic hyperplasia are the 5q– syndrome and cases with abnormalities of chromosome 3.

37.2.2.1 The 5q– syndrome

In general, the platelet count in MDS with thrombocytosis rarely exceeds $1000 \times 10^9/l$. The main subtype of MDS presenting with an increased platelet count is the 5q– syndrome. This syndrome is primarily a cytogenetic and clinical entity, associated with a favorable prognosis despite the requirement for regular RBC transfusions and complications resulting from iron overload. The risk of progression to AML and the incidence of infection, thrombosis and hemorrhage are low. Although the constellation of macrocytic anemia, a moderately increased platelet count ($> 1000 \times 10^9/l$) and the presence of hypolobulated megakaryocytes (Figure 37.2) in an elderly female suggests the 5q– syndrome, the diagnosis is less than straightforward for the following reasons:

1. None of the above-mentioned features is specific to the 5q– syndrome. Increased platelet counts have been described in association with RARS, and hypolobulated megakaryocytes similar to those seen in 5q– have been reported in MDS patients with both normal karyotypes and other cytogenetic abnormalities (Figure 37.3). Only when nuclear hypolobulation is present in nearly all megakaryocytes can the 5q– syndrome be suspected.
2. Some patients with the 5q– syndrome may not have all of the typical features. The peripheral blood picture may be that of a mild pancytopenia (with macrocytosis) instead of macrocytic anemia and moderate thrombocytosis.
3. The interstitial del(5q), either as an isolated finding or in association with other cytogenetic abnormalities, is one of the most common chromosomal aberrations in high-grade MDS and AML.
4. There has been variability in the criteria applied to the diagnosis of 5q– syndrome, whereby cases with excess blasts have also been included. This adds to the difficulty of comparing results between institutions and diminishes the prognostic significance of the diagnosis. In view of the favorable prognosis of the 5q– syndrome, current opinion is to restrict the definition to cases of primary refractory anemia with del(5q) as the sole cytogenctic abnormality.

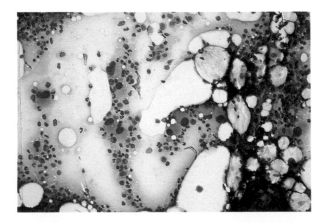

Figure 37.2 5q– syndrome in a 90-year-old female. Nearly all megakaryocytes are hypolobulated. The bone marrow in this patient is normocellular with increased megakaryocytes and a reversed M:E ratio

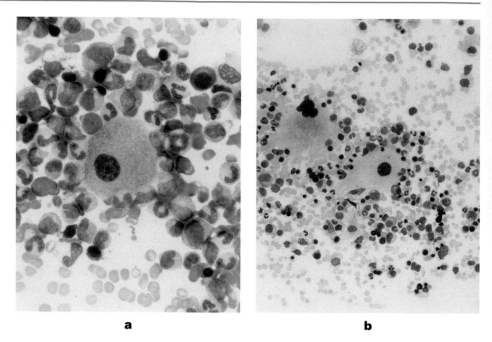

a   b

Figure 37.3 (a) One of the many monolobed megakaryocytes in a patient receiving G-CSF for peripheral blood stem cell harvest. The patient had Hodgkin's disease without bone marrow involvement. (b) A monolobed megakaryocyte in a case of RARS with del(7q) abnormality

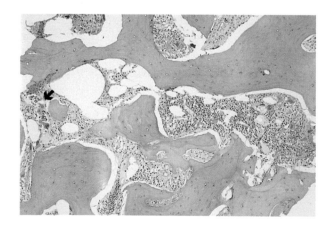

Figure 37.4 Late phase of AMM, showing scattered foci of increased megakaryocytes (arrow). Loose fibroblastic proliferation and new bone formation are also apparent, resulting in thickened bony trabeculae

37.3 Increased megakaryocytes and a leukoerythroblastic picture

The main diagnostic consideration in a leukoerythroblastic blood picture with megakaryocytic hyperplasia is AMM (see Section 38.2.2). The bone marrow in the late phase of AMM is composed predominantly of megakaryocytes, as the fibrosis gradually replaces other hematopoietic elements (Figure 37.4). The combination of a leukoerythroblastic blood picture and megakaryocytic hyperplasia can also occur as a transient rebound phenomenon during bone marrow recovery after chemotherapy, especially in children.

Bihyperplasia/panhyperplasia pattern

A hypercellular marrow with increased proliferation of more than one cell line is more commonly associated with an MPD than a reactive process, especially in the adult age group. Combined erythroid and megakaryocytic hyperplasia can also occur in some myelodysplastic syndromes, such as RARS or the 5q− syndrome.

In panhyperplasia, the hematopoietic elements from all three lineages are increased but the relative proportion of erythroid and myeloid precursors is maintained within the normal range. The most common combinations seen in bihyperplasia are: (1) megakaryocytic and erythroid hyperplasia; or (2) megakaryocytic and myeloid hyperplasia.

Bihyperplasia or panhyperplasia is a common finding in PRV and AMM. There is a substantial overlap in bone marrow morphology among the different MPDs, however. In evaluating a bone marrow specimen from an individual patient, it may be extremely difficult to distinguish PRV, ET and the early stage of AMM.

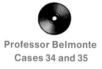

Professor Belmonte
Cases 34 and 35

A brisk bone marrow response to a variety of stimuli (e.g. thalassemia, some cases of HIV infection and an underlying malignancy secreting GM-CSF-like substances) can result in a benign hyperplastic picture simulating an MPD (Figure 38.1). A physiologic 'panhyperplasia' is normal in infants and young children. Therefore, bihyperplasia and panhyperplasia can only be properly evaluated when the clinical information and laboratory findings are known.

38.1 Bihyperplasia or panhyperplasia with a peripheral blood pattern of erythrocytosis

A hyperplastic marrow associated with peripheral erythrocytosis suggests PRV in the proliferative phase. Depleted iron stores secondary to excessive erythropoiesis and accentuated by repeated venesection is a helpful feature in the diagnosis. For the most part, the bone marrow is of limited value in distinguishing PRV from other MPDs, however. The diagnostic work-up for PRV is covered in Chapter 6.

Professor Belmonte
Case 36

In PRV, the hypercellular marrow contains an increased number of megakaryocytes, an M:E ratio varying from normal to decreased, normal maturation in both the erythroid and myeloid series, and usually no increase in bone marrow reticulin (Figure 38.2). None of these features is diagnostic for PRV. The same pattern is also observed in many cases of ET. The megakaryocytes in PRV

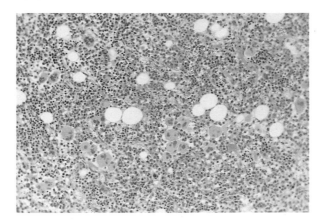

Figure 38.1 Hyperplastic bone marrow with increased proliferation of all three cell lines in an HIV-positive patient. The bone marrow picture is indistinguishable from that of a myeloproliferative disorder

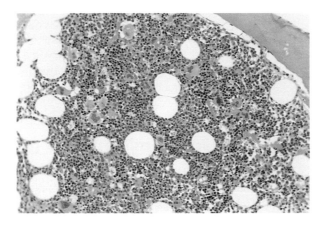

Figure 38.2 Hypercellular marrow with increased megakaryocytes and a reversed M:E ratio in a case of PRV

are often enlarged with hyperlobulated nuclei, another feature that overlaps with the typical findings in ET.

In about 40% of patients, PRV presents with panhyperplasia and increased reticulin. This picture is indistinguishable from that of the cellular phase of AMM. The reticulin fibrosis appears to have no prognostic significance, however. Although the spent phase of PRV is invariably accompanied by marked reticulin fibrosis, an increase in reticulin at the time of diagnosis does not necessarily imply imminent progression to the spent phase.

Although PRV usually presents with a markedly hypercellular marrow, normocellularity has been reported in 10–15% of the patients at the time of diagnosis. The normocellular appearance in such cases does not have any prognostic significance since the clinical course is similar to that observed in patients with hypercellular marrows. Follow-up bone marrow analysis in this subset of patients will usually reveal a typical hypercellular marrow.

38.2 Bihyperplasia/panhyperplasia with a peripheral leukoerythroblastic picture

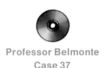

**Professor Belmonte
Case 37**

A vigorous regenerative response following chemotherapy may occasionally result in a hypercellular marrow with increased proliferation of erythroid and megakaryocytic elements, with one or more of the peripheral counts still lagging behind. The blood film in such cases usually reveals brisk polychromasia, circulating intermediate myeloid precursors and NRBCs, reflecting stressed hematopoiesis.

A leukoerythroblastic picture with basophilia points toward CML, AMM or the spent phase of PRV (also known as PPMM). A few circulating blasts are usually detectable. While CML typically presents with a higher WBC count ($>50 \times 10^9$/l) and fewer circulating NRBCs than AMM and PPMM, the latter two disorders can manifest a marked leukocytosis similar to that of CML. The three conditions share other features such as frequent giant platelets. The finding of abundant teardrop cells points toward AMM or PPMM, whereas a preponderance of small hypolobulated megakaryocytes in the bone marrow supports the diagnosis of CML. The most reliable distinguishing feature between CML and the other two conditions is the presence of the (9;22) translocation by standard cytogenetics or molecular genetics.

38.2.1 Post-polycythemic myeloid metaplasia (PPMM)

The diagnosis of PPMM cannot be made morphologically since the blood and bone marrow findings, as well as the massive splenomegaly, are indistinguishable from the findings in AMM. The diagnosis is made in the context of a well-documented history of PRV. The onset of the spent phase usually occurs 7–8 years after the initial diagnosis. The erythrocytosis of the proliferative phase is replaced during the spent phase by a progressive decrease in hemoglobin into the anemic range. The spent phase is associated with an increased risk of subsequent acute leukemia, especially in patients treated with alkylating agents.

38.2.2 Agnogenic myeloid metaplasia (or idiopathic myelofibrosis)

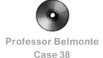

**Professor Belmonte
Case 38**

The diagnosis of AMM can be difficult because of overlapping hematological and clinical manifestations with other MPDs, including CML, ET and PRV. Furthermore, AMM and PPMM share bone marrow fibrosis, splenomegaly, extramedullary hematopoiesis and a leukoerythroblastic blood picture with abundant teardrop cells and basophilia.

The peripheral blood manifestations in AMM are discussed in Section 4.2. Although a leukoerythroblastic picture is typical, the WBC count, hemoglobin level and platelet count can vary widely. The variability in peripheral blood findings mirrors the variability in the bone marrow morphology of AMM. The bone marrow manifestations in AMM have been divided into three categories which appear to correspond to the early, intermediate and late stages of the disease. In general, as the disease progresses, reticulin and collagen fibrosis increases while the number of hematopoietic elements decreases.

In the cellular phase of AMM, there is a markedly hypercellular marrow with bihyperplasia or a trilineage proliferation (Figure 38.3) and diffuse reticulin fibrosis. Hematopoietic maturation is usually normal although some cases may display left-shifted myeloid maturation. Megakaryocytes are large with nuclear hyperlobulation.

Later in the course of AMM, the hematopoietic elements are normocellular but there is obvious collagen fibrosis. The predominant elements are megakaryocytes.

In the late stage of AMM, the hematopoietic elements are hypocellular with a few residual islands of megakaryocytes, extensive collagen fibrosis and neo-osseous formation (osteosclerosis). On biopsy sections, the megakaryocytes appear squeezed, stretched and distorted by the surrounding dense fibrosis (Figure 37.4).

The bone marrow in the latter two stages is indistinguishable from that seen in PPMM. A metastatic, poorly differentiated carcinoma with extensive fibrosis can closely mimic the end-stage bone marrow of AMM as well.

The mechanism causing fibrosis in AMM is not yet fully elucidated. Several megakaryocytic-derived growth factors are presumably involved, including platelet-derived growth factor (PDGF), transforming growth factor-β (TGF-β) and epidermal growth factor (EGF). Either an increase in synthesis or an abnormal release of PDGF from megakaryocytes could induce fibroblastic proliferation in AMM. The synthesis and activity of PDGF and EGF are influenced by TGF-β, which also facilitates the synthesis and accumulation of extracellular matrix. Platelet TGF-β is significantly increased in AMM in contrast to normal individuals and patients with ET.

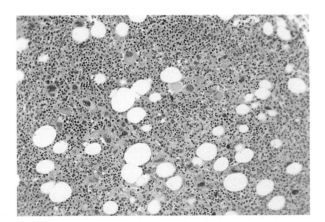

Figure 38.3   Bone marrow with panhyperplasia in AMM. There is also severe reticulin fibrosis (see Figure 33.2b). Cytogenetic and molecular studies revealed no bcr-abl rearrangement. The peripheral blood had a leukoerythroblastic pattern with moderate thrombocytosis but no erythrocytosis

Because of the extreme variability in the survival of patients diagnosed with AMM, a number of studies have been carried out to search for clinical and laboratory features that have prognostic value. The findings have varied, partially reflecting the difficulty in diagnosing AMM. In general, it appears that the size of the spleen and its rate of growth do not influence prognosis, whereas increasing age, anemia (Hgb $< 10\,g/dl$), and leukocytosis (WBC $> 12 \times 10^9/l$) are associated with a poor prognosis. The prognostic significance of thrombocytopenia, circulating blasts and cytogenetic abnormalities are not firmly established. The most frequently cited cytogenetic abnormalities include del(13q), del(20q) and partial trisomy 1q. Trisomy 8 and trisomy 21 occur less commonly.

38.3 Bihyperplasia/panhyperplasia with a peripheral blood thrombocytosis pattern

The differential diagnosis of bihyperplasia in the bone marrow along with a marked thrombocytosis ($1000 \times 10^9/l$) includes ET, reactive conditions (e.g. inflammatory disorders, underlying malignancies, post-chemotherapy rebound thrombocytosis) and the early stages of AMM, CML or PRV. Platelet morphology is of limited value in differential diagnosis, since giant platelets can be found in any of these conditions.

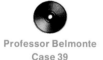

Professor Belmonte
Case 39

Most reactive conditions are associated with a normocellular bone marrow. The cellularity can be greater than 80% in reactive thrombocytosis, however. Although the number of megakaryocyte clusters present overlaps between reactive thrombocytosis and MPDs, the formation of sheets of megakaryocytes is suggestive of an MPD.

When considering the differential diagnosis between ET, PRV and the early stages of AMM, normal iron stores and absent reticulin fibrosis point toward the diagnosis of ET if the causes of reactive thrombocytosis have been excluded.

38.4 Bihyperplasia and peripheral cytopenias

Bihyperplasia (erythroid and megakaryocytic) along with peripheral cytopenias may occasionally be seen with brisk bone marrow regeneration following chemotherapy before the peripheral counts recover (Figure 38.4). Macrocytic anemia, and bicytopenia or pancytopenia together with bihyperplasia in the bone marrow can also occur in some low-grade MDSs (Figure 38.5). The bone marrow is hypercellular with an increased number of megakaryocytes and a decreased M:E ratio. Dyserythropoiesis and cytologic abnormalities in megakaryocytes are often present. Most cases represent RARS or the 5q– syndrome.

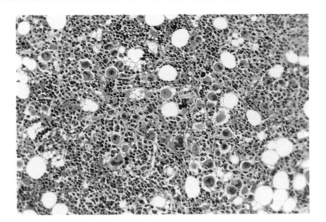

Figure 38.4 Hypercellular marrow with increased megakaryocytes and a reversed M:E ratio in a patient recovering from high-dose chemotherapy. The patient was still mildly anemic and leukopenic

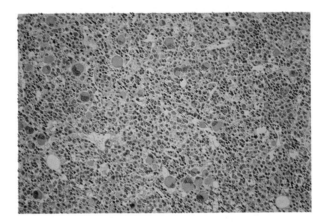

Figure 38.5 Hypercellular marrow with increased megakaryocytes and a reversed M:E ratio in therapy-related MDS (following autologous bone marrow transplantation for follicular lymphoma). The preponderance of early erythroid precursors on the biopsy section simulates the morphology of leukemic blasts

Bone marrow lymphocytosis/ plasmacytosis pattern

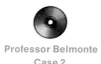

Professor Belmonte
Case 2

The upper limits of normal for plasma cells and lymphocytes have been set at 10% and 20%, respectively, in nonhypocellular bone marrows in adults. Care should be taken to perform the differential on good quality material so that blood contamination does not falsely elevate the lymphocyte count. An artifactual mild bone marrow lymphocytosis can occur when the manual differential is performed on aspirate smears prepared at the bedside using the 'push' technique.

In children, the upper limit of normal for lymphocytes is higher than in adults. Lymphocytes usually constitute about 30–35% of the nucleated cells in bone marrows of children, but can be as high as 50% in some instances. Many of the cells enumerated as 'lymphocytes' are actually hematogones, however.

The term 'lymphocyte' is used to designate cells that are present in the blood and bone marrow under normal conditions. Plasmacytoid lymphocytes and large granular lymphocytes are included in this category. In disorders such as CLL/ SLL, Waldenstrom's macroglobulinemia and LPC lymphoma-leukemia, the neoplastic cells are morphologically similar to their benign counterparts and are enumerated as lymphocytes in the bone marrow differential.

On blood films and bone marrow aspirate smears, it is possible to distinguish small lymphoma cells (most commonly FCC lymphoma and MCL) from small lymphocytes based on a combination of cytologic features. Furthermore, lymphoma cells can almost always be differentiated from CLL cells by their distinctive immunophenotype (see Section 27.4). Infiltration of the bone marrow by small lymphoma cells is discussed in Chapter 40.

On biopsy sections, where cytologic details are altered by fixation and processing, it is much more difficult to separate small lymphoma cells from lymphocytes. Chronic lymphocytic leukemia and MCL are difficult to diagnose on the biopsy alone since the H&E cytology of these disorders can overlap and the pattern of infiltration is not a distinguishing feature. For these reasons, small lymphoma cells and lymphocytes are designated together by the more generic term 'small lymphoid cells' in biopsy sections.

A severe bone marrow lymphocytosis or plasmacytosis on the aspirate smears invariably corresponds to a malignant process. Lesser degrees of lymphocytosis can be found in both benign and malignant conditions, however. In addition, the finding of fewer than 20% lymphocytes in the bone marrow does not exclude a malignant process (e.g. a low level of involvement by SLL).

Similarly, a diffuse or interstitial infiltrate of small lymphoid cells in biopsy sections points to a neoplastic process, whereas a focal lymphoid aggregate can be either benign or malignant. Diagnostic difficulty often arises when the bone marrow lymphocytosis is mild and/or the infiltration consists of a few focal lymphoid aggregates. This difficulty is further compounded when the material for evaluation is incomplete (e.g. biopsy sections only) and/or unaccompanied by adequate clinical and laboratory data.

The evaluation of bone marrow lymphocytosis or plasmacytosis should include:

1. Peripheral blood film examination.
2. FCM immunophenotyping, especially if the patient has unexplained peripheral lymphocytosis. Circulating monoclonal lymphoid cells may be readily detected by FCM immunophenotyping even when an absolute lymphocytosis is not present.
3. Adequate clinical information (including constitutional symptoms, autoimmune disease, lymphadenopathy and organomegaly).
4. The results of pertinent laboratory studies (e.g. an immunoelectrophoresis in patients with suspected CLL, LPC lymphoma-leukemia/Waldenstrom's macroglobulinemia and plasma cell dyscrasias).

39.1 Bone marrow lymphocytosis with peripheral absolute lymphocytosis

The main diagnosis to consider when there is lymphocytosis in both the blood and bone marrow is an LPD, either CLL, the most common adult leukemia in the Western world, or LPC lymphoma-leukemia. These diseases rarely occur before age 40, and affect males more commonly than females. The diagnoses of CLL and LPC lymphoma-leukemia are best established by peripheral blood examination together with FCM immunophenotyping (see Section 27.5). A preponderance of plasmacytoid lymphocytes points toward LPC lymphoma-leukemia.

The degree of lymphocytosis on aspirate smears usually mirrors the extent of neoplastic involvement observed on the corresponding biopsy sections. The proportion of lymphocytes may vary from one aspirate smear to another, however, particularly when the involvement consists of a few lymphoid aggregates (Figure 39.1) on the biopsy sections.

In LPC lymphoma-leukemia cases with marked differentiation toward the plasma cell stage, the plasmacytoid features can be appreciated on the biopsy sections. In addition, the bone marrow in lymphoplasmacytoid disorders often contains an increased number of mast cells. This is not a diagnostic feature, however, since increased mast cells can also occur in FCC lymphoma, Hodgkin's disease and acute leukemia.

In both CLL and LPC lymphoma-leukemia, the extent of bone marrow involvement correlates with the stage of the disease. Diffuse involvement indicates either progressive or advanced disease (Figure 39.2). Extensive bone marrow involvement in these disorders is invariably associated with heavy reticulin fibrosis, resulting in aspicular aspirates. In such instances, the biopsy touch imprints should be examined instead, since the lymphocytosis on the hemodilute aspirate is actually from the blood.

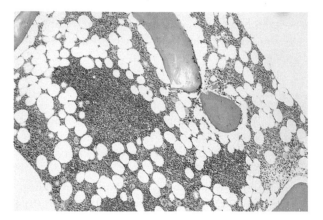

Figure 39.1 Two sizable lymphoid aggregates in a case of CLL (nodular pattern of infiltration)

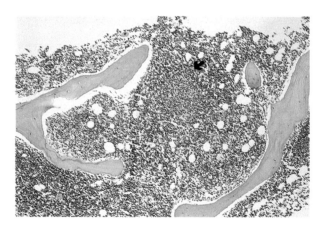

Figure 39.2 Chronic lymphocytic leukemia, showing diffuse infiltration by small lymphoid cells. A small proliferation center (arrow) is present

39.1.1 Chronic lymphocytic leukemia

According to National Cancer Institute (NCI) recommendations, a bone marrow sample is not an absolute requirement for the diagnostic work-up of CLL if the peripheral absolute lymphocytosis demonstrates the pathognomonic antigenic profile of CLL, i.e. weak CD20, weak surface immunoglobulin, plus expression of CD5 and CD23 (see Section 27.5.1). A bone marrow examination may be considered if the peripheral lymphocytosis is mild. The authors use an absolute lymphocyte count of $4 \times 10^9/l$ as the threshold instead of $5 \times 10^9/l$ proposed by the NCI.

A bone marrow lymphocytosis of at least 30% in a normocellular or hypercellular marrow has also been suggested as a criterion for the diagnosis of CLL. This feature is rather redundant once the peripheral blood and FCM results have established the diagnosis, however (Section 8.2.1).

In CLL, the infiltrate is composed mostly of small lymphocytes with occasional prolymphocytes (Figure 39.3). If there are 11–55% prolymphocytes, then the diagnosis is CLL with increased prolymphocytes (CLL/PL). A few plasmacytoid lymphocytes are often present.

Clinical and laboratory features have been used to stratify CLL into various stages. A system simpler than the existing Rai and Binet systems has been recently recommended by the NCI Working Group. This system separates patients into three risk groups: (1) low risk with only blood and bone marrow lymphocytosis; (2) intermediate risk with lymphocytosis, lymphadenopathy and/or organomegaly (spleen and/or liver); and (3) high risk with lymphocytosis and Hgb < 11 g/dl and/or platelets < 100 × 10^9/l.

The blood lymphocyte doubling time, pattern of bone marrow infiltration, and β_2 microglobulin level have also been used as prognostic factors. A long doubling time (> 12 months), nondiffuse infiltration and low β_2 microglobulin levels are features associated with a better outcome.

Chromosomal abnormalities are less widely used as prognostic indicators because cytogenetic analysis is not routinely performed in CLL. There is no unique genetic marker of CLL. The most commonly reported abnormalities involve chromosomes 12 (trisomy), 13q14, 14q32 in the vicinity of the heavy

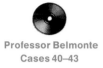

Professor Belmonte
Cases 40–43

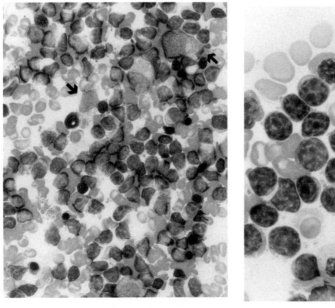
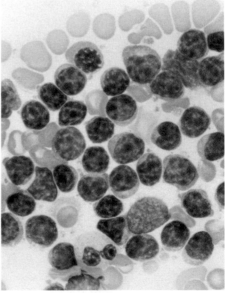

a   b

Figure 39.3 Chronic lymphocytic leukemia. (a) An infiltrate of lymphocytes with a few prolymphocytes (arrow). (b) 'Chunky' nuclear chromatin in the small lymphocytes of CLL

chain gene, 6q or 11q. Except for translocations involving 13q14, the presence of cytogenetic aberrancies is associated with a poorer prognosis. The karyotypic abnormality usually remains stable during the course of the disease. The appearance of complex karyotypic changes often heralds transformation to an aggressive large cell lymphoma (Richter's syndrome).

Disease progression in CLL is accompanied by humoral and cellular immune defects. Consequently, hypogammaglobulinemia is present in virtually all patients with advanced disease. The progressive reduction in immunoglobulins contrasts with the increasing number of B lymphocytes in the blood and bone marrow, implying that the neoplastic population in CLL is composed of 'inactive' B cells.

The CD5$^+$ B lymphocytes in CLL are different from normal CD5$^+$ B cells. In addition to low levels of surface immunoglobulin, other abnormalities have been reported, including high expression of bcl-2 (which accounts for the long lifespan of the tumor cells) and defects in antigen-receptor-mediated functions (resulting in impaired cell to cell interaction).

Experimental evidence suggests that CLL is a disorder of B cells in a state of functional anergy. In addition to the inability to mount an effective antibody response against infectious agents, CLL patients also have impaired delayed hypersensitivity reactions and an inverted peripheral blood CD4:CD8 ratio.

There appears to be an association between autoimmunity and CLL. Patients with systemic autoimmune disorders, such as refractory anemia or Sjogren's syndrome, have elevated numbers of CD5$^+$ B cells, which normally comprise only a small portion of the B cells in the blood and lymphoid organs. Although patients with CLL do not have an increased incidence of systemic autoimmune disease, autoantibodies against RBCs and/or platelets are detectable in many patients, independent of the stage of the disease. In most instances, the autoantibodies are not clinically significant since only a small proportion of patients actually develop AIHA or ITP. Autoantibodies in CLL are usually of the polyreactive type, with low affinity for several different antigens. The light chain and heavy chain isotypes of the autoantibodies are not restricted to those found on the malignant cells, which suggests that they are not produced by the leukemic clones.

39.1.2 LPC lymphoma-leukemia

Benign plasmacytoid lymphocytes are larger than small round lymphocytes. Similarly, neoplastic plasmacytoid cells in LPC neoplasms are larger than the cells in CLL. The plasmacytoid cells in LPC lymphoma-leukemia (Figure 39.4) have moderate cytoplasm of varying degrees of basophilia (Figure 39.5) depending on the extent of differentiation toward the plasma cell stage (see Section 8.2).

The diagnosis of LPC lymphoma-leukemia can be difficult. The difficulties arise mainly from the presence of morphologic artifacts and the lack of a distinctive antigenic profile. The most common artifacts on blood and bone marrow smears are hairy and villous projections secondary to slow drying (see Section 1.4). Systematic correlation of different laboratory studies such as the lymph node biopsy and immunoelectrophoresis improves reproducibility in the diagnosis of LPC lymphoma-leukemia.

Professor Belmonte
Cases 44 and 45

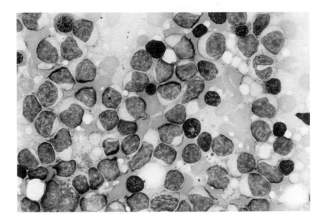

Figure 39.4 Bone marrow imprint in a case of lymphoplasmacytoid lymphoma-leukemia, showing plasmacytoid lymphocytes with a moderate amount of pale cytoplasm. A small nucleolus can be seen in some cells. The morphology is less easily appreciated in the bone marrow than in the corresponding peripheral blood because of the higher cell density

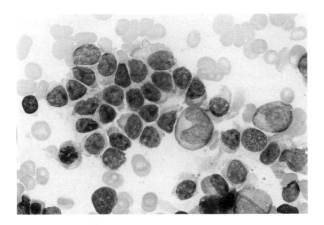

Figure 39.5 Lymphoplasmacytoid lymphoma-leukemia: the neoplastic cells in this case are more basophilic than those in the case shown in Figure 39.4

The spectrum of hematological manifestations in LPC lymphoma-leukemia is similar to that seen in CLL/SLL, in that the predominant presentation can be either bone marrow/peripheral blood disease or lymph node disease. Either manifestation can be accompanied by splenomegaly. Many patients have monoclonal immunoglobulin in the serum during the course of their disease, but this may not be detectable unless sensitive techniques are used. The morphologic findings in LPC lymphoma-leukemia and its relationship to Waldenstrom's macroglobulinemia are presented in Section 39.2.1.

Because of the hairy and villous projections (Figure 39.6), LPC lymphoma-leukemia has often been called splenic lymphoma with villous lymphocytes (SLVL). Except for the so-called characteristic cytoplasmic villi, the features

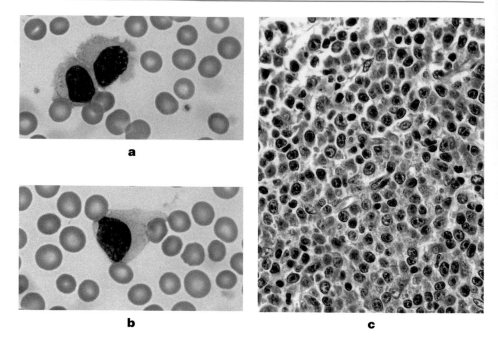

Figure 39.6 Peripheral blood films and bone marrow biopsy from a case of LPC lymphoma-leukemia. (a) Blood smear left to dry slowly: artifactual hairy projections are present on both the neoplastic plasmacytoid lymphocyte and a large granular lymphocyte. (b) Neoplastic plasmacytoid lymphocyte on the quickly dried blood film. Note that the stain is not quite optimal, imparting a more condensed appearance to the nuclear chromatin. (c) The plasmacytoid differentiation is evident on the bone marrow biopsy

of SLVL described in the literature are similar, if not identical, to those of LPC lymphoma-leukemia/Waldenstrom's macroglobulinemia and include the following:

- The affected patients are predominantly elderly males.
- The lymphocyte count varies from normal to markedly increased.
- The neoplastic cells are larger than the cells in CLL, with a round nucleus, clumped chromatin, distinct nucleolus, and moderate cytoplasm. In addition, published photographs often show an eccentric nucleus in SLVL.
- The bone marrow demonstrates prominent lymphoplasmacytic differentiation. The infiltration can be nodular, interstitial, diffuse or mixed and bone marrow disease is usually accompanied by splenomegaly.
- Splenic involvement starts in the white pulp with subsequent spilling into the red pulp. Lymphadenopathy can be present.
- A B-cell phenotype is present with moderate surface immunoglobulin intensity and frequent expression of CD11c. The phenotypic profile is not distinctive, however. Some cases may be CD5[+] and rare cases express CD103.
- A monoclonal gammopathy is a frequent finding, although at a concentration lower than that established for Waldenstrom's macroglobulinemia.
- Rare cases transform into Richter's syndrome.

Splenic lymphoma with villous lymphocytes has also been called 'splenomegalic immunocytoma with circulating hairy cells'. The term immunocytoma is synonymous with LPC lymphoma.

39.2 Bone marrow lymphocytosis without peripheral lymphocytosis

In adults, a marked bone marrow lymphocytosis (e.g. 50% or more lymphocytes) on aspirate smears or biopsy touch imprints is straightforward morphologic evidence of a lymphoid malignancy. Bone marrow lymphocytosis without peripheral lymphocytosis is a feature of SLL and Waldenstrom's macroglobulinemia. The same picture can be seen with CLL or LPC lymphoma-leukemia following treatment. Chemotherapy and monoclonal antibody therapy often cause clearing of the peripheral lymphocytosis even when the bone marrow response is less striking. Low numbers of circulating neoplastic cells in these conditions can easily be detected by multiparameter FCM immunophenotyping.

In the differential diagnosis of SLL and Waldenstrom's macroglobulinemia, other small cell lymphomas need to be considered. The neoplastic population in some cases of MCL or FCC lymphoma may be composed of monotonous small lymphoid cells with smooth round nuclear contours on air-dried preparations (Figure 39.7). Small lymphoma cells with such an apparently benign cytology can be easily overlooked and enumerated as lymphocytes in the bone marrow differential. Correct identification can usually be readily achieved by FCM immunophenotyping (see Sections 27.5.3, 27.6, 40.4.1 and 40.4.2).

39.2.1 Small lymphocytic lymphoma and Waldenstrom's macroglobulinemia

As discussed in Section 27.5.1, CLL and SLL are but one disease. The distinction is essentially a semantic issue based on the initial site(s) of presentation (bone marrow and peripheral blood vs. lymph node). There appears to be no difference in the biological behavior of this disease between patients who present predominantly with lymphadenopathy and those with lymphocytosis. Since the extent of bone marrow involvement mirrors the peripheral blood lymphocytosis, it is not surprising that the bone marrow infiltration in SLL is focal or multifocal, whereas interstitial (Figure 39.8) or diffuse infiltration is more common in CLL.

A similar relationship exists between Waldenstrom's macroglobulinemia and LPC lymphoma. Both conditions affect predominantly middle aged to elderly males. Many patients presenting with nodal LPC lymphoma have bone marrow involvement and detectable monoclonal IgM or IgA in the serum, although usually at a concentration lower than that arbitrarily set for Waldenstrom's. Conversely, many patients with Waldenstrom's macroglobulinemia develop hepatosplenomegaly and lymphadenopathy during the course of their disease. In either condition, the WBC count is often normal, with or without a relative lymphocy-

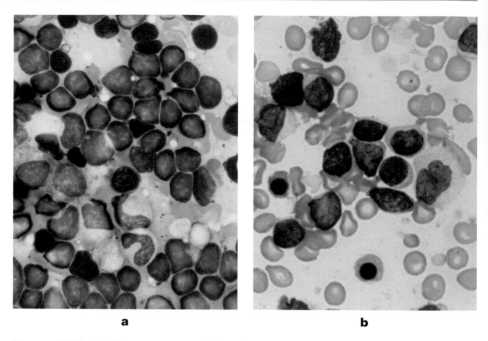

Figure 39.7 (a) Monotonous small lymphoma cells with round and regular nuclear contours in an FCC lymphoma, initially misinterpreted as SLL/CLL. Note that the neoplastic cells have a smooth nuclear chromatin. (b) Mantle cell lymphoma composed predominantly of neoplastic cells with round nuclear contours. Nuclear indentation is present in a rare cell

tosis (see Section 8.2.2). In a substantial number of patients, however, an elevated WBC count with absolute lymphocytosis is present at diagnosis or develops as the disease progresses. Similar to CLL/SLL, a small proportion of Waldenstrom's patients develop high-grade NHL, usually with immunoblastic morphology (Richter's syndrome).

Both LPC lymphoma and Waldenstrom's macroglobulinemia share the same morphology, namely a neoplastic population with a preponderance of plasmacy-

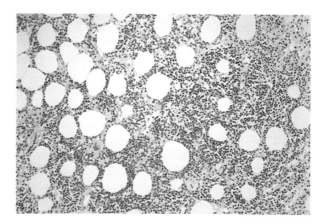

Figure 39.8 Interstitial infiltration in CLL

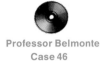

toid lymphocytes admixed with a lesser number of small round lymphocytes, plasma cells and transformed lymphoid cells (immunoblasts). Immunoblasts are few in number (well below 10% in the authors' experience) and may exhibit variable degrees of nuclear abnormalities (Figure 39.9). An increasing proportion of immunoblasts implies a more aggressive course. Cytoplasmic inclusions (Russell bodies), which may overlay the nucleus (Dutcher bodies), are sometimes detectable, especially in lymph node sections where a much larger number of cells are available for examination. Immunologically, plasmacytoid lymphocytes demonstrate a variable density of surface and cytoplasmic immunoglobulins depending on the degree of differentiation toward the plasma cell stage. With increasing differentiation, surface immunoglobulin progressively decreases and cytoplasmic immunoglobulin becomes more abundant.

Because of their identical features, it is logical to consider LPC lymphoma-leukemia and Waldenstrom's macroglobulinemia together as one disease entity with variable levels of monoclonal protein (IgM or IgA) in the serum. The disease can present in any of the following ways:

- Involvement of the solid lymphoid organs only, i.e. lymphadenopathy and/or organomegaly, with or without a monoclonal serum immunoglobulin. This presentation is analogous to SLL and localized plasmacytoma.
- Involvement of the bone marrow but no peripheral lymphocytosis, similar to SLL.
- A leukemic presentation, analogous to CLL.

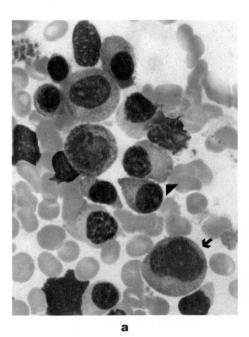
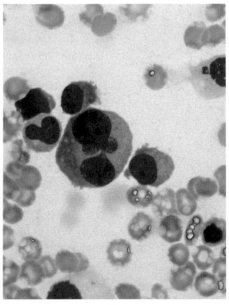

a **b**

Figure 39.9 Bone marrow aspirate smear from a case of Waldenstrom's macroglobulinemia. (a) Plasmacytoid lymphocytes with basophilic cytoplasm (arrowhead) and occasional immunoblasts (arrow). (b) One immunoblast with bizarre nuclear morphology

Patients with high levels of monoclonal immunoglobulin (i.e. the classical description of Waldenstrom's macroglobulinemia) develop symptoms of hyperviscosity such as visual impairment and fleeting neurologic disturbances. The plasma viscosity level does not necessarily reflect the severity of the hyperviscosity syndrome. In addition, aggregates of IgM polymers can precipitate as cryoglobulins, which, if they have wide thermal amplitude, can lead to intravascular hemolysis. Nonspecific binding of IgM to platelets, clotting factors and fibrin contributes to the bleeding diathesis. Unlike multiple myeloma, renal manifestations are uncommon since the polymers are too large to filter through the glomeruli, and the levels of calcium and uric acid are not increased.

39.2.2 Focal lymphoid aggregates and/or mild bone marrow lymphocytosis

Aspiration of a benign or malignant lymphoid aggregate can yield sheets of lymphocytes present on some but not all of the aspirate smears. The pattern of lymphoid infiltration on the corresponding biopsy sections can be helpful in determining the nature of the mild bone marrow lymphocytosis. An interstitial pattern, with or without focal aggregate(s), points toward a malignant lymphoid process.

The finding of a few focal lymphoid aggregates, with or without mild bone marrow lymphocytosis, can pose diagnostic difficulties since this morphologic manifestation is shared by both benign and malignant conditions (Figure 39.10). FCM immunophenotyping can be crucial in making the correct diagnosis.

Caution should be exercised when rendering a morphologic interpretation of a focal infiltrate as a benign lymphoid aggregate in patients with known LPD/NHL, either on the diagnostic staging marrow or on the follow-up marrow after chemotherapy. Retrospective studies in CLL have shown that among the patients considered to be in complete remission, those with a lymphoid nodule relapse quickly, implying that the focus represents residual disease rather than a benign lymphoid aggregate.

The size and number of lymphoid nodules on biopsy sections cannot be relied upon with absolute certainty to resolve the diagnostic dilemma between a benign aggregate and a malignant infiltrate. The level of the H&E section can affect the size of an aggregate. In addition, finding only a few (one to three) small aggregates does not exclude malignancy.

The cytology of the cells in the aggregate can also be misleading. The traditional description of a benign lymphoid aggregate is that of a small, well-circumscribed nodule composed of mature-appearing lymphocytes without nuclear irregularities. Disorders such as SLL/CLL have a similar morphology, however. In addition, nuclear irregularities can easily result from fixation and processing (Figure 39.11).

The reactive lymphoid aggregates in the bone marrow of HIV patients may be large and poorly circumscribed, containing a variable number of transformed lymphoid cells. These features can be easily misinterpreted as malignant. The morphologic differential diagnosis is rendered more difficult since AIDS patients are known to have a higher risk of developing NHL. These difficulties further

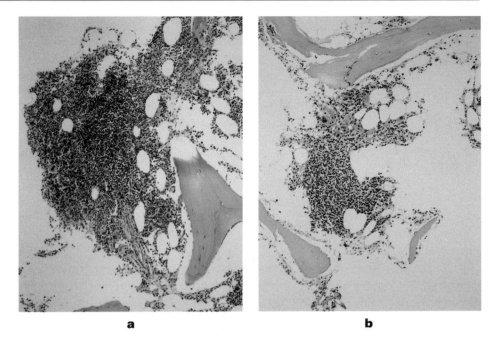

a   **b**

Figure 39.10 Bone marrow biopsies from two different patients, illustrating morphologic similarities (size, circumscription) between a benign lymphoid aggregate (a) and
a single focus of residual mantle cell lymphoma (b)

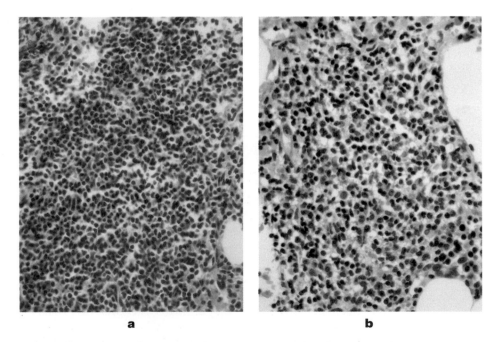

a   **b**

Figure 39.11 Bone marrow biopsies from two different patients (shown in Figure
39.10). Small lymphoid cells with round to irregular nuclei are present in both the
benign lymphoid aggregate (a) and the residual focus of mantle cell lymphoma (b)

stress the need to integrate multiparameter FCM immunophenotyping in the evaluation of lymphoid infiltrates in the bone marrow.

The frequency of benign lymphoid aggregates increases in autoimmune disorders as well as in older subjects. The elderly also have a higher incidence of LPD/ NHL, however. In the absence of immunophenotyping data and/or adequate clinical information, it is preferable to render a morphologic interpretation of 'focal lymphoid aggregate' rather than 'benign lymphoid aggregate' or 'nodular lymphoid hyperplasia'.

A morphologic feature helpful in identifying benign lymphoid aggregates is the presence of a well-defined germinal center surrounded by a complete mantle cuff (Figure 39.12). This finding is seen mainly in females with underlying autoimmune disorders or drug-related illness.

39.3 Lymphocytosis composed of large granular lymphocytes

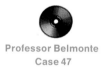

Professor Belmonte
Case 47

Increased numbers of LGLs are better appreciated in the peripheral blood (Figure 39.13) than in the bone marrow. The distinction between reactive and neoplastic LGL proliferations can be difficult when the peripheral blood LGL count is only mildly elevated and the cells appear normal cytologically. The diagnosis requires a multiparameter work-up including FCM analysis (see Sections 28.1 and 28.3), especially since neoplastic LGLs can be agranular by light microscopy (Section 8.2.3).

In LGL leukemia, the degree of bone marrow involvement is variable and does not correlate with the number of LGLs in the peripheral blood. In advanced or aggressive disease, a diffuse infiltrate of LGLs with abundant pale cytoplasm and widespread increased reticulin fibrosis can mimic the appearance of HCL in the bone marrow biopsy (Figure 39.14).

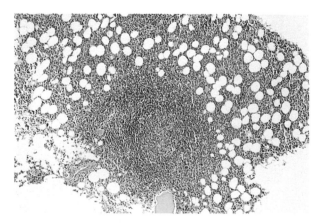

Figure 39.12 A sizable benign lymphoid aggregate with a mantle cuff and germinal center in a young adult female with rheumatoid arthritis

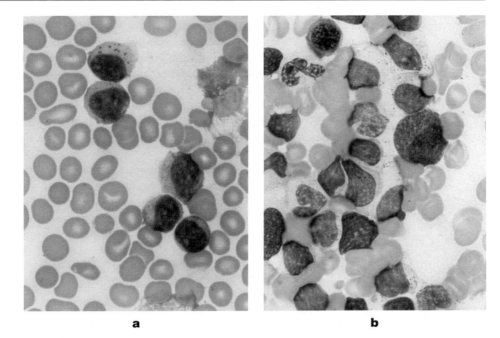

a   b

Figure 39.13   Peripheral blood (a) and bone marrow (b) films in a case of LGL leukemia. The bone marrow infiltration does not mirror the marked peripheral blood involvement (WBC count 50 $\times$ 10^9/l, 90% LGLs)

39.4 Bone marrow plasmacytosis

The number of plasma cells in a normal bone marrow is usually well below the established threshold of 10%. A focal distribution of plasma cells or an increase in reticulin fibrosis can result in lower plasma cell counts on aspirate smears than on biopsy sections. Therefore, evaluation of bone marrow plasmacytosis requires the availability of both an aspirate and a biopsy.

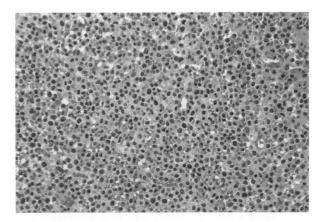

Figure 39.14   Aggressive LGL leukemia with a packed bone marrow. Neoplastic cells with ample pale cytoplasm are present, reminiscent of those in hairy cell leukemia (compare with Figure 40.37)

A marked bone marrow plasmacytosis or the presence of sheets of plasma cells (Figure 39.15) is straightforward morphologic evidence of a malignant plasma cell proliferation, even when the plasma cells appear cytologically normal. The diagnosis is more difficult when the proportion of normal-appearing plasma cells is only mildly increased and infiltration is slight in the biopsy, because these features can be found in both reactive and malignant plasma cell proliferations. Since bone marrow involvement in multiple myeloma may consist of only scattered foci, an arbitrary percentage of plasma cells cannot be applied as a discriminatory criterion either.

Scattered multifocal involvement in multiple myeloma can lead to sampling problems. Therefore, the absence of plasmacytosis does not imply absence of disease. Neither the presence of binucleated or trinucleated plasma cells nor the lack of a plasma cell predilection for vascular structures can be relied upon to differentiate a reactive plasmacytosis from multiple myeloma. In addition, other morphologic subtypes of plasma cells, such as the Mott cell, flame cell or Dutcher body, are of no diagnostic significance.

In mild to moderate plasmacytosis, a helpful morphologic feature favoring a neoplastic process is sizable plasma cell nodules displacing normal hematopoietic elements on the biopsy sections (a 'mass effect'). The most useful cytologic feature to diagnose a neoplastic plasma cell proliferation is the presence of immature-appearing plasma cells (plasmablasts) characterized by a less condensed nuclear chromatin and conspicuous nucleoli (Figures 39.16 and 39.17). Scattered plasmablasts are better appreciated on air-dried preparations than biopsy sections. When plasmablasts are present, the bone marrow meets the definition of the 'mononuclear cell infiltration pattern' rather than the 'lymphocytosis/plasmacytosis pattern'.

When plasmablasts and/or 'invasive' plasma cell nodules are absent, the distinction between multiple myeloma and reactive plasmacytosis is best made by laboratory studies rather than morphologic evaluation. Serum and urine immu-

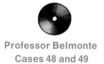

Professor Belmonte
Cases 48 and 49

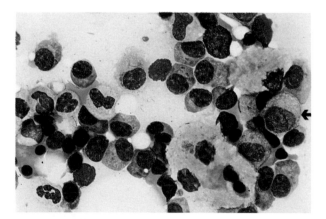

Figure 39.15 Multiple myeloma composed of mature-appearing plasma cells containing immunoglobulin crystals. Two macrophages are visible, with phagocytosis of immunoglobulin crystals. An occasional immature-appearing plasma cell (arrow) is present

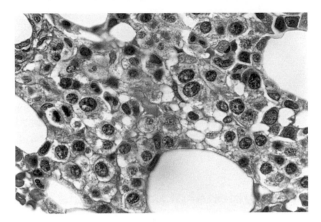

Figure 39.16   Plasmablasts on a biopsy section (100× oil objective)

noelectrophoresis, and the determination of clonality by FCM immunophenotyping (see Section 29.1) or immunostaining for cytoplasmic light chains on tissue sections are the most reliable tests.

In tissue sections, monoclonal plasma cells may be accompanied by extracellular amyloid deposits that appear homogeneous, eosinophilic and amorphous, usually associated with blood vessel walls. Staining of amyloid with Congo red yields a characteristic apple green birefringence when examined under polarized

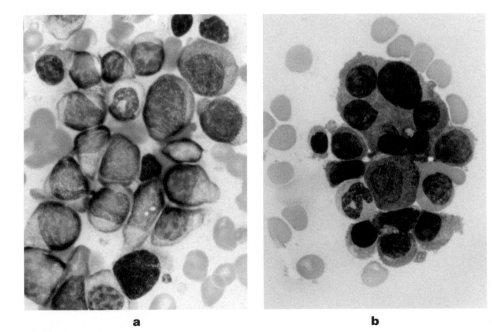

| a | b |

Figure 39.17   Bone marrow aspirates from two different cases of multiple myeloma. (a) Neoplastic population composed predominantly of plasmablasts with a high nuclear/cytoplasmic ratio, dispersed nuclear chromatin and visible nucleoli. (b) A bizarre multinucleated plasmablast. In this case, the bone marrow contained 5% plasmablasts and 1% plasma cells

light. The ultrastructural cross β-pleated sheet configuration of amyloid fibrils accounts for its optical and staining properties.

In amyloid deposits associated with monoclonal plasma cell proliferations (primary amyloidosis), the fibrils are composed of the variable region of the monoclonal light chain. Most cases involve the lambda light chain. Depending on the organs involved, the major clinical manifestations can include nephrotic syndrome, congestive heart failure, and hepatosplenomegaly. A bleeding diathesis is common since the amyloid protein can bind with factor X, causing an acquired factor X deficiency.

39.4.1 Polyclonal plasmacytosis

The most common causes of a reactive plasmacytosis are chronic infections, especially HIV (Figure 39.18), and autoimmune disorders such as rheumatoid arthritis. Up to 15–35% plasma cells can be found in the bone marrow in these conditions. Occasionally, the plasmacytosis is so striking as to mimic multiple myeloma morphologically. The reactive plasma cells can be enlarged and are occasionally binucleated or trinucleated. The serum immunoelectrophoresis in reactive plasmacytosis often demonstrates polyclonal hypergammaglobulinemia.

Professor Belmonte
Case 50

Systemic polyclonal immunoblastic proliferations have been reported as unusual florid reactive conditions. They are characterized by an extensive proliferation of plasma cells and immunoblasts involving the peripheral blood, bone marrow and several other organs. The underlying etiology is presumed to be infectious in origin. Because of the diffuse/interstitial pattern of infiltration on biopsy sections and the presence of abundant immunoblasts, this rare process can be misinterpreted morphologically as multiple myeloma or immunoblastic lymphoma. The correct diagnosis can be established based on the clinical history of an infection and the demonstration of polyclonality, either by FCM analysis or immunohistochemistry. Molecular studies are of limited value because clonal gene

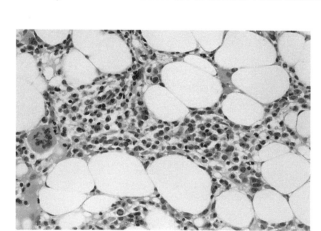

Figure 39.18 Interstitial infiltrate of mature-appearing plasma cells in an HIV-positive patient with reactive plasmacytosis. The bone marrow contained 35–40% plasma cells. The plasma cells were polyclonal. There was also a polyclonal hypergammaglobulinemia

rearrangements have been reported in rare proven cases of viral infection and may be absent in multiple myeloma.

39.4.2 Monoclonal/neoplastic plasma cell proliferations

The finding of monoclonal plasma cells in the bone marrow indicates a plasma cell dyscrasia irrespective of the number of plasma cells present. In addition to peripheral blood/bone marrow examination and FCM immunophenotyping (or immunohistochemical staining), the subclassification of a plasma cell dyscrasia into various categories including MGUS or multiple myeloma requires additional laboratory studies and clinical follow-up. The routine diagnostic work-up for plasma cell dyscrasias should include serum and urine immunoelectrophoresis with immunoglobulin quantitation, a large chemistry panel (including serum calcium, creatinine, alkaline phosphatase, LDH, C-reactive protein, and β_2 microglobulin), a skeletal survey (preferably by magnetic resonance imaging), and determination of the plasma cell labeling index. In addition to their role in diagnosis, some of these parameters are also of prognostic significance.

The spectrum of plasma cell dyscrasias ranges from stable, harmless monoclonal gammopathy to fatal plasma cell leukemia (PCL). The current classification of monoclonal plasmacytosis includes MGUS, solitary plasmacytoma, the various grades of myeloma (smoldering, indolent and overt) and PCL. Primary amyloidosis can occur in the background of any of these conditions.

The most common monoclonal (M) immunoglobulin produced in plasma cell dyscrasias is IgG. Monoclonal IgA occurs in 20–25% of patients with multiple myeloma. The level of the M protein reflects the size of the monoclonal plasma cell proliferation. Serial quantitation of the M component is therefore useful for monitoring the disease course, including response to therapy or progression from MGUS to overt multiple myeloma.

In most instances, the M protein is secreted as an intact molecule with both heavy and light chain components. The neoplastic plasma cells in some patients may produce light chains only, however, or an excess of light chains in addition to the whole immunoglobulin molecule. Because of their low molecular weight, the light chains are filtered through the kidney and ultimately excreted in the urine. Therefore, in light chain multiple myeloma, the serum immunoelectrophoresis may demonstrate only hypogammaglobulinemia and no detectable M protein. The production of heavy chains only (resulting in heavy chain disease) and the absence of an M component in multiple myeloma (i.e. nonsecretory multiple myeloma) are infrequent occurrences. In nonsecretory myeloma, M protein is synthesized by the neoplastic cells as indicated by the presence of monoclonal cytoplasmic immunoglobulin. Its release is impaired, however, presumably because of a block at the level of the Golgi apparatus.

39.4.3 Monoclonal gammopathy of undetermined significance (MGUS)

The diagnosis of MGUS is a clinical diagnosis that requires follow-up over a long period. The diagnostic criteria for MGUS are shown in Table 39.1.

Table 39.1 Diagnosis criteria for MGUS

- A serum monoclonal spike (<3 g/dl if IgG, <2 g/dl if IgA).
- If a urine light chain is present, it should not exceed 1 g per 24 hours.
- Less than 10% bone marrow plasma cells.
- No lytic bone lesions.
- No symptoms associated with myeloma (mainly no anemia, no renal failure and a normal calcium level).

Despite established criteria, the distinction between MGUS and early multiple myeloma can be problematic, since the level of the M protein and the number of plasma cells can be low in the very early stage of myeloma.

The incidence of MGUS increases with age, and approximates 3% among individuals older than 70 years. The patients may or may not have other associated medical conditions (e.g. chronic inflammation or an autoimmune disorder). About 15–30% of the cases progress to myeloma over a 10-year period. Therefore, in patients clinically diagnosed as having MGUS, serial quantitation of immunoglobulins should be carried out, initially at 6 months from diagnosis and yearly thereafter.

39.4.4 Solitary plasmacytoma of bone

Solitary plasmacytoma of bone is defined as a single lesion identified on magnetic resonance imaging with or without a serum M-band. The most commonly involved site is the spine. The criteria for MGUS shown in Table 39.1 also apply to this condition. The cellular composition of the plasmacytoma is variable, ranging from mature plasma cells to a preponderance of plasmablasts.

There exists a close relationship between this disorder and the subsequent development of overt myeloma. The age of onset for solitary plasmacytoma is usually in the sixth decade whereas myeloma occurs mainly in the seventh decade. The majority of patients with solitary plasmacytoma ultimately develop disseminated disease. In half of the patients, this progression occurs within a median of 3 years. Based on large studies, only 10% of the patients are apparently cured. These findings suggest that solitary plasmacytoma of bone is a premyelomatous condition, necessitating careful long-term follow-up of the patient.

39.4.5 Multiple myeloma

The diagnosis of multiple myeloma requires the correlation of morphologic, radiologic and laboratory findings. Instead of a complex scheme of major and minor criteria, the current minimal criteria for myeloma include bone marrow plasmacytosis or plasmacytoma, and one of the following:

- A monoclonal serum protein of at least 3 g/dl if IgG or 2 g/dl if IgA.
- Monoclonal light chain in the urine, at least 1 g per 24 hours.
- Lytic bone lesions.

The focal nature of bone marrow involvement in multiple myeloma can lead to sampling problems. Consequently, the number of plasma cells in the specimen can be normal. The percentage of plasma cells in such cases does not necessarily correlate with the overall tumor burden.

Since rare cases of multiple myeloma (about 1%) have no detectable M protein, the finding of cytologically abnormal plasma cells and immunologic confirmation of monoclonality become important diagnostic clues when the usual criteria are not present.

In addition to the degree of plasmacytosis, the morphologic diagnosis of myeloma relies on cytologic abnormalities in plasma cells on air-dried preparations and the pattern of infiltration on biopsy sections. The cytology of the neoplastic cells can vary considerably. Normal-appearing plasma cells, large multinucleated cells with more than three nuclei, and plasmablasts may all be present within the same case. The morphology of the large cells can be indistinguishable from that seen in immunoblastic lymphoma and the distinction between myeloma with numerous plasmablasts and bone marrow involvement by immunoblastic lymphoma is not always clear-cut (Figure 39.19). In addition, neoplastic cells with a markedly increased nuclear/cytoplasmic ratio may also simulate the appearance of leukemic blasts. Cytoplasmic vacuoles or crystalline inclusions of accumulated immunoglobulins may also be present. These are of no diagnostic significance, however.

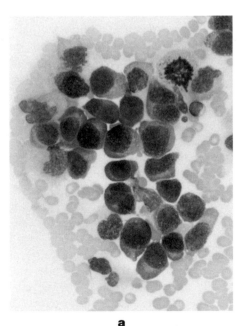 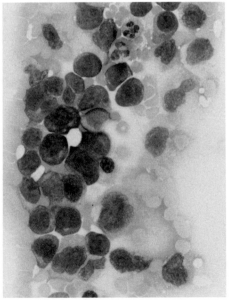

a   b

Figure 39.19 Morphologic similarities between a plasmablastic multiple myeloma (a) and an immunoblastic lymphoma (b) with diffuse bone marrow involvement in an HIV-positive patient. The first patient had a large IgG kappa spike and multiple osteolytic lesions. The second patient had extensive lymphadenopathy but no monoclonal spike or osteolytic lesions

It appears that an increase in plasmablasts is associated with an adverse clinical outcome. Using this feature to predict prognosis can be problematic, however, because of the variability in the distribution of plasmablasts in the bone marrow and the subjective recognition of these immature-appearing cells. Nevertheless, multiple myeloma composed virtually entirely of plasmablasts follows an aggressive clinical course.

On biopsy sections, the bone marrow in multiple myeloma is normocellular or hypercellular, depending on the extent of the neoplastic infiltration. The pattern of the infiltrate can be focal, interstitial, diffuse or mixed. A subtle interstitial plasma cell infiltrate can be highlighted by immunostaining for cytoplasmic immunoglobulin light chains. Reticulin fibrosis can accompany the plasma cell infiltrate.

39.4.5.1 Clinical subtypes of multiple myeloma

Multiple myeloma is further subdivided into various clinical phases (smoldering, indolent and overt) based on the extent of disease and its rate of progression. Smoldering myeloma is similar to MGUS in that there are no myeloma-related symptoms and no bony lesions, but with a monoclonal spike of more than 3 g/dl and a mild bone marrow plasmacytosis (<20% plasma cells). Smoldering myeloma usually remains stable for at least 5 years without therapy. In indolent myeloma, the bone marrow contains 20–30% plasma cells, and there are a few bony lesions. Anemia can be present at diagnosis. This condition progresses to overt myeloma within a few years. Since the plasma cell content varies greatly between bone marrow samples and does not necessarily reflect the extent of the disease, the diagnoses of smoldering and indolent myeloma should be made clinically rather than on a purely morphologic basis.

Overt multiple myeloma is accompanied by symptoms related to bone demineralization, bone marrow failure and increasing M protein production, which result in vertebral compression fractures, hypercalcemia, pancytopenia and impaired renal function. The renal insufficiency is caused by several factors, including precipitation of the light chains in renal tubules, elevated calcium and uric acid levels, and infiltration by amyloid deposits. The immunoglobulins produced by the neoplastic cells do not have a normal antibody function. Furthermore, normal plasma cell functions are suppressed, resulting in a reduction of normal immunoglobulins. These factors account for the defective immune response in myeloma.

In rare instances, the patients present with osteosclerotic rather than lytic lesions. Osteosclerotic myeloma with an IgA lambda monoclonal protein is often associated with the POEMS syndrome characterized by polyneuropathy, organomegaly, endocrine abnormalities (e.g. amenorrhea), M-protein, and skin changes (e.g. hyperpigmentation).

The neoplastic cells in multiple myeloma express high levels of several adhesion molecules including CD56, CD44, CD49d, and CD49e. This may account for the absence of peripheral blood involvement until the very terminal phase of the disease, when PCL can develop, defined as greater than 20% plasma cells and at least $2 \times 10^9/l$ plasma cells in the peripheral blood (see Section 5.7).

In rare instances, the terminal phase of multiple myeloma may 'transform' into a high-grade immunoblastic lymphoma involving extramedullary sites. The lymphoma carries a plasma cell phenotype, i.e. down-regulated expression of both CD45 and pan-B-cell markers, and monoclonal cIg. CD30 may also be expressed.

39.4.5.2 Assessment of prognosis in multiple myeloma

The complex traditional staging system, which incorporated the clinical and laboratory parameters (Hgb, serum calcium and creatinine levels, serum and urine M protein levels, and the number of lytic lesions), is slowly being replaced by other prognostic factors. The three main prognostic factors include: (1) the plasma cell labeling index, an indicator of the tumor growth rate; (2) β_2 microglobulin, which reflects the tumor burden; and (3) C-reactive protein, an indirect measurement of IL-6 activity. A high labeling index, elevated β_2 microglobulin and increased C-reactive protein are associated with a poor prognosis.

Aggressive disease is also associated with cytogenetic abnormalities. No specific genetic marker has been found for multiple myeloma. Abnormalities of chromosomes 1, 6, 11, 13, and 14 have been reported, with t(11;14) being the most common. By FCM analysis a high percentage of cases demonstrate DNA aneuploidy, however.

Mononuclear cell infiltration pattern

The mononuclear cell (MNC) infiltration pattern covers neoplastic conditions with one of the following characteristics:

1. An increased percentage of blasts.
2. Excessive proliferation of mast cells.
3. Neoplastic hematopoietic cells for which there is no known benign counterpart in the blood and bone marrow (e.g. hairy cells, follicular center cells).

Disorders composed of cells which are morphologically indistinguishable from their benign counterparts (e.g. small lymphocytes, plasmacytoid lymphocytes) are discussed in Chapter 39.

Traditionally, hematopoietic malignancies that initially manifest in the peripheral blood and/or bone marrow are referred to as 'leukemias', whereas the designation 'lymphoma' is used for those tumors which start in the lymph nodes, spleen or extranodal solid tissue. A given disease may have one name when it presents with lymph node involvement and another name when it is first detected in the bone marrow (e.g. Burkitt's lymphoma and ALL-L3). With our increased understanding of hematopoietic malignancies, these disorders should be viewed biologically rather than based on the predominant site of involvement.

40.1 Approach to the morphologic evaluation of a mononuclear cell infiltrate

Characterization of an MNC infiltrate in the bone marrow requires a multiparameter approach including:

1. Morphologic evaluation of the peripheral blood and bone marrow with review of any previous bone marrow specimens and/or samples from other sites (e.g. lymph nodes).
2. FCM immunophenotyping.
3. Cytogenetics and, where applicable, molecular genetics.

It is prudent to have FCM immunophenotyping results available when evaluating an MNC infiltrate. When an efficient immunophenotyping laboratory is located on-site, the FCM results should be available on the same day as the bone marrow procedure.

If the initial morphologic evaluation of an MNC infiltrate takes place before the FCM results are known, it is judicious to follow a systematic approach to formulating a preliminary differential diagnosis. This should take into account the distribution of the population (uniform vs. heterogeneous), the cell size, the nuclear characteristics of the majority of the cells (chromatin, nucleolus, nuclear contours), specific cytoplasmic characteristics, cytochemical stains and, if the biopsy sections are available, the pattern of the infiltrate.

The diameter of a normal RBC (7–8 μm) or the size of the nucleus of a normal 'resting' lymphocyte serves as an internal ruler to estimate the size of mononuclear cells. The nucleus of a small round lymphocyte is slightly larger than the diameter of a normal RBC. In assessing the size of a neoplastic cell, consider the number of RBCs that will fit into the nucleus of that cell. If one and a half to two RBCs fit into the nucleus, it is considered 'small'. If between two and three RBCs fit into the neoplastic cell, it is 'medium'. If three or more RBCs will fit into the nucleus of a neoplastic cell, the cell is 'large'. Since neoplastic populations are rarely mono-tonous, the authors consider that a two-level morphological classification of cell size is much more reproducible than a three-tier classification. Therefore, in the following discussion, populations that are 'small to medium' are considered 'small', and populations that are 'medium to large' are considered 'large'.

On air-dried preparations, features that point toward a malignant process include an extensive infiltrate, the presence of nuclear irregularities, and a large cell size. Some cytoplasmic features may provide diagnostic clues (e.g. Auer rods). In the assessment of nuclear irregularities, ensure that the cells in question are not monocytes, and the irregularities are V-shaped (i.e. deep sharp indentations) instead of U-shaped (Figure 40.1). Nuclear irregularities with a U shape can be EDTA or centrifugation artifacts.

40.2 Biopsy sections

In biopsy sections, an MNC infiltrate can be focal, paratrabecular, interstitial, diffuse, or a combination of any of these patterns. A focal infiltrate may be benign or malignant. Any pattern other than focal suggests a malignant pro-cess. The interstitial and diffuse patterns are not specific to any subtype of MNC infiltration. Features such as frequent mitotic figures, apoptosis and necrosis also suggest malignancy.

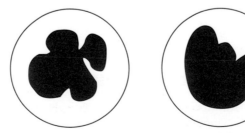

Figure 40.1 Schematic drawing comparing a nucleus with a sharp nuclear V-shaped indentation (right) versus a U-shaped nuclear irregularity (left). U-shaped irregularity can be real, but it can also be artifactually induced by delayed processing

40.2.1 Focal/multifocal pattern

Another term for a focal pattern is nodular. The infiltrate may be composed of one or more aggregates. Focal refers to a single aggregate, and multifocal is used when more than one aggregate is present. The term 'multifocal' is preferred to the layman's term 'patchy', which has been used inconsistently to designate either a multifocal infiltrate or interstitial involvement.

In a focal infiltrate, the aggregate should not obliterate the space between two widely separated bony trabeculae to a large extent (Figure 39.10). In other words, a very large focus of infiltration with resulting increased cellularity is more correctly referred to as diffuse involvement.

The cellular composition of a focal infiltrate (nodule) may provide a clue as to its nature. If the aggregate is composed mostly of large cells, then the process is nearly always neoplastic. The distinction between a benign and malignant infiltrate is more problematic when the nodule is composed of either small cells or a mixed lymphohistiocytic infiltrate. Mixed lymphohistiocytic nodules in the marrow may represent involvement by Hodgkin's disease, certain peripheral T-cell lymphomas or a so-called abnormal immune response.

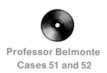

**Professor Belmonte
Cases 51 and 52**

In Hodgkin's disease, careful examination of multiple sections, together with immunostaining for CD30 and CD15, will invariably reveal the presence of diagnostic Reed-Sternberg cells or mononuclear Hodgkin's cells. A much less infrequent pattern of Hodgkin's disease involvement in the bone marrow is interstitial infiltration by scattered Reed-Sternberg/Hodgkin's cells without any associated fibroblastic reaction. The aspirate smears in such instances often contain identifiable Reed-Sternberg/Hodgkin's cells.

In aggregates composed of small lymphoid cells, features such as size, contour, and the number of nodules have been proposed in an attempt to discriminate benign from malignant processes. In general, the larger the size of the nodules and the higher the number of foci, the more likely it is that the infiltrate represents a malignant disorder, especially if the patient has known low-grade NHL. There is a high degree of overlap, however. Both low-grade NHL and benign lymphoid aggregates occur with increased frequency in the older age group. The size and, in some cases, the number of aggregates may be affected by the level of the sections.

Since fixation and decalcification of biopsy sections can cause nuclear irregularities in small lymphoid cells, the nuclear shape cannot be relied upon as an indicator of malignancy (Figure 39.11). The malignant nature of a focal infiltrate can be confirmed if neoplastic cells are detectable in the peripheral blood.

40.2.2 Paratrabecular pattern

A paratrabecular pattern is relatively specific for bone marrow involvement by FCC lymphoma (Figure 40.2). Since the paratrabecular pattern is a useful marker of FCC lymphoma, this pattern must be distinguished from a pseudo-paratrabecular appearance (Figure 40.3). A paratrabecular infiltrate molds along the length of the bony trabeculae. In contrast, a pseudo-paratrabecular infiltrate is

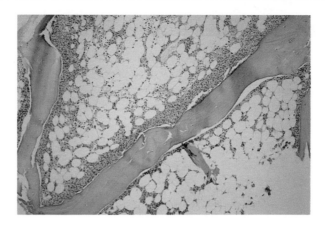

Figure 40.2 Paratrabecular infiltration in FCC lymphoma. The infiltrate 'hugs' the length of the bony trabeculae

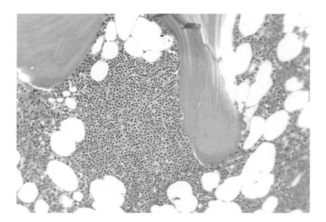

Figure 40.3 A pseudo-paratrabecular nodule in LPC lymphoma-leukemia. Although the infiltrate is apposed to the trabeculae, most of it projects as a nodule into the medullary space. Compare this pattern with the paratrabecular pattern in Figure 40.2

actually a nodular aggregate, partially against the trabeculae, but with most of the infiltrate projecting into the medullary space.

The pseudo-paratrabecular appearance is usually seen in biopsies obtained shortly after chemotherapy for small cell LPD/NHL when there was previous nodular involvement of the marrow. Along with a variable reduction in the neoplastic infiltrate secondary to chemotherapy, there is a decrease in normal hematopoietic elements and some dropout of the stroma. Because of this, residual nodules of lymphoma may partially lie against the bony trabeculae. A pseudo-paratrabecular appearance can also result from distortion of the biopsy secondary to faulty technique.

40.2.3 Interstitial pattern

In an interstitial pattern, the MNC infiltrate is admixed with normal hematopoietic elements, with no excessive encroachment on the fatty component (Figure 39.8). The cellularity is therefore not severely altered. The interstitial pattern is most commonly observed in low-grade malignancies, such as CLL/SLL.

40.2.4 Diffuse pattern

A bone marrow with diffuse involvement by neoplastic cells is always hypercellular, with marked to complete obliteration of the normal hematopoietic elements and fat cells. The diffuse pattern can be extensive, spanning across several bony trabeculae, or limited within a large marrow area bordered by two bony trabeculae.

40.2.5 Combined patterns

The common combinations include nodular and interstitial, interstitial and diffuse, paratrabecular and nodular, and paratrabecular and diffuse.

40.3 The MNC infiltrate is composed of mast cells, in nodules or sheets

Mast cells are most easily recognized on air-dried Romanovsky-stained preparations by their characteristic ovoid to spindle appearance and abundant coarse purple granules. The granules leach out during tissue processing. Therefore, mast cells are virtually undetectable on H&E sections of normal bone marrow.

The normal bone marrow contains an extremely low number of mast cells (<0.01% of the bone marrow cells, based on FCM enumeration). A number of clonal hematological disorders such as aplastic anemia, AML and LPC lymphoma-leukemia/Waldenstrom's macroglobulinemia are associated with an increased number of mast cells which, on the aspirate smears, are mainly found within the stromal particles (Figure 40.4). On bone marrow biopsies stained with Giemsa or toluidine blue, increased mast cells in lymphoproliferative disorders appear as scattered, darkly stained polygonal or spindle cells rather than forming mast cell nodules.

In bone marrow mastocytosis, nodules or sheets of mast cells infiltrate the marrow (Figure 40.5). The mast cells in bone marrow mastocytosis are invariably larger than normal mast cells. Because of the focal distribution of the nodules, and the associated increase in reticulin fibers, the abnormal mast cells may be missed on aspirate smears.

Abnormal mast cells can be identified with FCM analysis by the characteristic combination of high FSC and SSC, intense CD117, and expression of CD33,

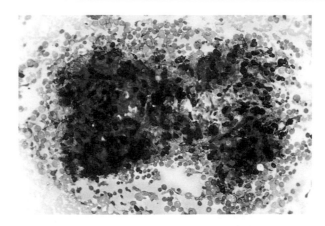

Figure 40.4   Markedly increased mast cells in AML-M5a

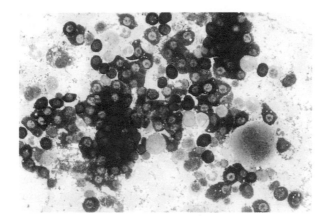

Figure 40.5   Sheets of polygonal mast cells in systemic mastocytosis

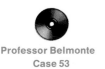

Professor Belmonte
Case 53

CD13, CD2 and CD25. The last two markers are not expressed on normal mast cells. On H&E-stained biopsies, nodules of mast cells may superficially mimic the appearance of granulomata, especially if the mast cells are spindle-shaped (Figure 40.6). Similarly, because of leaching out of the granules during tissue processing, ovoid mast cells can appear to have abundant pale cytoplasm, thus simulating the morphology of hairy cells. On biopsy sections stained with Giemsa or CAE, the mast cell infiltrate can be identified by the characteristic purple or deep red granules, respectively. Note that the CAE stain does not work on B5-fixed sections. In addition to fibrosis, the mast cell infiltrate is usually associated with osteosclerosis of the adjacent bony trabeculae.

Bone marrow mastocytosis is nearly always a manifestation of systemic mast cell disease (SMCD), a rare disorder with involvement of skin, liver, spleen and lymph nodes. The protean symptomatology of SMCD is related to the organs involved and the products released from mast cell granules (e.g. histamine and prostaglandins). The current classification includes indolent SMCD, aggressive

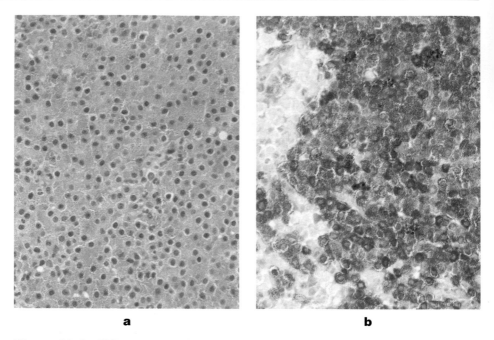

a   b

Figure 40.6 Diffuse mast cell infiltration on H&E (a) and Giemsa (b) stained bone marrow biopsy sections

SMCD, mast cell leukemia, and mastocytosis coexisting with hematologic disorders. In the latter group, the patient's clinical manifestations and prognosis are mainly those of the associated hematological malignancy. The diagnosis of the hematological malignancy should take precedence over SMCD in such instances.

The distinction between indolent and aggressive SMCD requires clinical and laboratory correlation and follow-up. In general, patients with cutaneous disease have a better prognosis than those with liver and spleen involvement, in whom the reported median survival is less than 1 year. The bone marrow involvement in indolent SMCD has been described as low, with a focal distribution. Low numbers of circulating mast cells are detectable in some cases of SMCD. In contrast, abundant mast cells in the peripheral blood (> 30%) are the hallmark of the rare mast cell leukemia.

40.4 A relatively uniform MNC infiltrate composed predominantly of small cells

In an MNC infiltrate composed of small cells, the nuclear chromatin is nearly always condensed or homogeneous (i.e. mature-appearing), the nucleoli inconspicuous (or apparently absent) and the cytoplasm not abundant. These are cytologic features strongly suggestive of a lymphoid lineage. The main differential diagnosis is between lymphoid malignancies, a benign lymphocytic infiltrate and, less frequently, nonhematopoietic metastases (e.g. extensive involvement by small cell carcinoma). The presence of nuclear molding is an important clue that the infiltrate is nonhematopoietic (see Chapter 41).

On blood films and bone marrow aspirates, small lymphoid cells with deeply indented nuclei are a reliable cytologic feature of malignancy. These nuclear irregularities have been referred to as 'cleaved' or 'convoluted'. It is preferable to avoid using this morphological terminology indiscriminately since the terms 'cleaved' and 'convoluted' may infer 'follicular small cleaved cells' and 'convoluted lymphoblasts', respectively. The clefting may be seen to transect the nucleus, resulting in a 'buttock' appearance. Although the name 'buttock cells' has been associated with FCC lymphoma, these cells are not unique to this entity (Figure 5.33).

The main differential diagnosis of an infiltrate composed of small (to medium) cells with a variable degree of nuclear irregularity and inconspicuous nucleoli includes NHL of the small cell type and, less commonly, an ALL composed of relatively small lymphoblasts with scant cytoplasm (i.e. ALL-L1 by the FAB classification). The chromatin texture can overlap between these two categories of disease (Figure 40.7). Nuclear irregularities are usually minimal in small lymphoblasts, however. Although the cytology in ALL can simulate that of CLL or NHL, the severe thrombocytopenia and anemia that are usually present in ALL constitute important clues suggesting the diagnosis. The patient's age can be helpful since small cell (low-grade) NHL is a rare occurrence in childhood.

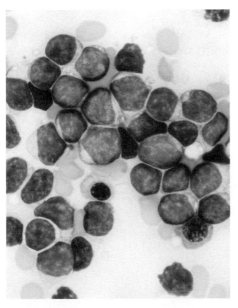 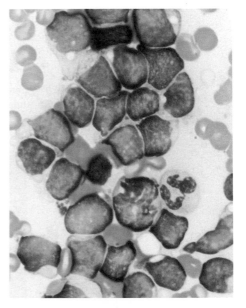

a   b

Figure 40.7 Overlapping morphologic features in ALL in a 10-year-old child (a) and NHL in a 60-year-old female (b). (a) Lymphoblasts with small to medium cell size, condensed nuclear chromatin and no visible nucleoli. (b) An NK-like T-cell lymphoma with extensive bone marrow, lymph node and skin involvement at presentation. The neoplastic population is composed predominantly of small to medium-size cells. The chromatin is not condensed. This case was initially misinterpreted as ALL

In the Western world, the two most common subtypes of NHL composed of small lymphoid cells with indented nuclei are FCC lymphoma and MCL. Cellular heterogeneity, a feature better appreciated on air-dried preparations than on biopsy sections, is more common in MCL than in FCC lymphoma. This feature is also seen in cases of FCC in transformation to large cell lymphoma, however (Figure 40.8). With well-prepared and optimally stained blood films and aspirate smears, it is possible in many cases to discern subtle differences in the nuclear chromatin between these two disorders. The chromatin is usually homogeneous (reminiscent of one smooth coat of paint) in FCC lymphoma (Figure 40.9) but clumped in MCL (Figure 40.10). The differential diagnosis can be resolved based on the FCM immunophenotyping results (see Sections 27.5.3 and 27.6). Alternatively, the pattern of the infiltrate on the biopsy can be a helpful feature to

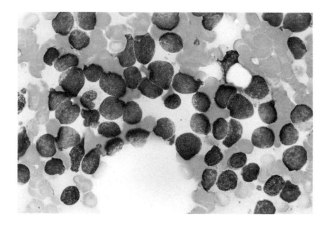

Figure 40.8 Bone marrow imprint, illustrating a heterogeneous population of small, medium and large cells in FCC lymphoma transforming into a large cell lymphoma

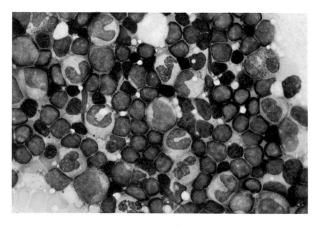

Figure 40.9 FCC lymphoma: small lymphoma cells with homogeneous chromatin and round nuclear contours are visible. Cells with nuclear indentations are rare in this case

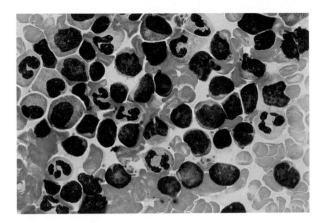

Figure 40.10 Mantle cell lymphoma: the neoplastic population is composed mostly of small and medium-size cells with detectable nuclear irregularities. The chromatin texture is more heterogeneous than that usually seen in FCC lymphoma

separate the two disorders. A paratrabecular pattern, by itself or in combination with other patterns, is highly suggestive of FCC lymphoma.

40.4.1 Follicular center cell lymphoma

The subclassification of FCC lymphoma is based on the lymph node biopsy or, less commonly, a biopsy from an extranodal site. The current classification scheme includes three grades (I, II, III), based on the number of large cells. During the natural history of FCC lymphoma, the number of large cells increases and the lymph node pattern changes from follicular to diffuse, i.e. a progression from FCC I to diffuse large cell lymphoma (DLCL).

The majority of cases of FCC lymphoma are FCC I, i.e. the neoplastic follicles in the lymph node are composed predominantly of small cells. Reproducibility of the FCC II diagnosis has been problematic, mainly because of the lack of agreement on the relative proportion of large cells needed for this diagnosis. FCC III is the least common subtype, presumably because this stage is transient and quickly progresses to a DLCL. FCC I and II are considered low grade, and FCC III is intermediate/high grade. DNA cell cycle analysis (performed along with FCM immunophenotyping) is an objective way of separating low-grade and high-grade NHL. The typical FCM immunophenotyping results in FCC lymphoma can be summarized as follows: mature B-cell phenotype, CD10$^+$, bcl-2$^+$, and monoclonal surface light chain (see Section 27.6). Note that immunoreactivity for bcl-2 is not restricted to FCC lymphoma.

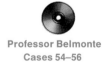

Professor Belmonte
Cases 54–56

The reported incidence of bone marrow involvement in FCC lymphoma ranges from 30 to 60%. The true incidence is likely to be higher. With routine use of multicolor FCM immunophenotyping, it is possible to detect very low levels of involvement, where the NHL component accounts for less than 5% of the total hematopoietic cells and multiple biopsy levels are apparently negative. In the context of the clinical history, the detection of rare lymphoma cells can also be achieved on aspirate smears if a very thorough examination is carried out by an experienced microscopist (Figure 40.11).

No criteria have been proposed to establish a diagnosis of FCC in transformation in the bone marrow. The authors have observed that, in such cases, the number of large lymphoma cells exceeds 25–30% of the total lymphoma cells, a finding similar to that applied to the grading of FCC lymphoma in lymph nodes. A more objective method to document FCC in transformation is by FCM cell cycle analysis to determine the S-phase fraction of the neoplastic population. An S-phase fraction above 5% usually indicates intermediate- or high-grade disease.

In positive biopsy sections, involvement by FCC lymphoma usually manifests as multiple paratrabecular infiltrates composed predominantly of small lymphoid cells. Because reticulin fibrosis can interfere with the aspiration of neoplastic cells, FCC involvement can be obvious on the biopsy but apparently absent on the aspirate smears. In most of these apparently negative aspirates, FCM analysis and/or a careful examination of the smears can actually reveal a low number of lymphoma cells.

Extensive diffuse infiltration is seen mainly with advanced disease, often in leukemic phase (Figure 5.31). The cellular composition of the marrow infiltrate can remain unchanged even if the disease in the lymph nodes has progressed from FCC I to FCC III or DLCL. This situation has traditionally been referred to as

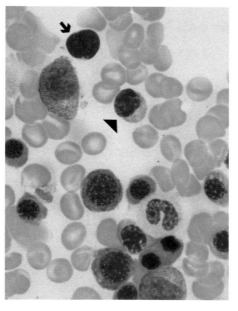
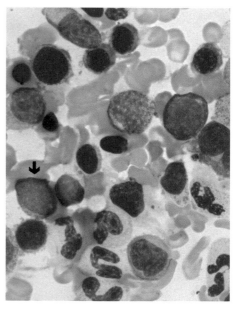

a   b

Figure 40.11   (a), (b) Bone marrow aspirate smears in an FCC lymphoma with a low level of bone marrow involvement. Occasional small lymphoma cells (arrow) can be recognized based on nuclear indentation. Compared to the normal lymphocyte (arrowhead), the small lymphoma cells have an inappropriately high nuclear/cytoplasmic ratio. Morphologically, detectable lymphoma cells approximate 5% in this case. By FCM immunophenotyping, the neoplastic FCC cells accounted for 9% of all bone marrow cells

'discordant' morphology, and may reflect differences in the ability of small lymphoid cells and large cells to circulate/disseminate. The phenomenon is characteristically seen in FCC lymphoma, and is therefore a useful clue to separate the category of DLCL arising in an FCC lymphoma from the group of *de novo* DLCL. In a small number of patients, the progression from low grade to high grade can be documented on sequential bone marrow studies. Morphologic features supportive of transformation include increased mitoses, easily detectable apoptotic figures (Figure 40.12), and conspicuous numbers of large cells. The bone marrow smears (and blood film) demonstrate increased cytologic heterogeneity within the neoplastic population (Figure 40.8).

The cytogenetic abnormality characteristic of FCC lymphoma is t(14;18)(q21;q32) whereby the *bcl*-2 proto-oncogene on chromosome 18 is juxtaposed to the heavy chain gene (*IgH*) joining segment on chromosome 14. This leads to increased transcription of the *bcl*-2 gene and overexpression of bcl-2 protein. The balance between bcl-2 and other proteins involved in the regulation of programmed cell death is altered, rendering the affected cells resistant to apoptosis. Bcl-2 protein can also be increased in other hematopoietic neoplasms without t(14;18).

In about 70% of FCC lymphoma, the breakpoints on 18q21 are clustered within a major breakpoint region in the 3′ untranslated region of the *bcl*-2 gene. In 15–25% of cases, the breakpoints lie within a minor cluster region 20–30 kb distal from the *bcl*-2 gene. By PCR analysis, these breakpoints can be detected in the blood or bone marrow of most patients with FCC lymphoma, including those with clinical stage I and II disease. This technique is currently used

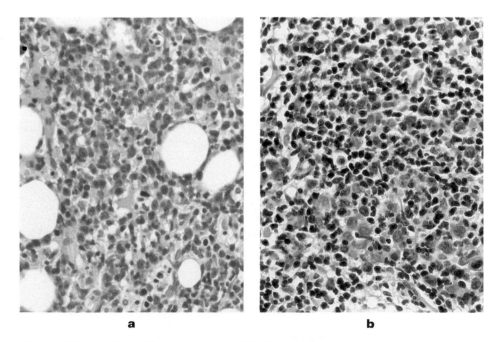

a   b

Figure 40.12 Two different cases of FCC in transformation. (a) Apoptotic figures within the infiltrate. (b) Increased proportion of large cells

in assessing patient response to various therapeutic regimens and as a marker for minimal residual disease. Note, however, that detectable *bcl*-2 rearrangements have been reported in benign lymphoid tissue with overt follicular hyperplasia, as well as in circulating B cells of healthy blood donors when PCR is performed on concentrated B-cell preparations.

40.4.2 Mantle cell lymphoma

The diagnosis of MCL cannot be made in the blood or bone marrow based on morphologic features alone. The nuclear irregularities and heterogeneous cell size distribution of the cells in MCL are shared by other B-cell and T-cell lymphomas. On biopsy sections, the pattern of infiltration (focal, interstitial or diffuse) is nondiagnostic and nuclear irregularities may or may not be present (Figure 40.13). Therefore, it is helpful to correlate the marrow findings with those from the extramedullary sites of involvement. Several patterns of involvement can be seen in the lymph node, i.e. mantle zone, nodular or diffuse. The diffuse pattern appears to be associated with a poorer outcome.

The lymph node morphology, in cases with diffuse involvement by MCL, can be mimicked by ALL/lymphoblastic lymphoma. In institutions where separate departments review lymph nodes and bone marrows (a common practice in Europe), ALL/lymphoblastic lymphoma in the lymph node and the so-called 'blastic' variant of MCL can be confused with each other. If FCM immunophenotyping is performed, this error can be avoided.

In the bone marrow and/or peripheral blood, MCL can be diagnosed based on the combination of the FCM results and the cytologic appearance of the neoplastic cells. The typical findings include a monoclonal B-cell proliferation, CD5$^+$ and CD23$^-$, with small to medium cells and nuclear irregularities on air-dried smears (Figures 5.35 and 40.10).

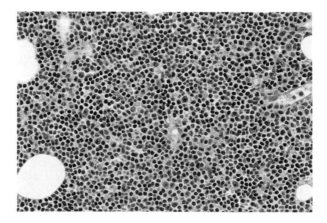

Figure 40.13 Diffuse infiltration by small lymphoid cells with round to minimally irregular nuclei in a mantle cell lymphoma. The morphologic features are similar to those seen in CLL and other malignancies of small lymphoid cells

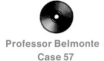

Positive staining for cyclin D1 on paraffin-embedded tissue is another helpful diagnostic feature in MCL (Figure 40.14). Since the immunoreactivity on fixed tissue can be affected by processing, the diagnosis cannot be excluded based on the absence of cyclin D1 expression. It is important to interpret the significance of positive cyclin D1 staining in the context of laboratory studies and other FCM results (especially CD5 and CD23).

Overexpression of cyclin D1, t(11;14), and *bcl*-1 rearrangements have been documented, albeit infrequently, in other lymphoid malignancies (e.g. B ALL, CLL, PLL, LPC lymphoma-leukemia and multiple myeloma). In addition, up-regulated cyclin D1 is found in a high number of HCL cases. The underlying molecular mechanism in HCL is unknown, since these cases do not have detectable abnormalities involving chromosome 11q23.

MCL is no longer viewed as an indolent disease. The reported overall survival in MCL is poorer than that in other low-grade lymphomas. This most likely results from cyclin D1 overexpression. Cyclin D1 is one of the several nuclear proteins involved in the control of the cell cycle. The interaction of cyclin D1 with its associated cyclin-dependent kinase allows cells to get through the first checkpoint of the G_1-phase beyond which cells are committed to divide. Therefore, up-regulated cyclin D1 leads to dysregulated cellular proliferation and genomic instability.

The gene encoding cyclin D1 is located on chromosome 11q23, 120 kb from the *bcl*-1 proto-oncogene. In MCL, the translocation between the *bcl*-1 locus on 11q23 and the *IgH* gene on 14q32 leads to increased transcription of this gene. In most instances, the breakpoints occur within a 2 kb major translocation cluster region of the *bcl*-1 locus. Breakpoints can occur outside the major translocation cluster, however. Consequently, only 50–70% of cases of MCL have detectable *bcl*-1 rearrangements with the currently available molecular probes.

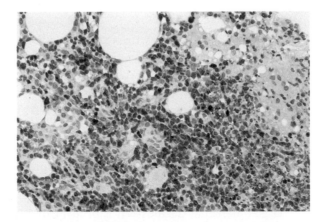

Figure 40.14 Cyclin D1 immunostaining on a biopsy section in MCL. Positive nuclear staining of variable intensity is present in many but not all of the tumor cells

40.4.3 Sezary syndrome

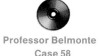

The diagnosis of Sezary syndrome requires a correlation of the clinical presentation, the skin biopsy findings and the cerebriform cytology of the neoplastic cells. Sezary cells are easier to detect in the blood than in the marrow (see Section 5.10). Bone marrow involvement in Sezary syndrome can be slight (Figure 40.15) despite a high number of circulating Sezary cells. The advanced stage of the disease may manifest as transformation to a high-grade lymphoma at any of the involved sites (skin, lymph nodes and bone marrow). The peripheral blood involvement may not reflect this transformation.

The transformation of Sezary syndrome to high-grade lymphoma is often accompanied by CD30 expression, which may lead to diagnostic confusion with CD30$^+$ anaplastic large cell lymphoma.

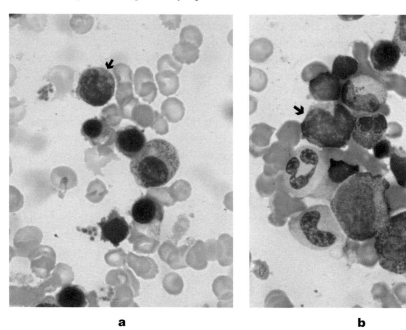

a   b

Figure 40.15   Bone marrow aspirate in Sezary syndrome. (a) A rare small Sezary cell (arrow). (b) A rare large Sezary cell (arrow)

40.5 The MNC infiltrate is relatively uniform and composed predominantly of large cells

In most cases, the presence of a conspicuous number of large cells is highly suggestive of a malignant process, such as an acute leukemia, certain types of LPD, high-grade NHL or a metastatic 'undifferentiated' tumor. In view of the large differential diagnosis, it is prudent to refrain from rendering an interpretation based solely on morphologic features. An exception is the presence of Auer rods, since this feature is virtually pathognomonic for AML (Figure 40.16).

Ensure that the Auer rods are long and sharp since immunoglobulin crystals (in rare cases of NHL/LPD) may be mistaken for Auer rods. Bundles of Auer rods are characteristic of AML-M3 (Figure 40.17). The presence of a few cytoplasmic azurophilic granules is not evidence of myeloid origin, since azurophilic granules can be found in ALL (Figure 40.18) and some high-grade NHL (Figure 40.19).

The morphology of large MNCs on air-dried preparations is often nondescript, i.e. round to irregular nuclei, prominent nucleoli and moderate to ample blue cytoplasm. In the context of hematopoietic malignancies, the combination of coarse, condensed to reticulated chromatin and a prominent nucleolus suggests that the neoplastic cells are large mature lymphoid cells, either high-grade NHL cells or prolymphocytes. The quality of the nuclear chromatin in large MNCs can be easily affected by suboptimal staining, however. The appearance of lymphoma cells can overlap with that of myeloblasts (Figure 40.20), leading to a misdiagnosis of large cell NHL as AML. The differential diagnosis of large MNCs is even more difficult on biopsy sections, where the features are less distinct.

On well-prepared material, some cytologic features of large MNCs may offer clues to narrow down the differential diagnosis and/or guide the subsequent work-up:

- Large cells with a low nuclear/cytoplasmic ratio, abundant pale gray agranular cytoplasm, ovoid to reniform nuclei and reticulated chromatin (Figure 5.14). These are features highly suggestive of hairy cells.
- Deep blue cytoplasm and an eccentrically located nucleus with coarse reticulated chromatin and a prominent single nucleolus (i.e. transformed cells with plasmacytoid appearance). These are cytologic features seen in immunoblasts (Figure 40.21). On H&E sections the cytoplasm appears amphophilic. The plasmacytoid appearance can easily be obscured on thick biopsy sections. Although a presumptive interpretation of bone marrow involvement by immunoblastic lymphoma may be rendered, it is important to recognize that some nonhematopoietic tumors (e.g. melanoma, round cell sarcoma) and cer-

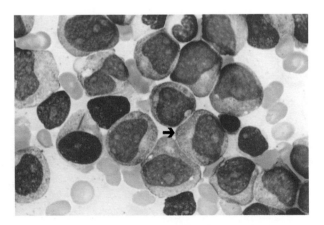

Figure 40.16 A sharp Auer rod in a myeloblast in AML-M2. Note the large azurophilic granules (pseudo Chediak-Higashi) in some of the blasts (arrow)

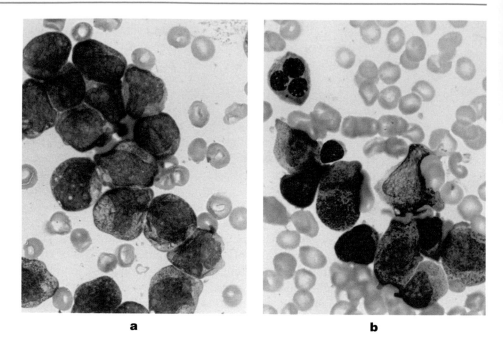

a   b

Figure 40.17   AML-M3 from two different patients. (a) Blasts with bundles of Auer rods overlying the nuclei. (b) Hypergranulated blasts and a trinucleated erythroid precursor with karyorrhexis

tain cases of AML-M5a can have a similar cytologic appearance (Figure 40.22).

• Deep blue cytoplasm, abundant sharp cytoplasmic vacuoles and reticulated to coarse chromatin. These are features considered to be morphologically consistent with Burkitt's cells (Figure 40.23). This cytology can be seen in some mature T-cell malignancies and the round cell subtypes of rhabdomyosarcoma. Note that precursor-B ALL cells can contain multiple vacuoles (Figure 5.27b) and may therefore be misidentified as Burkitt's cells.

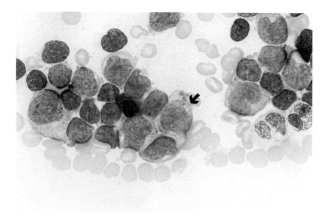

Figure 40.18   A heterogeneous population of blasts in a case of T-ALL in a 10-year-old girl. Some of the blasts contain azurophilic granules (arrow)

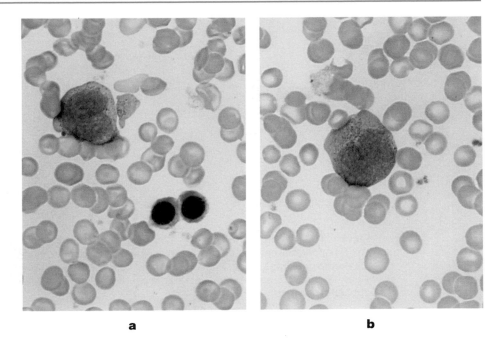

a   b

Figure 40.19 (a), (b) Scanty bone marrow aspirate from a case of high-grade B-cell lymphoma. Two large lymphoma cells can be seen with abundant azurophilic granules, reticulated chromatin and visible nucleoli. Nuclear indentation is evident in one cell (a)

It can be problematic to differentiate a metastatic tumor from a high-grade lymphoid malignancy unless there is evidence of tight cluster formation and gigantic cell size. In addition, nonhematopoietic tumor cells can circulate in low numbers in the blood. Therefore, in the absence of appropriate clinical history, it is best to rely on immunophenotyping results to establish the identity of a large MNC infiltrate.

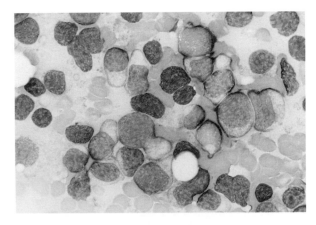

Figure 40.20 High-grade B-cell lymphoma: large lymphoma cells with nondescript morphology are present, initially misinterpreted as blasts

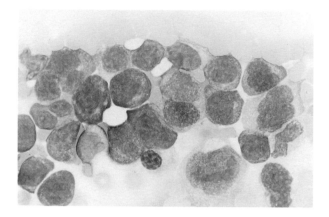

Figure 40.21 High-grade B-cell lymphoma in an HIV-positive patient, showing large lymphoma cells with moderate to deeply basophilic cytoplasm. Some have a plasmacytoid appearance. The chromatin is coarser than in those cells seen in Figure 40.20. Monoclonal surface and cytoplasmic light chains were detectable by FCM immunophenotyping

When large mononuclear cells are present on bone marrow aspirates and/or touch imprints, MPO cytochemistry and NSE stains are necessary. In addition, a comprehensive FCM immunophenotyping panel should be performed. The remaining discussion is based primarily on the phenotype of the large MNCs. Using this multiparameter approach, the large MNCs can be classified into three general categories: myeloblasts, lymphoblasts and large lymphoma cells.

40.5.1 Proliferations of myeloblasts

Auer rods, definitive proof of myeloid differentiation, can be seen in any type of AML except AML-M0 and AML-M7. In the absence of Auer rods, myeloblasts are recognized by: (1) MPO, detectable either cytochemically or immuno-

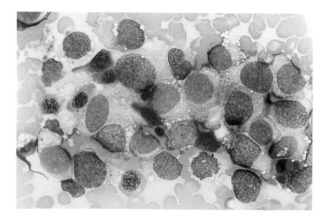

Figure 40.22 Neoplastic cells with a pronounced plasmacytoid appearance in a metastatic amelanotic melanoma

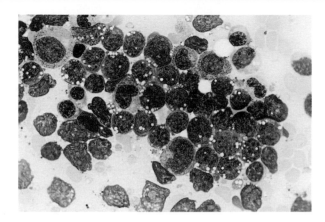

Figure 40.23   Burkitt's lymphoma in the bone marrow of an HIV-positive patient

logically; and/or (2) expression of CD13/CD33 and no evidence of other line-age-associated markers (see Section 22.2). Positive staining for MPO cytochemistry has been defined by the FAB criteria as reaction in at least 3% of the critical cells. The positive reaction can range from a few stained granules to dense and diffuse staining of the cytoplasm. Rarely, when the neoplastic cells are negative for all routine markers, the myeloid phenotype can be proved by a positive MPO reaction at the electron microscopic level.

Certain morphologic features, such as a 'hand mirror' appearance or the presence of a few cytoplasmic azurophilic granules, are not helpful in proving a myeloid phenotype. Azurophilic granules can be found in about 10% of ALL cases (Figure 40.18), some of which can be Sudan black-positive (Figure 32.4). A cytoplasmic tail, which imparts the hand mirror morphology, occurs in AML, ALL and large cell NHL.

A bone marrow differential on at least 200 cells (preferably 500 cells) is necessary to subclassify disorders with an increased percentage of myeloblasts. Furthermore, the percentage of blasts in the peripheral blood must be considered along with the bone marrow blast count. If the bone marrow is the only material available for examination, distinction between an advanced MDS, an MPD, and the early relapse of AML can be problematic. If only a bone marrow biopsy is examined, the differential diagnosis is further complicated, since the cytologic details which allow the distinction between blasts and intermediate myeloid precursors are lost with fixation, decalcification and processing of the core.

The finding of myeloblasts with irregular nuclei does not necessarily infer monocytic differentiation. Positive NSE activity is reliable evidence of monocytic differentiation when performed by the ANBE procedure, however. A positive ANBE reaction is normally seen as diffuse positivity but, in a small number of cases, positive staining is centered in the Golgi area of the leukemic blasts. Expression of CD64 is also presumptive evidence of monocytic differentiation.

The FAB group has established 30% blasts in the bone marrow as the definition of AML and CML in myeloid blast crisis (CML-MBC). The authors, along with many others, also accept the presence of 30% blasts in the peripheral blood as a criterion for acute leukemia, even if the blast count in the bone marrow falls short of the 30% cut-off. Myeloperoxidase and NSE reactivity are key features in the FAB classification of the various subtypes of AML. Knowledge of the clinical history is also important to separate AML from CML-MBC.

The traditional FAB classification of AML has little prognostic significance or therapeutic implications except for the category of AML-M3. Although the FAB terminology is still widely used, it is expected that a biological approach to the classification of AML will be applied based on the wealth of current knowledge.

The FAB classification of AML begins with an evaluation of the percentage of erythroid precursors present in the marrow. Disorders with less than 50% erythroid precursors are covered in Sections 40.5.1.1–40.5.1.6. Acute myeloid leukemia with greater than 50% erythroid precursors (AML-M6) is covered in Section 40.5.1.8.

40.5.1.1 Myeloblasts with bundles of Auer rods (AML-M3)

Bundles of Auer rods are pathognomonic of AML-M3. This is one of the rare instances where the diagnosis of a specific subtype of acute leukemia can be rendered based solely on morphology. The neoplastic population is usually a mixture of blasts with numerous Auer rods, blasts packed with coarse azurophilic granules (also referred to as abnormal or hypergranular promyelocytes), and a small number of hypogranular or agranular blasts. The majority of the cells have a round nuclear contour and maturation is minimal. The erythroid component is markedly decreased and, contrary to previous beliefs, there may be dyserythropoietic features such as nuclear/cytoplasmic asynchrony and nuclear lobulation (Figure 40.17).

Care should be taken to avoid misdiagnosing a hypercellular marrow with markedly left-shifted myelopoiesis (i.e. a maturation arrest picture) as AML-M3. G-CSF therapy, when it results in hypergranularity and myeloid hyperplasia (Figure 40.24), can cause diagnostic confusion with AML-M3, especially when G-CSF is given as part of the induction regimen for another AML subtype.

Other characteristics of AML-M3 include intense MPO activity in virtually all neoplastic cells and the absence of HLA-DR expression. The typical immunophenotype is $CD13^+$, $CD33^+$, $HLA-DR^-$ and $CD34^-$ (see Section 22.2). The cells are negative for NSE.

The cytoplasmic granules in AML-M3 (including those not visible by light microscopy) contain procoagulants that lead to DIC in nearly all patients, especially during induction chemotherapy. Coagulation abnormalities indicative of DIC include prolonged prothrombin and thrombin times, increased fibrin degradation products and decreased fibrinogen.

The pathognomonic translocation in AML-M3, t(15;17)(q21;q11), fuses the *PML* gene on chromosome 15q with the retinoic acid receptor alpha (*RARα*) gene on chromosome 17. The breakpoints within the *RARα* gene are relatively constant, whereas those on the *PML* gene can occur at three different sites, yielding the short, long and variable forms of the *PML-RARα* fusion transcripts. The short isoform appears to be associated with a higher WBC count, M3v morphology, and the presence of additional cytogenetic abnormalities (trisomy 8 being the most common), which confer a worse prognosis.

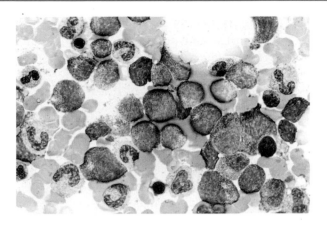

Figure 40.24 G-CSF-associated hypergranulation in intermediate myeloid precursors, which may be confused with the hypergranulated blasts in AML-M3

Three other translocations have been identified in a small number of cases of APL: t(15;17)(q35;q21), t(11;17)(q13;q21) and t(11;17)(q23;q21). In t(11;17) (q23;q21), the *PML* gene is fused with the *PLZF* (promyelocytic leukemia zinc finger) gene, resulting in the *PLZF-RARα* chimera. AML-M3 with this translocation is resistant to all-trans retinoic acid (ATRA) therapy.

The abnormal fusion protein (PML-RARα or PLZF-RARα) interferes with the normal interaction between retinoic acid receptors and physiological ATRA. As a result, cellular differentiation is inhibited. Pharmacological doses of ATRA can overcome the inhibitory effect of the *PML-RARα* chimera. Biochemical interactions between PLZF-RARα and other regulatory proteins render ATRA ineffective, however.

Because ATRA induces terminal differentiation in M3 blasts, the therapy does not result in bone marrow aplasia. During ATRA therapy, all maturation stages between promyelocytes and neutrophils appear in the bone marrow, and circulating mature granulocytes carry detectable *PML-RARα* rearrangements. Although AML-M3 is sensitive to ATRA at presentation, at relapse most cases are resistant to further ATRA therapy.

Molecular detection of the transcripts by RT-PCR assays has been applied to assess minimal residual disease. Currently, persistent detection of PML-RARα at greater than the 10^{-3} level is considered a good predictor of relapse. At the 10^{-5}–10^{-6} level, the clinical significance of the results is controversial, however, since, with this sensitivity, the transcripts are detectable in nearly all AML-M3 patients in continuous remission. A promising approach is 'real-time automated quantitative PCR', which compares the number of transcripts obtained from a follow-up marrow sample to the number in the diagnostic specimen from the same patient.

40.5.1.2 MPO-positive, NSE-negative and no evidence of maturation

If the bone marrow is replaced by a relatively uniform population of blasts, which are MPO-positive and NSE-negative, the differential diagnosis is between one of two disorders:

1. **AML-M3v** (Figure 5.9). A leukemic blast population with markedly twisted nuclei, and dusty purple cytoplasm is characteristic of AML-M3v. This variant accounts for about 25% of APL. The cytoplasm may be agranular and deeply basophilic in some cells. Rare blasts with dense coarse azurophilic granules or Auer rods can be identified in most cases if a careful review is performed. Because of the marked nuclear lobulation, AML-M3v may be misinterpreted as AML with monocytic differentiation if other studies are not performed. After ATRA therapy, the leukemic blasts in relapsed AML-M3v appear virtually agranular, further simulating the appearance of cells with monocytic differentiation (Figure 40.25).

   At the ultrastructural level, the neoplastic cells in AML-M3v are packed with primary granules that are of a size below the resolution of light microscopy. AML-M3v shares the clinical and laboratory characteristics of typical AML-M3 described above. The few minor differences include leukocytosis and abundant circulating malignant cells in AML-M3v, in contrast to the low WBC count and rare circulating blasts in AML-M3. The abundance of circulating cells is associated with a higher risk of DIC and early hemorrhage. Although some cases of AML-M3v may express HLA-DR, its expression is markedly down-regulated when compared to other subtypes of AML.

2. **AML-M1**. In contrast to the markedly twisted nuclei of M3v blasts, the blasts in AML-M1 display a nondescript cytology with no distinguishing morphologic features (Figure 40.26). The majority of AML-M1 blasts have medium to large nuclei, round to irregular nuclear contours, one or more distinct nucleoli and scant to ample agranular blue cytoplasm. Such cells have been named 'type I blasts' by the FAB group, but the morphology can be shared by large lymphoma cells.

   The cytoplasm of some AML-M1 blasts may contain a few azurophilic granules (i.e. FAB 'type II blasts'), vacuoles or, occasionally, Auer rods. Vacuoles are more often seen in relapsed disease. In most cases, there is virtually no differentiation beyond the blast stage (blasts comprises 90% or

Professor Belmonte
Case 60

Professor Belmonte
Cases 61 and 62

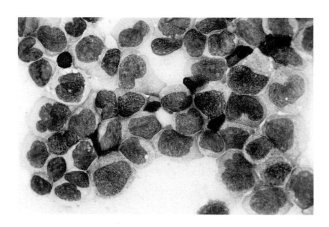

Figure 40.25 AML-M3v: markedly hypogranular blasts with ovoid to reniform nuclei are present, reminiscent of monocytic differentiation

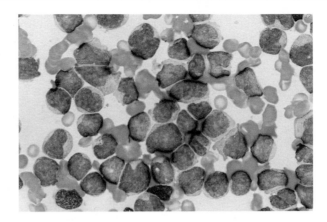

Figure 40.26 AML-M1: blasts with nondescript features (scant to abundant pale blue cytoplasm, round to irregular nuclei, dispersed chromatin and visible nucleoli) are present. There is no evidence of maturation

more of NEC). This morphology is also shared by AML-M0 which, if immunophenotyping is not done, can only be diagnosed as acute leukemia.

40.5.1.3 MPO-positive, NSE-negative and evidence of maturation

The differential diagnosis of myeloid leukemias that are negative for NSE and show evidence of maturation includes AML-M2, AML-M2Eo and AML-M4E. The first thing to look for is bone marrow eosinophilia with abnormal eosinophilic precursors characterized by a mixture of eosinophilic and large purple granules. Whereas bone marrow eosinophilia is seen in both AML-M2Eo and AML-M4E, the presence of abnormal eosinophils is a diagnostic criterion for AML-M4E (Figure 40.27). Peripheral blood eosinophilia is uncommon in either disorder. In contrast to normal eosinophils, the abnormal eosinophils in AML-M4E are CAE-positive.

The blasts in AML-M2, AML-M2Eo and AML-M4E share the same nondescript morphology described above for AML-M1. The blast count is less than 90% of bone marrow NEC. Qualitative abnormalities in myeloid cells, such as nuclear/cytoplasmic asynchrony, nuclear lobulation, hypogranulation and hyposegmentation, suggest that the maturing cells are derived from the leukemic clone. Other features of these subtypes are as follows:

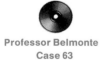

Professor Belmonte
Case 63

1. **AML-M4E.** In AML-M4E, the morphologic evidence of monocytic differentiation is not always clear-cut in the bone marrow. Most cases of AML-M4E are NSE-negative. The distinctive morphologic feature in AML-M4E is abnormal eosinophilic precursors, which correlate with abnormalities in chromosome 16. These abnormalities include inv(16)(p13;q32), t(16;16) (p13;q32) and del(16)(q22). Both inv(16) and t(16;16) result in the fusion of the core binding factor beta gene (*CBF*β) on chromosome 16q22 with the myosin smooth muscle heavy chain gene (*MYH11*) on chromosome 16p13. Because of complex rearrangements, the *CBF*β/*MHY11* fusion transcripts

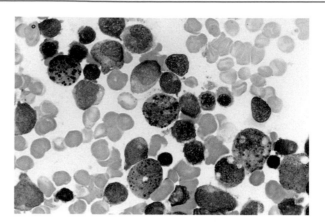

Figure 40.27 AML-M4E: blasts and abnormal eosinophils with prominent basophilic granules can be seen

are heterogeneous. Therefore molecular detection of inv(16) and t(16;16) for monitoring minimal residual disease still remains a challenge.

AML-M4E has a higher remission rate than AML-M4 with standard AML chemotherapy. However, there is a higher frequency of meningeal involvement at relapse.

2. **AML-M2** and **AML-M2Eo**. In general, Auer rods are more common in AML-M2 and AML-M2Eo (Figure 40.28) than other subgroups of AML. Rarely, Auer rods may be present in mature granulocytes as well as blasts. Other qualitative abnormalities described in these FAB subtypes include MPO-deficient neutrophils and giant granules that impart a pseudo-Chediak-Higashi appearance (Figure 40.29).

Since an MDS commonly precedes AML-M2, the cytogenetic abnormalities associated with this FAB subtype are heterogeneous. In children and young adults, a significant number of cases demonstrate t(8;21)(q22;q22). There is a particularly high association between this translocation and the M2Eo subtype. The presence of t(8;21) suggests a *de novo* presentation of the disease since this translocation is extremely rare in secondary AML. Cases with t(8;21) can also demonstrate positivity for CD19.

The (8;21) translocation results in the fusion of the *AML* gene on chromosome 21q22 to the *ETO* gene on chromosome 8. The breakpoints within both of these genes are relatively uniform from patient to patient. Therefore, in cases with t(8;21), the *AML1/ETO* fusion transcript can be reliably and consistently detected by an RT-PCR assay. The clinical usefulness of the assay for MRD detection is controversial, however, since persistent *AML1/ETO* transcripts are detectable with sensitive techniques in patients with long follow-up in continuous complete remission.

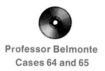

**Professor Belmonte
Cases 64 and 65**

40.5.1.4 NSE-positive and evidence of maturation

NSE positivity indicates monocytic differentiation. Clinically, monocytic leukemias manifest with increased lysozyme in the serum and urine, and exhibit a

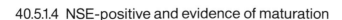

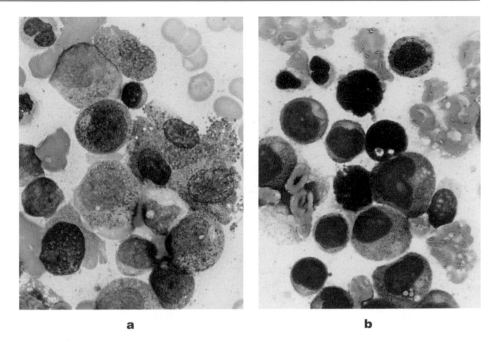

a   b

Figure 40.28   Bone marrow aspirate smears from a case of AML-M2Eo stained at two different laboratories on the same day. (a) A mixture of blasts, myeloid precursors and eosinophils (optimal stain). (b) Suboptimally stained smear with extreme darkening of the eosinophilic granules. Because of this artifact, the case was initially misinterpreted as AML-M4E. Cytogenetic studies revealed t(8;21)

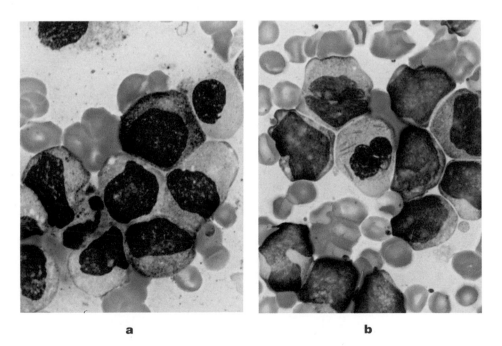

a   b

Figure 40.29   AML-M2 with pseudo-Chediak-Higashi anomaly (a) and numerous Auer rods in a neutrophil (b)

tendency toward extramedullary involvement. A monoblastic crisis of a pre-existing MPD may demonstrate the same features as a *de novo* monocytic leukemia.

The extent of the monocytic component in the bone marrow is used as a criterion to separate acute myelomonocytic leukemia (AML-M4) from acute monocytic leukemia (AML-M5b). According to FAB criteria, the NSE stain is positive in at least 80% of NEC in AML-M5b (Figure 40.30). NSE positivity ranges from 20 to 79% in AML-M4. The MPO stain is positive in AML-M4, but it can be negative in AML-M5b. The peripheral blood presentation in AML-M4 can be similar to AML-M5b if promonocytes and monocytes predominate.

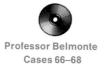

**Professor Belmonte
Cases 66–68**

The bone marrow appearance in AML-M4 can mimic that of AML-M2, as the monocytic component is not always morphologically apparent and promonocytes can be mistaken for intermediate myeloid precursors. However, the FAB group has established two secondary criteria for monocytic differentiation in lieu of a finding of at least 20% positive cells on an NSE stain. The two additional criteria are a peripheral blood monocyte count of at least $5 \times 10^9/l$, and lysozyme in the serum or urine elevated threefold compared to normal.

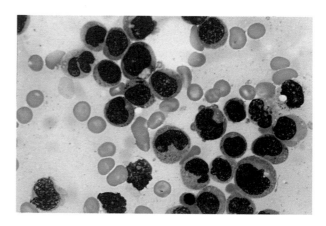

Figure 40.30   AML-M5b, exhibiting a mixture of blasts, promonocytes and monocytes

40.5.1.5 NSE-positive and virtually no evidence of maturation

**Professor Belmonte
Cases 69 and 70**

When NSE is present in at least 80% of NEC in the bone marrow and there is no morphologic evidence of maturation, the diagnosis is AML-M5a (acute monoblastic leukemia). This subgroup differs from AML-M5b only in the degree of monocytic maturation. Since it may be difficult to separate monoblasts from promonocytes, the distinction between AML-M5a and AML-M5b may be problematic. The two subtypes have not been shown to differ biologically, however. Similar to AML-M5b, the MPO stain is often negative in AML-M5a. In typical AML-M5a, the blasts exhibit an owl's eye nucleus with voluminous, vacuolated blue cytoplasm (Figure 40.31). In many cases, however, the cytologic features of monoblasts overlap with those seen in myeloblasts and large NHL cells with immunoblastic morphology (Figure 40.32).

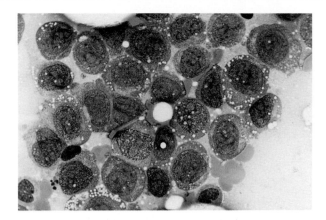

Figure 40.31   AML-M5a, exhibiting blasts with ample cytoplasm, abundant cytoplasmic vacuoles and conspicuous nucleoli

Monocytic leukemias are associated with abnormalities of chromosome 11, including del(11)(q23), t(9;11)(p22;q23), t(6;11)(q27;q23) and t(11;19)(q23;p13). The correlation is highest among infants. Translocations involving chromosome 11q23, which also occur in ALL and therapy-related AML associated with topoisomerase II inhibitors, result in the rearrangement of the *MLL* ('mixed lineage leukemia') gene. Irrespective of the lineage of the acute leukemia, an 11q23 trans-

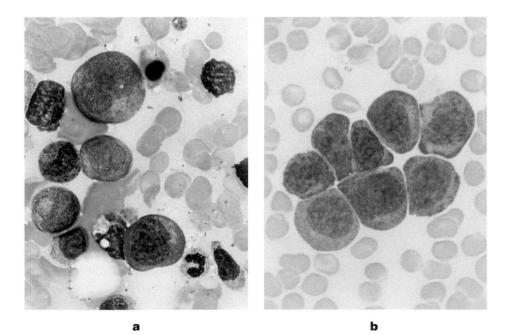

a   b

Figure 40.32   Morphologic similarities between blasts (a) and large lymphoma cells (b). (a) AML-M5a (in relapse); (b) B-immunoblastic lymphoma

location confers a poor prognosis, and is associated with hyperleukocytosis and early involvement of the central nervous system. Currently at least 20 partner chromosomes are involved in *MLL* translocations. Therefore, identification of an *MLL* rearrangement alone may not be sufficient to predict the clinical behavior.

40.5.1.6 Both MPO-negative and NSE-negative

Prior to the availability of monoclonal antibodies, cases of AML which were negative for both MPO and NSE were either misclassified as ALL or categorized as 'undifferentiated acute leukemia'. This category encompasses AML with minimal differentiation (AML-M0), acute megakaryoblastic leukemia (AML-M7) and acute mixed lineage leukemia. The great majority of these can now be identified by FCM immunophenotyping.

A pure myeloid phenotype with absence of other lineage markers defines AML-M0 (see Section 22.2). Expression of platelet glycoproteins CD41 and CD61 by the leukemic cells is supportive evidence of a megakaryocytic lineage (see Chapter 24). If the leukemic blasts demonstrate no apparent lineage differentiation despite an extensive FCM panel, ultracytochemistries for myeloperoxidase and platelet peroxidase are helpful.

Further characterization of these subtypes is as follows:

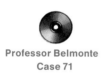

**Professor Belmonte
Case 71**

1. **AML-M0**. The leukemic blasts in AML-M0 have a nondescript morphology and express myeloid antigens (CD13, CD33) and/or demonstrate reactivity with MPO antibody. Occasional cases may present with a mediastinal mass, thus mimicking the clinical presentation of ALL/lymphoblastic lymphoma. In AML-M0, peroxidase positive granules are present at the electron microscopic level (Figure 5.6), despite the negative MPO cytochemistry.

**Professor Belmonte
Case 72**

2. **AML-M7** (Figures 40.33 and 40.34). The morphology in AML-M7 varies from case to case, ranging from predominantly large cells with nondescript cytology to a heterogeneous population of medium and large cells. The medium-size cells have condensed chromatin and mimic typical lymphoblasts. The diagnosis can be suspected if the leukemic population in the peripheral blood is accompanied by morphologically recognizable immature-appearing (monolobed) megakaryocytes, or there is evidence of platelets budding off from the leukemic blasts (Figure 40.35). Megakaryoblasts may be weakly positive for ANAE but are negative for ANBE.

   Severe marrow fibrosis is common in AML-M7, probably related to the release of platelet-derived growth factor by the malignant cells and abnormal megakaryocytes. FCM immunophenotyping in these cases is best done on cell suspensions made from fresh core biopsies or on blasts from the peripheral blood. Note that marked reticulin fibrosis also occurs in other subtypes of acute leukemia, although less frequently.

The terminology concerning AML-M7 (acute megakaryoblastic leukemia) and closely related disorders has been the subject of great confusion. The related disorders have been designated acute myelofibrosis, acute myelodysplasia with myelofibrosis, and malignant myelosclerosis. In all of these disorders, the following characteristics have been described:

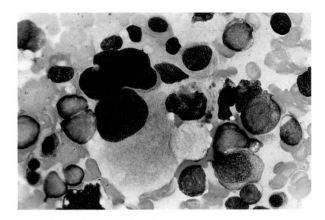

Figure 40.33   AML-M7, exhibiting a blast with nondescript features and a monolobed megakaryocyte. By FCM immunophenotyping, the blasts in this case coexpressed CD34 and CD41. Myeloid and lymphoid antigens were not expressed

- Peripheral pancytopenia, with a variable percentage of circulating blasts, and nonspecific RBC abnormalities (e.g. macrocytes, elliptocytes).
- A hypercellular marrow with extensive reticulin fibrosis, resulting in scanty aspirates or a 'dry tap'. This precludes both an accurate assessment of the blast content and adequate phenotypic characterization of the malignant cells.
- Qualitative abnormalities in the maturation of all three cell lines (including conspicuous numbers of abnormal megakaryocytes).
- A rapid downhill clinical course, with most cases terminating as acute megakaryoblastic leukemia.

The above features are also observed in *de novo* AML-M7, however. It appears that the plethora of terminology most likely reflects either minor differences in the clinical presentation, or is due to incomplete characterization of a given case because of the severe marrow fibrosis. For practical purposes, all of these related disorders can be considered together with AML-M7.

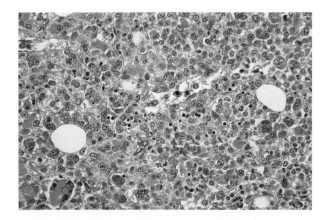

Figure 40.34   Sheets of blasts in a case of AML-M7. There is also marked reticulin fibrosis (not shown)

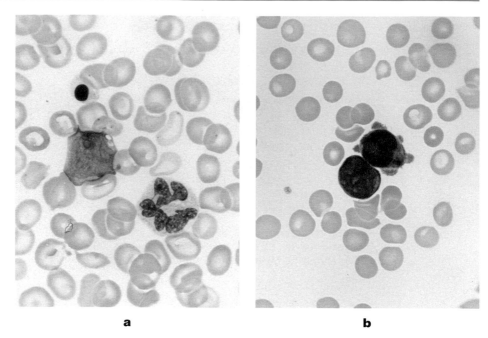

a   b

Figure 40.35 (a), (b) AML-M7 blasts in the peripheral blood of two different patients. The morphology is nondescript. In one case, the presence of an immature megakaryocyte with budding platelets (b) suggests that the accompanying blast may be of megakaryocytic lineage

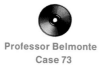

Professor Belmonte
Case 73

3. **Leukemias with mixed phenotypes**. Acute mixed lineage leukemias are discussed in Section 22.3. It is difficult to determine the clinical significance of these disorders since no uniform, stringent criteria have been established. Conceptually, acute mixed leukemia can be divided into biphenotypic leukemias, in which both myeloid and lymphoid antigens are present on the leukemic cells, and biclonal leukemias, in which there are two phenotypically different blast populations (i.e. coexisting myeloblasts and lymphoblasts). Biphenotypic leukemia is uncommon and accounts for no more than 3–5% of acute leukemias.

40.5.1.7 Myeloid blast crisis of CML (CML-MBC)

Professor Belmonte
Case 74

Since CML is a disorder of pluripotent stem cells, the blast crisis can be of any lineage differentiation. CML-MBC accounts for 70–80% of the blast crises. The bone marrow and peripheral blood appearance can be indistinguishable from AML-M1, M2, or M4. Basophilia, when present, is a helpful diagnostic clue, especially if no clinical information has been provided. Because increased eosinophilic precursors are frequently present in CML, CML-MBC can also mimic AML-M2Eo. Other forms of blast crisis (M3, M4Eo, M5 and M7) are rare. The blast crisis is usually heralded by additional cytogenetic abnormalities, most commonly an extra (9;22) translocation, an isochromosome for the long arm of chromosome 17, trisomy 8 or trisomy 19.

40.5.1.8 Erythroid preponderance (AML-M6)

The FAB criteria which define AML-M6 (Figure 40.36), also known as erythro-leukemia or Di Guglielmo's syndrome, are myeloblasts accounting for at least 30% of NEC in a bone marrow with erythroid preponderance. The majority of AML-M6 cases are therapy-related (i.e. secondary) AML and are therefore preceded by an MDS stage characterized by erythroid predominance, often with ring sideroblasts. Most cases of AML-M6 progress to AML-M1, M2, or M4. In contrast to the nondescript morphology of the blast component, the erythroid precursors in AML-M6 usually demonstrate a dramatic range of qualitative abnormalities including binucleation, multinucleation, karyorrhexis, nuclear lobulation and cytoplasmic vacuoles. Giant erythroid precursors with nuclear/cytoplasmic asynchrony (i.e. megaloblastic maturation) can be present. Note that diffuse or chunky PAS staining in the erythroid precursors is neither pathognomonic nor a diagnostic requirement for AML-M6.

**Professor Belmonte
Case 75**

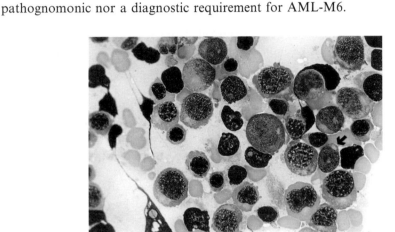

Figure 40.36 AML-M6, exhibiting blasts (arrow) surrounded by abundant erythroid precursors with nuclear/cytoplasmic asynchrony and nuclear lobulation. The bone marrow contained 80% erythroid precursors, 11% blasts and 9% maturing myeloid precursors

40.5.1.9 MDS and MPD

If blasts comprise 5–20% of the nucleated cells in the marrow (or there is erythroid preponderance and blasts are 5–20% of NEC), the bone marrow findings should be carefully correlated with the clinical history and peripheral blood data. The differential diagnosis includes RAEB, CMMoL and CML, which share the common features of hypercellularity and myeloid hyperplasia. In many of these cases, the hyperplastic marrow with a preponderance of intermediate myeloid precursors overshadows the increased percentage of blasts. In addition, megakaryocytes may be increased, creating an overall bone marrow picture of bihyperplasia. These disorders are discussed in Chapter 36.

The FAB classification designated the group of diseases with bone marrow blasts between 21 and 30% as RAEB-T (see Section 36.1.2). The distinction between RAEB-T and AML-M2 is not always clear-cut. The clinical behavior in many cases is similar to AML, and an AML regimen is used for this disorder in many institutions.

40.5.2 The large MNCs are mature lymphoid cells

Involvement of the bone marrow by large mature lymphoid cells can be divided into two broad categories:

1. Disorders with distinctive cytologic features, phenotypic profiles, and/or hematological presentations. These include HCL, PLL, Burkitt's lymphoma-leukemia and aggressive large granular lymphocyte leukemia. In these disorders, a preliminary interpretation may be safely made shortly after examination of the blood film, bone marrow aspirate or touch imprints.
2. Disorders without a distinctive cytology, including large cell NHL and the uncommon mature B-cell leukemia.

Large B-cell LPD/NHL can be diagnosed when there is monoclonal light chain expression, or if there is no detectable light chain expression and both CD34 and TdT are negative (see Section 27.1). Monoclonal cytoplasmic light chains indicate plasmacytoid differentiation.

Large MNCs are mature T cells if both CD34 and TdT are absent. In the T-cell lineage there is no equivalent to immunoglobulin light chains to indicate clonality. When both CD34 and TdT are negative, loss of a pan-T-cell marker suggests malignancy in the adult age group. In the Western world, B-lineage large cell LPD/NHL is more common than the T-cell counterparts.

40.5.2.1 Hairy cell leukemia

Hairy cell leukemia is an indolent disease with a constellation of highly characteristic clinical, phenotypic and morphologic features. Furthermore, HCL has become a 'curable' disease in view of the remarkable therapeutic advances during the last 10–15 years. For this reason, it is important to identify HCL correctly since it is exquisitely sensitive to 2-chlorodeoxyadenosine (2-CdA).

The FCM immunophenotyping pattern of HCL is diagnostic for the disorder, based on the combination of high forward scatter, bright CD20, bright CD11c, and expression of CD25 and CD103 (see Section 27.7). The characteristic cytology of hairy cells (Figure 5.14) is best appreciated on the peripheral blood film (see Section 5.4). Hairy cells are considered 'large' cells because of the voluminous pale gray cytoplasm that imparts a 'fried egg' appearance. The nuclei, which may be eccentrically located, are actually relatively small (2–2.5 times RBC size).

Because of marked reticulin fibrosis in HCL, bone marrow aspiration invariably yields a 'dry tap'. A good core biopsy and well-prepared imprints are critical for morphologic assessment. On the biopsy, the infiltration ranges from interstitial to diffuse. In most cases, the bone marrow is hypercellular. Because of the abundant cytoplasm of hairy cells, the 'fried egg' appearance is visible on fixed tissue and the infiltrate appears loosely packed (Figure 40.37). This morphology

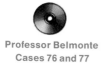

Professor Belmonte
Cases 76 and 77

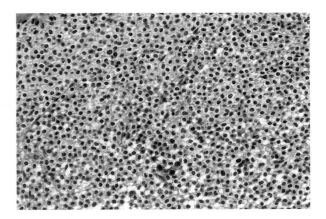

Figure 40.37   Hairy cell leukemia (diffuse infiltration)

can be mimicked by other disorders including LGL leukemia. Careful attention to the clinical presentation and the FCM immunophenotyping pattern should easily resolve the differential diagnosis.

A focal pattern of bone marrow infiltration is uncommon in HCL and is mainly seen with residual disease (Figure 40.38). The small foci of residual hairy cells can be highlighted by immunostaining with a paraffin-resistant pan-B-cell marker such as CD20c (L26).

The current therapy of choice for HCL is 2-CdA, which achieves a complete remission in approximately 90% of patients. Complete remission in HCL has been defined as no organomegaly, no circulating hairy cells, a morphologically negative bone marrow and a return of blood counts to 'normal' (i.e. Hgb at least 12 g/dl, neutrophils $> 1.5 \times 10^9/l$ and platelets $> 100 \times 10^9/l$). If complete remission has been achieved by these criteria, the finding of scattered hairy cells in the bone marrow by molecular techniques or L26 immunostaining does not appear to indicate impending recurrence.

40.5.2.2 Prolymphocytic leukemia

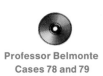

Professor Belmonte
Cases 78 and 79

The diagnosis of PLL is made in the peripheral blood, and a bone marrow aspirate/biopsy is usually not necessary (see Section 5.5.1). The distinction between B-PLL and T-PLL can be easily made by FCM immunophenotyping. In the bone marrow, because of the higher cell density, the neoplastic cells can appear smaller (shrunken), with morphologic artifacts including hair, villi or blebs. In contrast to HCL, the bone marrow is easily aspirated. Since the tumor burden in the marrow parallels that in the blood, bone marrow involvement is invariably extensive (Figure 40.39).

40.5.2.3 Burkitt's lymphoma-leukemia

Burkitt's lymphoma and ALL-L3 refer to same entity. Note that the FAB classification of ALL antedated our current immunologic understanding of leuke-

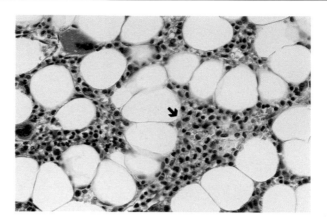

Figure 40.38 Residual hairy cell leukemia following interferon therapy. A small focus of hairy cell infiltration is apparent (arrow)

mias and lymphomas. Since the term 'lymphoblast' indicates immature lymphoid cells and Burkitt's cells are mature B cells, it is conceptually and semantically more correct to designate the disease as Burkitt's lymphoma-leukemia rather than 'lymphoblastic' leukemia. There is a higher prevalence of the disease in immunodeficient patients. Because Burkitt's lymphoma-leukemia has the highest S-phase fraction of all hematopoietic neoplasms, the patient often has bulky disease at presentation (e.g. an abdominal mass and/or organomegaly).

A presumptive diagnosis of Burkitt's lymphoma-leukemia can be made based on the finding of medium to large cells with deep blue cytoplasm, abundant sharp cytoplasmic vacuoles and stippled chromatin (Figure 40.23). This morphology may occur in PTCL, however (Figure 28.6). In some Burkitt's lymphoma-leukemia, the morphology is less distinctive and may overlap with large cell NHL with plasmacytoid differentiation.

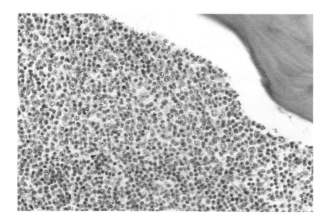

Figure 40.39 B-prolymphocytic leukemia (diffuse infiltration): the cytology of the transformed lymphoid cells on the biopsy section is not diagnostic for PLL, however

If DNA cell cycle kinetics are investigated along with FCM immunophenotyping, the combination of a mature B-cell phenotype (often CD10$^+$) and an extremely high S-phase in the 35–50% range, is virtually diagnostic of Burkitt's lymphoma-leukemia. Because of the high cell turnover rate, FCM studies need to be performed soon after the bone marrow has been collected, to avoid loss of viable tumor cells.

Prior to the era of immunophenotyping, the cytochemical stain Oil red O, which reacts with lipid-containing vacuoles, was used to identify Burkitt's cells. This procedure can be omitted since other subtypes of ALL and some nonhematopoietic malignancies may also be positive.

The pattern of peripheral blood involvement in Burkitt's lymphoma-leukemia is similar to that seen in other high-grade NHL, i.e. a low number of circulating cells in most cases. Bone marrow infiltration is extensive, however, with frequent mitotic and apoptotic figures. A 'starry sky' appearance secondary to scattered phagocytic macrophages may be apparent (Figure 40.40). These features can also be seen in other aggressive malignancies. On H&E sections the neoplastic cells are seen as medium-sized, with a sharp nuclear membrane, multiple distinct nucleoli and amphophilic cytoplasm.

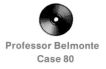

**Professor Belmonte
Case 80**

The cytogenetic abnormalities in Burkitt's lymphoma-leukemia have been well established. The three main translocations are t(8;14)(q24;q32), t(2;8)(p12;q24) and t(8;22)(q24;q11). These result in the juxtaposition of the c-*myc* oncogene to the heavy chain gene, kappa chain gene, and lambda chain gene, respectively. This leads to up-regulation of c-myc.

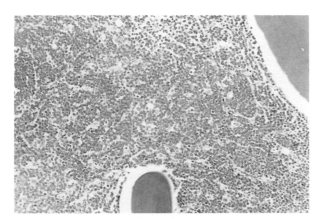

Figure 40.40   A 'starry sky' appearance in Burkitt's lymphoma

40.5.2.4 Aggressive large granular lymphocyte leukemia

The clinical presentation and immunophenotype of large granular lymphocyte disorders are discussed in detail in Section 28.4.

Aggressive NK and NK-like T-cell lymphoma-leukemias share similar morphologic features. The aggressive behavior is often reflected morphologically by a preponderance of large neoplastic cells (larger than normal LGLs), with moderate to ample cytoplasm and variable numbers of azurophilic granules. Some cases may be agranular. Ultrastructurally, electron-dense granules but no parallel tubular arrays have been reported. Nuclear irregularities may be present. The large cell size, visible nucleoli, and cytoplasmic granules may lead to a misidentification of these larger LGLs as monoblasts or immature monocytes (Figure 40.41).

Cases with leukemic manifestations have rapidly increasing WBC counts in addition to infiltration of the liver and spleen. The extent and pattern of bone marrow involvement are variable, ranging from interstitial to diffuse. As a rule, the neoplastic cells are more easily appreciated on the blood films or bone marrow smears than on the biopsy sections. The suggested work-up for these diseases is discussed in Section 28.2.

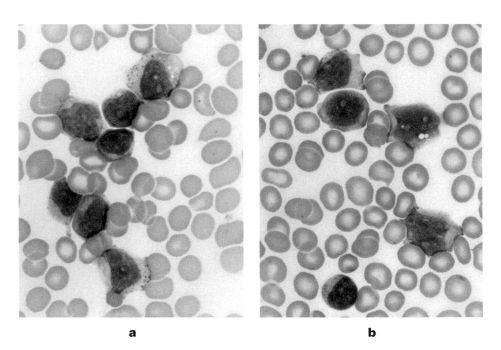

a   b

Figure 40.41 (a), (b) Peripheral blood in aggressive LGL leukemia. The neoplastic population is composed of medium and large cells. Many of the large cells do not have visible cytoplasmic granules (b). The appearance simulates that of AML blasts. FCM studies and molecular studies revealed an NK phenotype: coexpression of CD2, CD8 and CD57, absence of TdT, CD34 and other T cell markers (CD3, CD5, CD7, CD4, TCR$\alpha\beta$ and TCR$\gamma\delta$) and a germ line configuration of the TCR genes. The patient had hepatosplenomegaly and cutaneous involvement

40.5.2.5 Large cell NHL with either nondescript or immunoblastic cytology

In immunocompetent patients with LCL, involvement of the bone marrow at presentation is infrequent. Infiltration is more common late in the course of the disease or in immunocompromised patients with widespread disease at diagnosis. Involvement of the peripheral blood or bone marrow by LCL is a poor prognostic sign.

Large cell lymphoma infiltration in the marrow usually causes a 'mass effect', a pattern reminiscent of metastatic malignancies. The pattern of infiltration can be focal, paratrabecular, interstitial or diffuse. Necrosis (Figure 40.42) and apoptotic figures, features of aggressive disease, may be present. The involved areas can contain primarily tumor cells or may demonstrate a large reactive component composed of small lymphocytes, histiocytes, fibroblasts and increased vascularity, obscuring the neoplastic cells (Figures 40.43 and 40.44). Focal lesions with a large reactive component may simulate a granuloma (Figure 40.45). Although a prominent reactive component is associated with PTCL, it can also occur in large B-cell NHL. Irrespective of the bone marrow appearance, the subclassification of LCL into various histologic subtypes is based on the extramedullary sites of involvement. Immunophenotyping is necessary to determine the lineage of the tumor.

Flow cytometry immunophenotyping and a thorough examination of aspirate smears and touch imprints can detect low numbers of large lymphoma cells even when involvement is not readily apparent on the biopsy sections. The cytologic features of large cell NHL vary from case to case. On Romanovsky-stained air-dried preparations, as well as on the biopsy sections, the large cells may display a nondescript cytology (Figures 40.20 and 40.46), simulating the appearance of leukemic blasts. In such cases, immunophenotyping is crucial to establish the maturity and lineage of the neoplastic cells.

In some cases, it is possible to infer that the large cells are mature lymphoid cells based on a plasmacytoid appearance (Figure 40.21) with prominent nucleoli

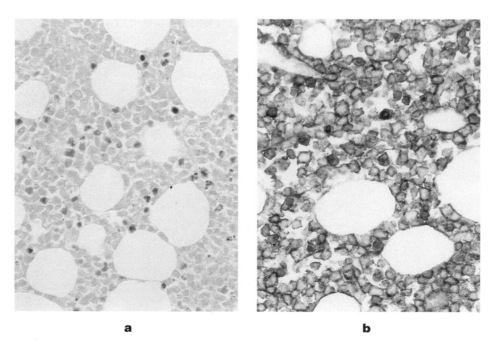

a   b

Figure 40.42 High-grade B-cell lymphoma with extensive necrosis. (a) An interstitial infiltrate of 'ghost' tumor cells and apoptotic figures. (b) Strong positive L26 reactivity

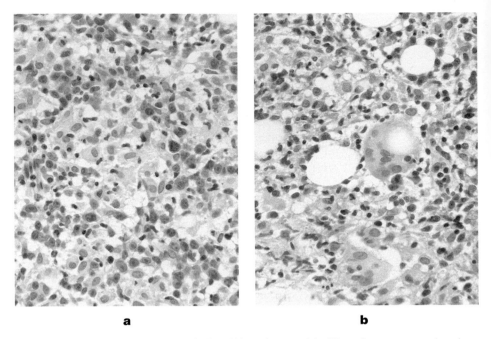

Figure 40.43 (a), (b) High-grade B-cell lymphoma with diffuse bone marrow involvement. The infiltrate contains a conspicuous number of benign histiocytes as well as multinucleated giant cells (b)

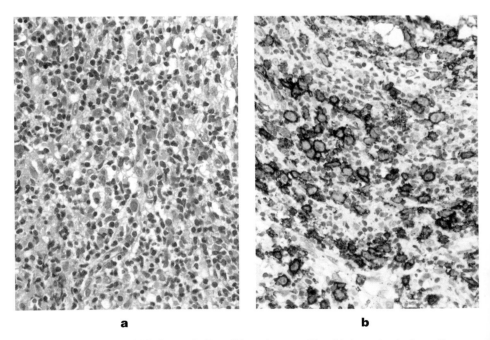

Figure 40.44 (a), (b) High-grade B-cell lymphoma with a high content of small reactive T cells. The medium and large neoplastic cells are highlighted with strong L26 reactivity. A subsequent lymph node biopsy revealed a diffuse large cell lymphoma without the high number of reactive T cells

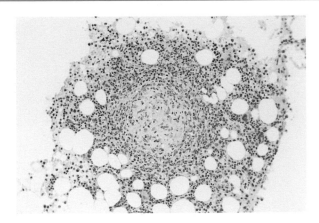

Figure 40.45 A 'granuloma-like' focus in a case of PTCL. Elsewhere on the biopsy section the infiltrate demonstrated a paratrabecular and interstitial pattern

and coarse chromatin (i.e. immunoblastic lymphoma). Expression of monoclonal cytoplasmic light chains is proof that the neoplastic cells are B immunoblasts.

Immunoblastic lymphoma is common in immunocompromised patients (e.g. iatrogenic immunosuppression or AIDS). In AIDS patients, the tumor cells tend to appear more heterogeneous with a variable number of binucleated or multi-nucleated giant cells. Some cases can also express CD30.

In addition to bone marrow involvement, LCL in AIDS patients has a high propensity for infiltration of extranodal sites such as the central nervous system or body serous cavities (giving rise to primary effusion lymphoma). Human herpes virus-8 (HHV-8) is often found in cases presenting as primary effusion lymphoma. Epstein-Barr virus has been demonstrated in a high proportion of AIDS LCL. The combination of EBV and/or HHV-8 infection, along with chronic antigenic stimulation (resulting in B-cell activation and proliferation), dysregulated cyto-

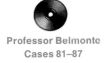

Professor Belmonte
Cases 81–87

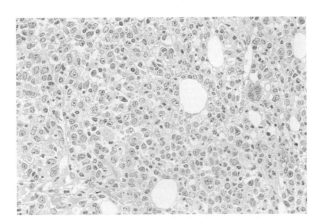

Figure 40.46 Diffuse involvement by a large B-cell lymphoma. The appearance of the transformed lymphoid cells is similar to that of leukemic blasts

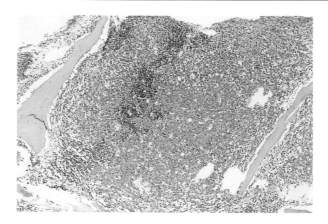

Figure 40.47 Richter's syndrome following long-standing CLL, showing diffuse infiltration by transformed lymphoid cells with a starry sky pattern. Note the residual small lymphoid cell infiltrate of CLL

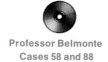

Professor Belmonte
Cases 58 and 88

kine production, and/or inadequate immune surveillance, is believed to account for the frequent development of lymphomas in AIDS patients.

Large cell lymphomas can occur *de novo* or can represent transformation from a known low-grade process (Figure 40.47) such as long-standing CLL, LPC lymphoma-leukemia/Waldenstrom's macroglobulinemia, FCC NHL or Sezary syndrome.

40.5.3 The MNC infiltrate is composed of large immature lymphoid cells

Immature lymphoid cells are identified by FCM immunophenotyping. An immature B-cell phenotype is seen in both precursor-B acute leukemia and hematogones (see Chapter 25). An immature T-cell pattern indicates that the proliferation is neoplastic (T ALL/lymphoblastic lymphoma). The morphologic features of ALL are discussed in Section 40.6.2.2 since, in most cases, the neoplastic population is heterogeneous.

40.6 The MNC infiltrate is of heterogeneous cell size

An MNC proliferation may be heterogeneous with a spectrum of cells ranging from small to large. Heterogeneity in cell size may be present in a variety of the hematopoietic neoplasms described above, including AML (especially subtypes M0, M1 and M7), MCL, FCC in transformation, peripheral T-cell lymphomas, Sezary syndrome, ATLL and CLL/PL (see Sections 5.5 and 39.1.1). The heterogeneity in cell size is better appreciated on air-dried smears where the cells are not crowded.

40.6.1 Heterogeneous cell size and cloverleaf nuclear irregularities ('flower' cells)

A mononuclear cell infiltrate with pleomorphic cytology and so-called 'flower' cells (best appreciated on the blood film) is virtually pathognomonic for ATLL.

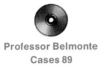

Professor Belmonte Cases 89

The diagnosis is made primarily in the peripheral blood (see Section 5.9). Bone marrow involvement, which ranges from focal to diffuse, often does not parallel the striking peripheral blood leukocytosis. Evidence of increased bone turnover can be seen, with increased numbers of osteoblasts and osteoclasts (Figure 40.48). This accounts for the commonly associated hypercalcemia. Presumably, the increased bone resorption is secondary to lymphokines secreted by the tumor cells.

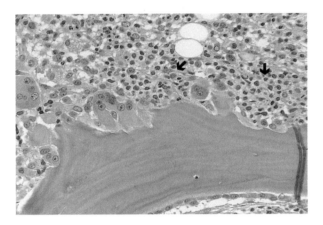

Figure 40.48   Bone marrow in a case of ATLL with a WBC count of 47×10^9/l and 90% neoplastic T cells. Prominent osteoclasts are associated with the subtle paratrabecular neoplastic infiltrates (arrow)

40.6.2 The heterogeneous MNCs are immature lymphoid cells

In adults, a proliferation of immature lymphoid cells in the bone marrow is virtually indicative of ALL/lymphoblastic lymphoma. In children, however, the diagnostic possibilities include both ALL/lymphoblastic lymphoma and increased hematogones. Hematogones are medium to large, with scant cytoplasm, coarse chromatin and regular nuclear contours (Figure 33.12).

40.6.2.1 Differential diagnosis between ALL and hematogones

The two helpful morphologic clues to distinguish lymphoblastic proliferations from hematogones are:

1. Heterogeneous MNCs in the peripheral blood, accompanied by significant anemia and thrombocytopenia, suggest ALL.

2. An MNC population that obliterates other hematopoietic elements in the bone marrow is unlikely to be hematogones.

The difficulty in differential diagnosis arises when the bone marrow contains 30–50% heterogeneous MNCs and the peripheral blood demonstrates no such cells, only mild to moderate thrombocytopenia and mild anemia (which may be nutritional). These features may be present in bone marrow either involved by lymphoblastic lymphoma or with increased hematogones, which are invariably elevated in ITP. Metastatic childhood tumors such as neuroblastoma also need to be considered.

Immunologically, hematogones are precursor B cells. With properly performed data analysis, FCM immunophenotyping can provide clues to separate benign precursor B cells from precursor-B ALL (see Section 25.4). If a diagnosis has not been firmly established and the possibility of increased hematogones has not been excluded, then a conservative 'watch and wait' approach may be indicated.

40.6.2.2 Acute lymphoblastic leukemia and lymphoblastic lymphoma

The FAB classification of ALL (which includes Burkitt's lymphoma-leukemia) was proposed prior to the era of monoclonal antibodies. In recent years, it has been shown that the classification bears little correlation with antigenic profiles, karyotypic abnormalities and prognosis. Therefore it is no longer necessary to categorize a given case as ALL-L1 or L2. For historical interest, the FAB criteria for distinguishing the L1 and L2 subtypes based on cell size, nuclear/ cytoplasmic ratio, nuclear outline and prominence of nucleoli are shown in Table 40.1. Since the cytologic appearance of lymphoblasts is easily affected by the quality of the smears, it is evident that good reproducibility is difficult to obtain in such a morphologic scoring system, despite the defined criteria.

Cytochemical stains are also of limited usefulness in the diagnosis of ALL. Block positivity with PAS is seen in many but not all ALLs. Focal acid phosphatase positivity located near the nucleus was believed to indicate T ALL. However, it has been shown that this reaction pattern does not correlate with immunophenotype and occurs in other leukemias. Azurophilic granules can be found in ALL (Figure 40.18) and rare cases of ALL are also positive for SBB (Figure 32.4) or ANAE, which may lead to an incorrect diagnosis of AML.

In most cases of ALL, the cell size is heterogeneous (Figure 40.49). Occasionally, ALL may present with a relatively monotonous population of small cells

---

Table 40.1 FAB scoring system for subclassifying ALL

A score of +1 is given for each of the first two criteria and a score of −1 is assigned for each of the last four.
A total score of 0 to +2 indicates ALL-L1, whereas −1 to −4 indicates ALL-L2.
1. High N/C ratio (defined as the cytoplasm occupying <25% of the cell area) in >75% of cells.
2. No nucleolus or one small nucleolus in >75% of the cells.
3. Low N/C ratio (defined as the cytoplasm occupying >20% of the cell area) in >25% of cells.
4. An irregular nuclear contour in >25% of cells.
5. A prominent nucleolus (or nucleoli) in >25% of cells.
6. Large cells (defined as twice the size of a small lymphocyte) make up >50% of cells.

with condensed chromatin. Such cases are easily mistaken for either benign lymphoid cells or a low-grade LPD/NHL if other parameters (e.g. severe anemia and thrombocytopenia, or the patient's age) are overlooked (Figure 40.7).

On biopsy sections, the cell size heterogeneity is less perceptible. The great majority of cases present with a hypercellular marrow and a lymphoblast population with stippled chromatin and small nucleoli (Figure 40.50). The number of mitoses and apoptotic figures is variable, reflecting the kinetic activity of the tumor. Other less common features include reticulin fibrosis, necrosis and bone resorption. In rare cases, the bone marrow is initially hypocellular. The patient presents with pancytopenia, mimicking the picture of aplasia. The interstitial blast infiltration is easily overlooked. This stage is transient, lasting for only a few weeks to several months. It is followed by a hypercellular marrow with the typical features of ALL.

The diagnosis and classification of ALL is currently based on FCM immunophenotyping. The immunologic subgroups are discussed in Sections 25.2 and 26.2. The clinical and hematological parameters at presentation, together with DNA content analysis and cytogenetics, allow an evaluation of the prognosis in a given case.

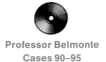

**Professor Belmonte
Cases 90–95**

The morphology and phenotype of CML in lymphoid blast crisis (CML-LBC) are indistinguishable from those of *de novo* ALL. Most cases of CML-LBC have a precursor-B phenotype. In addition to t(9;22), additional karyotypic abnormalities are invariably present.

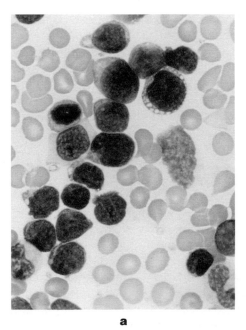

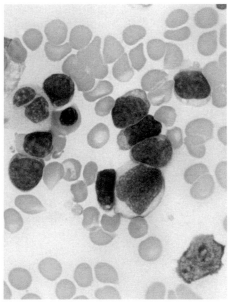

a b

Figure 40.49 A heterogeneous population of blasts in a case of T ALL. (a) An occasional blast with cytoplasmic vacuoles arranged in a 'pearl necklace' pattern. (b) Blasts, along with a hyposegmented and hypogranular neutrophil. Note that the pseudo-Pelger-Huët change in neutrophils is not limited to myeloid malignancies

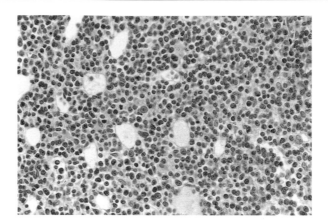

Figure 40.50 ALL/lymphoblastic lymphoma, showing diffuse bone marrow infiltration by small to medium-size lymphoid cells

T-cell acute lymphoblastic leukemia and lymphoblastic lymphoma are different presentations of the same disorder. The neoplastic cells in both diseases share a similar morphology and antigenic profile. Conceptually, lymphoblastic lymphoma begins in the lymph nodes and spreads to the bone marrow, whereas ALL follows the reverse pathway. Both the lymph nodes and bone marrow are involved at presentation in many instances, however. With a T ALL presentation, the bone marrow is virtually replaced by neoplastic cells, often with a decreased number of megakaryocytes. When the disease presents as lymphoblastic lymphoma, there may be a substantial proportion of normal hematopoietic elements and adequate numbers of megakaryocytes in the bone marrow. The pattern of involvement can be interstitial.

In addition to hematogones, the morphologic differential diagnosis of ALL includes small round cell tumors of childhood (e.g. neuroblastoma) and small cell carcinoma in adults (see Chapter 41). An important diagnostic clue to the nonhematopoietic nature of an MNC infiltrate is the presence of nuclear molding on aspirate smears.

Molecular analysis is of limited usefulness in the diagnosis and classification of ALL/LL since rearrangements of *TCRβ* can be found in about 30% of cases of precursor-B ALL, and a higher number of cases have a rearranged *TCRδ*. In addition, rearrangement of the heavy chain gene (*IgH*) can be present in T ALL. Furthermore, both *TCR* and *IgH* rearrangements can be found in some cases of AML.

Acute lymphoblastic leukemia has a bimodal age distribution, with the first peak in childhood (2–5 years) and a second peak around age 50. Age and the WBC count at presentation remain the most relevant prognostic factors. The low-risk group in childhood ALL has been recently defined as WBCs $< 50 \times 10^9$/l and age 1–9 years. Other useful factors for risk assessment include the initial response to induction therapy and the type of cytogenetic abnormality.

With high-resolution banding cytogenetics, about 90% of ALL cases demonstrate chromosomal abnormalities. Hyperdiploid cases are those with a DNA index of 1.16 or greater by FCM analysis, or more than 50 chromosomes by standard karyotyping. In ALL, there are nonrandom gains of chromosomes 21, 18, 17, 14, 10, 6, 4, and X. The good prognosis associated with hyperdiploidy has been attributed to the associated low WBC count, increased accumulation of methotrexate in the leukemic blasts, increased sensitivity to antimetabolites, and a propensity for spontaneous apoptosis. Hyperdiploidy is found in about 30% of cases of childhood precursor-B ALL, mainly in the age group of 2–10 years. The prognostic impact of hyperdiploidy in adults is less significant, mainly because of other coexisting unfavorable karyotypic abnormalities.

Cases with less than 45 chromosomes are defined as hypodiploid. Hypodiploid ALL is uncommon and is associated with a poor prognosis.

Most cases of diploid ALL are accompanied by a T-cell phenotype. It is unclear if these patients harbor clones with submicroscopic genetic changes. A pseudodiploid karyotype is seen in about 40% of ALL. This group comprises various chromosomal translocations, most of which are seen in precursor-B ALL. Pseudodiploid ALL occurs more often in adults than children. The prognosis depends on the underlying translocations.

The well-established translocations in ALL include:

1. Translocations in T ALL. They usually affect *TCR* loci such as the *TCRα/δ* genes and *TCRβ* gene on chromosomes 14q11 and 7q34, respectively, and are associated with high-risk features (high WBC count, mediastinal mass, lymphadenopathy and organomegaly). In some of the translocations, the *TAL*-1 gene on chromosome 1p32 is overexpressed when juxtaposed to a *TCR* locus. *TAL*-1 gene abnormalities may be submicroscopic and therefore not detectable by routine cytogenetics in 25–30% of cases.

2. The (12;21)(p13;q22) translocation, which results in the fusion of the *TEL* gene on chromosome 12p13 to the *AML1* gene on chromosome 21q22. This is currently the most common translocation in childhood precursor-B ALL (25% of cases) but it is infrequent in adult ALL. It is associated with a good outcome. Since the abnormality is not visible by standard analysis, detection is based on molecular probes such as FISH or RT-PCR. Recent data indicate that the *TEL-AML1* rearrangement occurs before birth, and that a second 'hit' is required to induce leukemic transformation. The *AML1* gene is also involved in the *AML1/ETO* fusion in the (8;21) translocation. In the *TEL/AML1* fusion, nearly the entire coding sequence of the *AML1* gene is preserved, including the transactivation domain. In contrast, in the *AML1/ETO* fusion the transactivation domain of *AML1* is lost. The mechanism of leukemogenesis may therefore be different in the two disorders.

3. A Philadelphia chromosome, present in 20% of adult ALL but only 4% of childhood ALL. This is associated with a poor prognosis. The molecular genetics of the Philadelphia chromosome are discussed in Section 18.4.

4. Other translocations which confer a poor prognosis. These include t(1;19)(q23;p13), which is associated with a high WBC count and a pre-B (i.e. cmu-positive) phenotype, and translocations involving chromosome 11. The (4;11)(q21;q23) translocation, found mainly in infants, results in re-

arrangements of the *MLL* gene and is associated with hyperleukocytosis. *MLL* gene rearrangements also occur in secondary AML following exposure to topoisomerase II inhibitors and in infants with AML.

The above chromosomal abnormalities can be applied to MRD detection by RT-PCR. The clinical utility remains to be proven, however. For ALL cases with a specific DNA motif, studies of MRD detection have concentrated on detecting specific PCR targets that include rearrangements of the *IgH* and *TCRγ* genes, kappa deletion rearrangements, and *TAL*-1 gene deletion.

40.7 Infrequent gigantic MNCs on aspirate smears and/or lymphohistiocytic infiltrate on biopsy sections

On aspirate smears or touch imprints, the finding of scattered single enormous mononuclear cells detectable at scanning magnification can indicate Hodgkin's disease, anaplastic large cell lymphoma (ALCL), and poorly differentiated non-hematopoietic tumors. On the biopsy, the finding of a lymphohistiocytic infiltrate raises the differential diagnosis between Hodgkin's disease, NHL and, possibly, a reactive process (so-called 'abnormal immune response'). A thorough immunophenotypic and molecular genetic work-up will help to distinguish between reactive lymphohistiocytic infiltrates and a malignant lymphoma. Most of the NHLs with a prominent lymphohistiocytic infiltrate are high-grade lymphomas (see Section 40.5.2.5).

Enormous MNCs may be mistaken for small megakaryocytes. A high nuclear/cytoplasmic ratio, sharp nuclear indentations, lack of fine purple cytoplasmic granules, and a more 'open' nuclear chromatin are helpful clues to distinguish giant neoplastic MNCs (especially Reed-Sternberg/Hodgkin's cells) from megakaryocytes (Figure 40.51). The morphology on the accompanying biopsy, FCM immunophenotyping, and/or paraffin immunostaining results can provide additional clues to identify the correct disorder. In the absence of specific features, a presumptive diagnosis can be made from the clinical history and/or the original diagnostic lymph node biopsy.

The morphologic distinction between Hodgkin's disease and ALCL can be difficult. Both diseases can demonstrate: (1) scattered enormous cells (mononuclear to multinucleated) on aspirate smears; and/or (2) a lymphohistiocytic infiltrate with large binucleated or multinucleated cells and associated fibrosis on biopsy sections. Lack of clinical information or an inappropriately small immunostaining panel can easily lead to misinterpretation.

40.7.1 Hodgkin's disease

Bone marrow involvement in Hodgkin's disease is often focal. For this reason, bilateral bone marrow biopsies have been traditionally advocated as a staging procedure. In addition, multiple levels of the biopsy should be examined to ensure the detection of any bone marrow involvement.

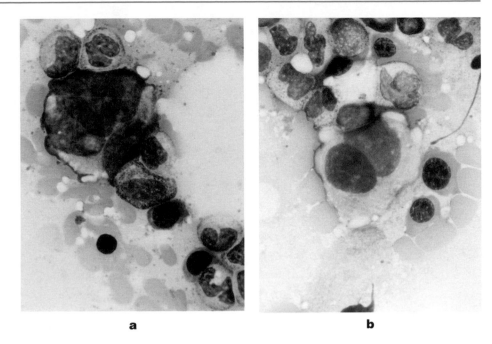

a   b

Figure 40.51 (a), (b) Occasional enormous neoplastic cells on the bone marrow aspirate smear from a case of Hodgkin's disease. One of the cells has the binucleated appearance of a Reed-Sternberg cell (b)

The required criterion for an initial diagnosis of Hodgkin's disease is the presence of typical Reed-Sternberg cells in a reactive background composed of lymphocytes, histiocytes, plasma cells and eosinophils. Because of increased reticulin fibrosis and fibroblastic proliferation, Reed-Sternberg cells are infrequent in bone marrow aspirates. The most characteristic feature of Reed-Sternberg cells on well-prepared H&E sections is the huge central eosinophilic nucleolus, with a diameter approximating at least half of that of the nucleus (Figure 40.52a). Variants of Reed-Sternberg cells may not demonstrate these nuclear characteristics. In LCL (including ALCL), the prominent nucleoli of 'Reed-Sternberg-like' cells rarely achieve the large size and degree of eosinophilia present in true Reed-Sternberg cells.

In some cases, the cellular background of focal lesions in Hodgkin's disease consists mostly of lymphocytes, masking the neoplastic cells (Figure 40.53). This may lead to misinterpretation as either low-grade NHL or benign lymphoid aggregates. Lesions with abundant histiocytes may be overlooked as granulomata.

In previously documented Hodgkin's disease, the requirements for bone marrow involvement are less stringent. The finding of mononuclear variants (i.e. Hodgkin's cells) within the appropriate reactive background is considered sufficient. Note that the morphologic subclassification of Hodgkin's disease is based on the lymph node biopsy and not on the bone marrow morphology.

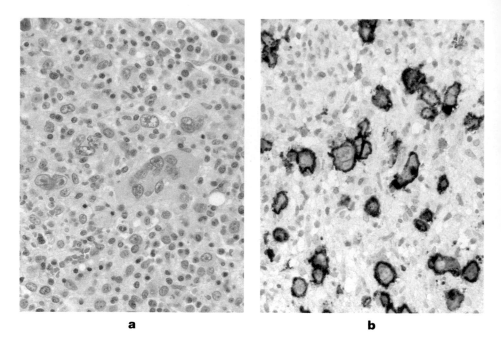

a   b

Figure 40.52 Diffuse bone marrow involvement by Hodgkin's disease in a young Mexican male. (a) Abundant Reed-Sternberg/Hodgkin's cells. (b) Strong CD30 positivity

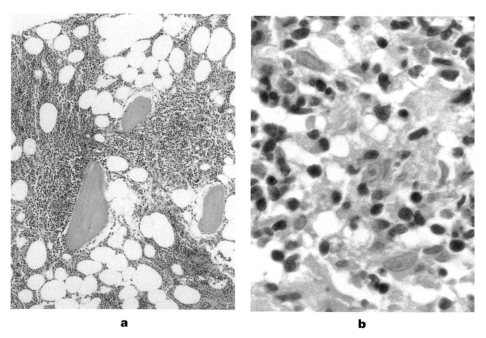

a   b

Figure 40.53 Focal involvement by Hodgkin's disease in a 33-year-old male. (a) The neoplastic foci contain a high number of small lymphoid cells obscuring the few Reed-Sternberg/Hodgkin's cells. This case was initially misinterpreted as low-grade lymphoma. Furthermore, an erroneous clinical history of FCC lymphoma was given on the request form. The correct diagnosis was made after re-review of the lymph node and bone marrow. (b) An occasional mononuclear Reed-Sternberg cell is visible with a prominent eosinophilic nucleolus (100× oil objective). Staining for CD30 was positive (not shown)

The detection of Reed-Sternberg/Hodgkin's cells is made easier with appropriate immunostaining on the biopsy. This is most helpful when the diagnostic cells are rare or scattered interstitially among normal hematopoietic elements. The battery of immunostains should include sufficient markers to exclude other diagnostic possibilities (e.g. ALCL), especially if the marrow was not submitted for FCM immunophenotyping. Since CD15 can be positive in a small number of $CD30^+$ non-Hodgkin's lymphomas, these two markers alone are insufficient to establish the diagnosis. An appropriate panel of immunostains should include at least LCA (CD45), L26 (CD20c), CD3, UCHL-1 (CD45RO), CD30, Leu-M1 (CD15), ALK-1, and EMA (epithelial membrane antigen).

The expected staining profile in the usual case of mixed cellularity or syncytial Hodgkin's disease is LCA^-, EMA^-, $L26^-$, $UCHL-1^-$, $ALK-1^-$, $CD30^+$ (Figure 40.52b), and $CD15^+$. The assessment of LCA negativity can be difficult because the surrounding small lymphoid cells are LCA^+. In many instances, the neoplastic cells are positive for CD30 but negative for CD15. The combination of $CD30^+/CD15^+$ or $CD30^+/CD15^-$ in the absence of LCA, EMA and all other lymphoid-associated markers is confirmatory for Hodgkin's disease. UCHL-1 and CD43 react with most ALCLs, but not Hodgkin's disease.

In patients with a history of Hodgkin's disease, the uninvolved marrow frequently demonstrates one or more of the following nonspecific changes: eosinophilia, hypercellularity with increased myeloid and/or erythroid precursors, and epithelioid granulomata. The hyperplastic marrow can simulate the picture of an MPD.

40.7.2 Anaplastic large cell lymphoma (CD30$^+$ LCL)

Anaplastic large cell lymphoma initially referred to LCL with CD30 expression and prominent sinusoidal involvement mimicking the pattern of metastatic carcinoma. The lymph node morphology is highly variable. On H&E sections, the tumor can be: (1) monomorphous, composed of large cells with abundant amphophilic cytoplasm (similar to LCL with plasmacytoid differentiation); or (2) heterogeneous, composed of large cells with multilobed or horseshoe-shaped nuclei, and frequent binucleated or multinucleated cells simulating Reed-Sternberg cells (Figure 40.54). The majority of $CD30^+$ ALCLs are of the monomorphous type (Figure 40.55). Therefore, the term 'anaplastic' is not always appropriate.

Over time, many authors have used the term ALCL to include any histologic subtype of NHL containing $CD30^+$ large cells, such as the LCL in AIDS patients, localized $CD30^+$ cutaneous lymphoma (an indolent disease), and NHL with a predominant reactive component (lymphocytes or histiocytes). This has resulted in a plethora of morphologic variants such as 'histiocyte-rich', 'sarcomatoid', 'Hodgkin's-related', 'small cell predominant', thereby rendering the diagnosis of ALCL less clearly defined.

Since CD30 is an activation marker and therefore relatively nonspecific, it is of limited usefulness in differential diagnosis. In addition to ALCL and Hodgkin's disease, CD30 expression can be found in transformed benign lymphoid cells in IM and in the transformation phase of MF/Sezary syndrome.

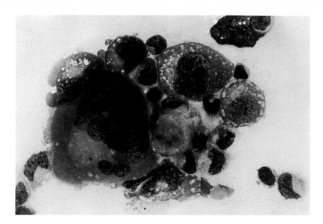

Figure 40.54 Anaplastic large cell lymphoma: an occasional tumor cell is enormous and multinucleated. By FCM immunophenotyping, the neoplastic cells demonstrated an aberrant T-cell phenotype (loss of surface CD3). Cytoplasmic CD3 was positive

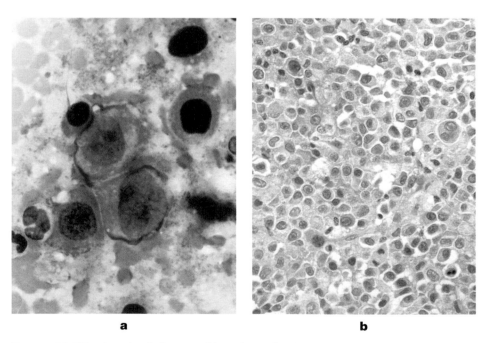

a   b

Figure 40.55 Anaplastic large cell lymphoma in a 16-year-old patient. (a) Plasmacytoid-appearing neoplastic cells on bone marrow imprints. (b) Diffuse infiltration by a relatively monomorphous population of tumor cells. An occasional cell is binucleated. The lymph node biopsy in this patient demonstrated a sinusoidal pattern of infiltration, and positive staining for CD30, EMA and ALK-1. Immunostaining with L26, polyclonal CD3 and LCA was negative

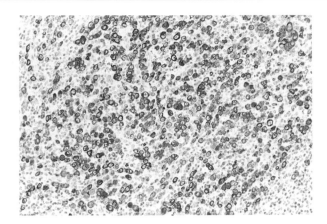

Figure 40.56 Immunostaining with ALK-1 antibody, showing diffuse involvement by anaplastic large cell lymphoma. The tumor cells are relatively monomorphous

The identification of t(2;5)(p23;q35) should help in redefining ALCL as a clinicopathological entity. Neither CD30 expression nor pleomorphic cytology predicts the presence of t(2;5). The translocation fuses the nucleophosmin gene (*NPM*) on chromosome 5 to the anaplastic lymphoma kinase gene (*ALK*) on chromosome 2, resulting in an *NPM-ALK* transcript detectable by RT-PCR and a protein detectable with the ALK-1 antibody (Figure 40.56). The majority of t(2;5) CD30$^+$ lymphomas are T-cell lymphomas which infrequently infiltrate the marrow.

It is important to apply a multiparameter approach to the diagnosis of ALCL to avoid misinterpreting ALCL as Hodgkin's disease or vice versa. An aberrant mature T-cell phenotype by FCM, when present, distinguishes ALCL with t(2;5) from Hodgkin's disease. Alternatively, immunostaining on paraffin-embedded tissue using the above recommended minimum battery of immunostains is helpful. UCHL-1 and CD43 react with most cases of ALCL but not with Hodgkin's

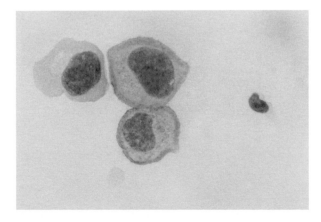

Figure 40.57 EMA reactivity in anaplastic large cell lymphoma (same patient as in Figure 40.54). Positive staining is seen in most of the tumor cells

disease. Since rare cases of ALCL may lack CD45 and other lymphoid markers, the most reliable markers to separate the two disorders are EMA reactivity (Figure 40.57) and evidence of t(2;5) by either immunohistochemistry (ALK-1), molecular analysis or cytogenetics.

CHAPTER 41

Foreign cell infiltration pattern

Involvement of the bone marrow by nonhematopoietic malignancies is much easier to recognize and diagnose than the classification of hematological disorders. A few pitfalls need to be avoided, however, especially when the metastasis is a poorly differentiated carcinoma or a non-epithelial tumor, since these can simulate the morphology of large cell hematopoietic malignancies. Rarely, patients with widespread nonhematopoietic malignancies present with a small number of circulating malignant cells (Figure 5.46), which can easily be mistaken for blasts, Burkitt's cells or large lymphoma cells.

When the bone marrow is aspirated with a strong vacuum force, it is nearly always possible to free metastatic tumor cells into the aspirate unless the tumor is embedded in sclerotic stroma. Since the tumor infiltration may be focal and the aspiration unsuccessful, it is important to obtain a satisfactory core biopsy and make routine touch preparations from the biopsy.

The most common metastatic solid tumors in the bone marrow include neuroblastoma in young children, and breast, lung and prostate carcinomas in adults. Other tumors, such as low-grade neuroendocrine tumors, renal cell carcinoma, melanoma, germ cell tumor, retinoblastoma, Ewing's sarcoma and rhabdomyosarcoma, have a lower propensity to spread to the bone marrow. Metastatic spindle cell sarcoma in the bone marrow is an extremely rare event. Immunostaining with appropriate markers can be performed on the biopsy if the location of the primary tumor is unknown, no clinical information is available, or when the diagnostic specimen is not available for review.

41.1 The morphology of metastatic tumors on aspirate smears

The distribution of metastatic tumor cells on bone marrow films depends on the cohesiveness of the tumor, and varies with the technique of spreading the bone marrow (see Section 32.5.2). On 'pull' preparations, metastatic clusters scatter toward the edges of the slide, around the periphery of the area where the particles are concentrated. On 'push' preparations, the tumor clumps are in the vicinity of individual spicules, at the feather-edge of the film.

In the bone marrow, metastatic carcinomas often form three-dimensional clusters. In many cases, the individual tumor cells are larger than any hematopoietic cells (except megakaryocytes). Glandular formation, nuclear molding, and/or sharp nuclear indentations may be present.

**Professor Belmonte
Case 96**

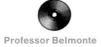

Note that in the rare cases of metastatic low-grade endocrine tumor, the tumor cells are bland-appearing without nuclear molding or indentations, and often form 'two-dimensional' clusters rather than piling up on each other.

In poorly differentiated carcinomas or small round cell tumors, the neoplastic cells are less cohesive and therefore manifest as single cells. Several morphologic features in such cases can cause confusion with malignant lymphoma and leukemia:

- The cell size may fall within the range of that seen in hematological malignancies.
- The tumor cells may have a high nuclear/cytoplasmic ratio and fine nuclear chromatin reminiscent of ALL.
- Deep basophilia and sharp cytoplasmic vacuoles mimicking Burkitt's cells may be present.
- If the tumor cells have ample cytoplasm with eccentric nuclei or cytoplasmic vacuoles, it may lead to a misinterpretation of plasmablasts, malignant monocytes, or LCL with plasmacytoid differentiation.

The first two features are mainly seen in neuroblastoma and small cell carcinoma of the lung (Figure 41.1), the two most common small round cell tumors involving the bone marrow. In these diseases, the aspirate smears in most instances demonstrate sheets of mononuclear cells. With a careful search, however, typical clumps of tumor cells with overlapping nuclei and nuclear molding are invariably present. Rosette formation may be evident. Involvement by

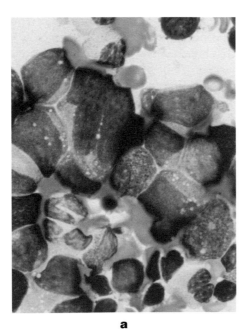 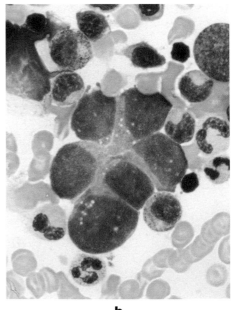

a   b

Figure 41.1 Neuroblastoma in a 2-year-old child. (a) Individual neoplastic cells with dispersed nuclear chromatin and cytoplasmic vacuoles. (b) A cluster of tumor cells with nuclear molding

retinoblastoma or medulloblastoma yields a similar morphology. The last two features in the list can be present in metastatic melanoma, rhabdomyosarcoma, renal carcinoma and some germ cell tumors (Figure 41.2). Granules of pigment, if present, are a helpful feature to identify melanoma cells. The detection of single metastatic tumor cells can be difficult in cases with low involvement.

41.2 The morphology of metastatic tumor on biopsy sections

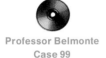

Professor Belmonte
Case 99

Tumor involvement on biopsy sections is obvious in the great majority of cases. Epithelial tumors appear as sheets and clusters, often with abortive glandular formation or occasional cytoplasmic vacuoles. They are accompanied by a variable degree of stromal reaction, including collagen fibrosis and new bone formation (Figure 41.3). Tumor necrosis may be present. The sclerotic process is particularly pronounced with breast or prostatic carcinoma. Occasional cases may mimic the appearance of AMM, with scattered strands of tumor cells and individual cells (which may be overlooked) entrapped in dense fibrosis. Immunostaining with a keratin cocktail will facilitate the identification of the neoplastic cells.

The stromal reaction is less intense in metastatic small round cell tumors of neuroendocrine origin. The extensive diffuse infiltrate closely simulates that of an acute leukemia, especially ALL. The finely stippled nuclear chromatin and the pattern of the crush artifacts (if present) are also similar to those associated with

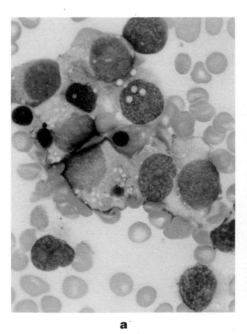
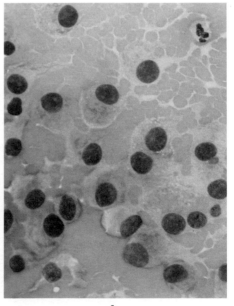

a   b

Figure 41.2 Metastatic tumors with plasmacytoid cytology in melanoma (a) and pheochromocytoma (b). Note the darkly stained melanin granules in some of the melanoma cells

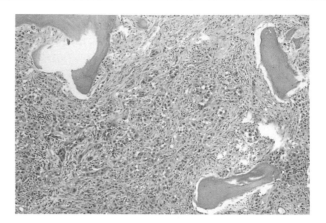

Figure 41.3   Metastatic adenocarcinoma with extensive collagen fibrosis

ALL. The tendencies for compact cluster formation (i.e. an organoid pattern, best appreciated at low power) and/or rosette formation are clues that the infiltrate is not of hematopoietic origin, however (Figure 41.4). Dot positivity with keratin immunostaining is a pathognomonic feature for small cell carcinoma of the lung. Perivascular pseudorosettes and PAS-positive vacuoles are typical findings in Ewing's sarcoma.

In addition to keratin, a battery of special stains is helpful in the classification of metastatic tumors on biopsy sections, especially if the primary site is unknown. The procedure is also useful for those rare cases with minimal involvement, in which the metastatic tumor cells may escape visual detection on routine H&E sections. Prostatic specific antigen and prostatic acid phosphatase are valuable in the detection of prostate carcinoma. HMB45 and S-100 can be used to detect malignant melanoma. Carcinoid tumors can be picked up with a chromogranin reaction. Neuron-specific enolase and vimentin are of limited diagnostic value because of low specificity. There exist no good antibodies to identify rhabdomyosarcoma. Myosin and myoglobin occur late in the differentiation of muscle cells and are not present in most embryonal rhabdomyosarcomas.

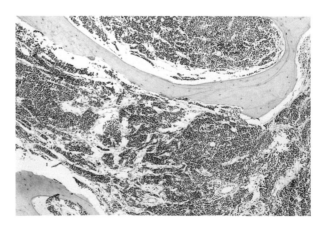

Figure 41.4   Organoid pattern in a metastatic retinoblastoma

41.2.1 Sarcomas involving the bone marrow

Spindle cell sarcomas are composed of more differentiated neoplastic elements than their round cell counterparts. With the exception of rhabdomyosarcoma and Kaposi's sarcoma, they rarely metastasize to the bone marrow.

Embryonal and alveolar rhabdomyosarcoma are composed mostly of undifferentiated round cells with no obvious muscle differentiation at the light microscopic level. On air-dried preparations, the tumor cells can exhibit a Burkitt's-like morphology or a plasmacytoid appearance. Follow-up bone marrow biopsies in a small round rhabdomyosarcoma can demonstrate more mature neoplastic muscle cells. Large polygonal cells with ample eosinophilic cytoplasm containing whorls of fibrils and strap cells with cross striations can be present (Figure 41.5). This most likely reflects a maturing effect secondary to chemotherapy.

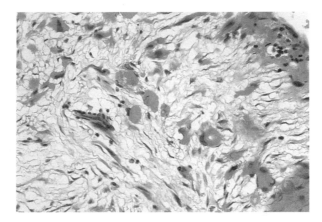

Figure 41.5 Scattered strap cells and polygonal rhabdomyoblasts in a follow-up bone marrow biopsy for metastatic rhabdomyosarcoma. In the initial diagnostic bone marrow biopsy (3 months earlier), the neoplastic population was composed of small round cells with no evidence of differentiation by light microscopy

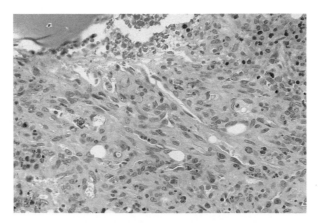

Figure 41.6 Kaposi's sarcoma in the bone marrow of an HIV-positive patient

Kaposi's sarcoma (KS) is a rare example of a spindle cell tumor that can spread to the bone marrow (Figure 41.6). Affected patients have advanced AIDS or widespread KS. The bone marrow diagnosis can be made based on the pathognomonic appearance of extensive involvement by spindle cells associated with slit-like spaces containing extravasated RBCs.

Granulomata/histiocytic proliferation pattern

The histiocytic-monocytic system has been traditionally divided into two major populations: monocytes/phagocytes (antigen-processing cells) and dendritic (antigen-presenting) cells. Results from *in vitro* studies on precursors cells obtained from bone marrow, cord blood and peripheral blood suggest that both of these subsets originate from a common intermediate precursor (CD14$^+$ and HLA-DR$^+$). Differentiation towards dendritic cells or monocytes/phago-cytes is influenced by microenvironmental factors including cytokines. Stimula-tion by GM-CSF, tumor necrosis factor-α, stem cell factor and IL-4 leads towards maturation into dendritic cells with acquisition of CD1a and co-stimu-latory molecules (CD40, CD60, CD86), and down-regulation of CD14. The presence of monocyte-CSF induces development into monocytes.

Antigen-processing cells (i.e. phagocytes) are characterized by abundant lyso-somal enzymes, which account for diffuse NSE positivity on air-dried prepara-tions and, both lysozyme and α-antitrypsin on fixed tissue. This group includes monocytes, macrophages, epithelioid histiocytes and multinucleated giant cells. Macrophages are large cells with a small central nucleus and inconspicuous nucleoli. Although difficult to recognize on bone marrow biopsies, macrophages are easily found on aspirates, concentrated within the spicules.

The phenotypic profile of phagocytic cells is not specific. The surface antigens expressed on these cells include CD4, CD11b, CD13 and CD33, CD14, CD25, and CD45. The intensity of CD4 and CD45 on phagocytes/monocytes is weaker than that on T cells.

Dendritic cells are involved in T-cell-mediated responses. The soluble antigen taken up by the dendritic cells is processed into immunogenic molecules and presented to T cells in association with HLA-DR and the co-stimulatory mole-cules necessary for T-cell stimulation and proliferation. Antigen uptake and pro-cessing are mainly performed by Langerhans' cells (the dendritic cells of the skin), whereas antigen presentation and T-cell stimulation are the responsibility of inter-digitating reticulum cells in lymph nodes.

Dendritic cells have abundant cytoplasm, round to folded nuclei, and are nor-mally not detectable in the bone marrow. They differ from monocytes/phagocytes phenotypically by the absence of CD11b, CD14 and CD68. CD45 and CD4 are expressed. Because of the small content of lysosomal enzymes, lysozyme and α-antitrypsin are absent. Similarly, NSE activity is absent or only focally detectable in the Golgi area. S-100 positivity facilitates the identification of these cells on tissue sections.

The subtle morphologic and phenotypic differences between interdigitating reticulum cells and Langerhans' cells mirror their functional differences. Co-sti-mulatory molecules are well expressed in interdigitating reticulum cells whereas

Birbeck granules (ultrastructural racquet-shaped organelles of unknown function) and the expression of CD1 are characteristic of Langerhans' cells.

Histiocytic/monocytic proliferations in the bone marrow mainly involve the monocyte/phagocyte subset. Apart from AML with monocytic differentiation and CMMoL, most of the histiocytic disorders are constitutional or reactive. Langerhans' cell histiocytosis involvement of the bone marrow is a rare occurrence.

42.1 Granulomata

Granulomata are aggregates of epithelioid histiocytes (Figure 42.1) that may be accompanied by multinucleated giant cells and/or a variable number of lymphocytes, plasma cells and eosinophils. A variety of foreign substances and infectious pathogens can induce granuloma formation. The most common conditions in which granulomata are found in the bone marrow include mycobacterial infection, infestation by fungal organisms and some unusual organisms (e.g. those causing leprosy, brucellosis), drug reactions, sarcoidosis, Hodgkin's disease and, less commonly, NHL. The diagnosis of sarcoidosis is primarily a clinical one.

In bone marrows involved with granulomata, the surrounding hematopoietic elements may demonstrate reactive changes such as increased erythroid precursors, eosinophilia or left-shifted myeloid maturation. The granulomata can appear tight and well defined with few inflammatory elements such as in sarcoidosis, or small and poorly defined. Poorly formed granulomata may be overlooked if only one level of the biopsy is examined.

Because of an associated increase in reticulin fibers, granulomata are rarely found on aspirate smears. If the granulomata are loosely formed, as in leishmaniasis, the aspirate may contain scattered histiocytes filled with intracellular organisms.

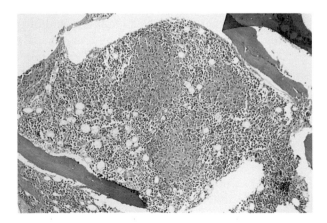

Figure 42.1   Granulomata in an HIV-positive patient

In Hodgkin's disease, the finding of sarcoid-like granulomata in the bone marrow may represent a host response and does not necessarily imply infiltration by Hodgkin's disease. Epithelioid clusters associated with T-NHL are more common in lymph nodes than in the bone marrow (Figure 40.45).

The routine work-up for bone marrow granulomata should include microbiological cultures of the aspirates in addition to the Ziehl-Nielsen and Gomori methenamine silver stains on the biopsy sections to detect acid-fast bacilli (AFB) and fungal organisms (Figure 42.2). Granulomata filled with organisms occur mainly in opportunistic infections in the context of severe immunosuppression.

42.2 Infectious granulomata and other bone marrow manifestations in AIDS

The diagnosis of AIDS is based on laboratory parameters, namely a positive HIV and a decreased number of T-helper cells (CD4$^+$ lymphocyte count < 200/μl), irrespective of the clinical symptomatology. Progressive cytopenias develop during the course of the disease.

The bone marrow manifestations in HIV-positive patients are extremely diverse, reflecting the complex effects of impaired immunity, infection and multi-

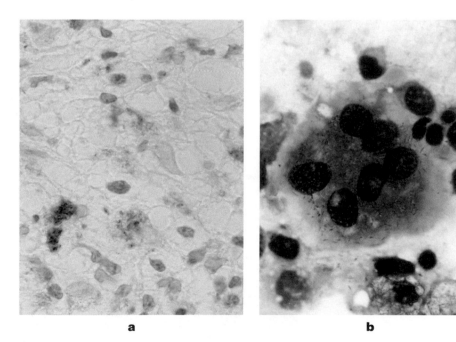

a   b

Figure 42.2 Bone marrow biopsy and aspirate from an HIV-positive patient. (a) Ziehl-Nielsen stain, showing numerous acid-fast bacilli (Mycobacterium avium intracellulare). (b) The organisms are visible on the aspirate smear inside the multinucleated giant cell

drug therapy. The main findings include granulomata, high-grade lymphoid malignancies, and a wide range of nonspecific abnormalities affecting both bone marrow stroma and hematopoietic elements.

The granulomata in the bone marrow of HIV patients are often ill-defined and loosely formed. Large confluent granulomata may be misinterpreted as 'histiocytic hyperplasia'. The principal organisms encountered in AIDS-associated granulomata include *Mycobacterium avium intracellulare* (MAI), *Leishmania donovani* and a variety of fungal organisms.

In contrast to the scarcity of bacilli in tuberculous granulomata, the granulomata in MAI infection are usually overladen with bacilli (Figure 42.2). This facilitates their identification (even at low-power magnification) on sections stained for AFB. In rare instances, the organisms can be seen in abundance on the air-dried preparations as azurophilic bacilli.

On air-dried preparations, *Leishmania donovani* (Figure 42.3) can be distinguished from *Histoplasma capsulatum* by the presence of a tiny kinetoplast, and the absence of any reaction to the Gomori silver stain which highlights the spores in histoplasmosis.

Candida, Histoplasma capsulatum, Cryptococcus neoformans, and *Pneumocystis carinii* are the typical fungal organisms found in AIDS (Figure 42.4). The development of effective prophylactic antibiotics and antifungal agents in recent years has markedly decreased the frequency of the above infections, however. The improved survival in AIDS is accompanied by a steady increase in the incidence

Professor Belmonte
Case 100

Professor Belmonte
Case 101

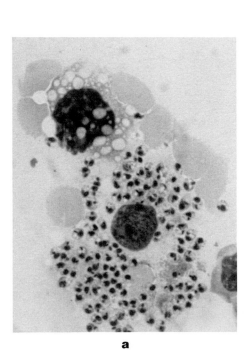
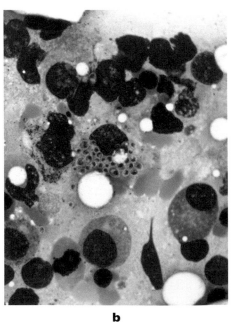

a
b

Figure 42.3 Bone marrow aspirates from two different HIV-positive patients. (a) A macrophage laden with Leishmania organisms. (b) A histiocyte laden with Histoplasma organisms

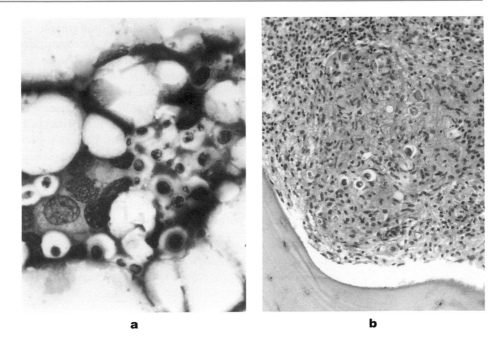

a   b

Figure 42.4 Bone marrow specimens from two different HIV-positive patients. (a) Intracellular and extracellular Cryptococcus organisms on the aspirate smear. (b) Granuloma with Coccidioides organisms: this patient lived in Arizona (USA), where this organism is endemic

of high-grade NHL, mainly Burkitt's lymphoma-leukemia (Figure 40.23) and large cell lymphoma with plasmacytoid differentiation (Figure 40.21).

Apart from specific involvement by infectious granulomata or lymphoid malignancies, the bone marrow morphology in HIV patients is somewhat nonspecific, consisting of one or more features of stromal injury, ineffective hematopoiesis, reaction to chronic viral infection and drug effects. The bone marrow ranges from hypocellular to hypercellular, with several of the following features:

- Stromal abnormalities, such as serous fat atrophy (Figure 34.3b), reticulin fibrosis and macrophages with hemophagocytosis (Figure 33.5a).
- Mild to moderate plasmacytosis and/or lymphoid aggregates. If the aggregates are large and contain transformed lymphoid cells, they may be confused morphologically with a malignant lymphoid infiltrate.
- Megakaryocytic abnormalities, including an ITP picture with increased megakaryocytes and peripheral thrombocytopenia. In many patients the number of megakaryocytes is either normal or decreased, however. The megakaryocytes are often small with nuclear hypolobulation. The abnormal morphology and deficient production of platelets are most likely related to the actual infection of megakaryocytes by HIV.
- Increased iron stores but decreased iron incorporation; a pattern similar to that seen in anemia of chronic disease.

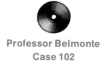

Professor Belmonte
Case 102

• Quantitative and qualitative abnormalities in erythroid and myeloid elements resulting from the combined effects of HIV infection, drug therapy and any concomitant infections. The bone marrow M:E ratio varies from decreased to markedly increased. In cases with an increased myeloid component, a variable degree of left-shifted maturation and 'dysplastic' features such as hypogranulation are found. The left shift, accompanied by large hypergranulated myeloid precursors, can be especially pronounced when concomitant G-CSF therapy is given to ameliorate the patient's peripheral neutropenia. In cases with erythroid preponderance or hyperplasia, 'dyserythropoietic' features such as nuclear/cytoplasmic asynchrony and binucleated or multinucleated erythroid cells are often present. In some HIV patients, the erythroid hyperplasia is compensatory to peripheral RBC destruction (e.g. oxidative hemolysis secondary to drug therapy).

Administration of antiretroviral agents of the nucleoside family (e.g. AZT, 3TC) and long-term administration of some antifungal and antiviral agents (e.g. amphotericin and gancyclovir) can induce myelosuppression. HIV patients also have increased susceptibility to parvovirus infection, resulting in profound red cell aplasia.

The peripheral cytopenias in HIV patients result from the combined effects of decreased production and shortened survival of the mature hematopoietic elements. The altered survival may be immune-mediated and associated with splenomegaly. The impaired hematopoiesis, secondary to depletion or inhibition of stem cells, may be due to infection of stem cells by HIV or dysregulated cytokine production and an altered bone marrow microenvironment. Hematopoiesis can also be altered by retroviral drug therapy or superimposed infection by CMV or hepatitis C.

42.3 Other types of phagocytic proliferations

In addition to granulomata, there are two broad groups of phagocytic proliferations: those seen in lysosomal storage diseases, and those associated with infection in patients with impaired immunity. In hereditary deficiencies of lysosomal enzymes responsible for glycolipid and glycoprotein degradation, the undegraded substrates accumulate in macrophages. Infections in patients with altered immunity often result in widespread hemophagocytosis.

42.3.1 Foamy histiocytes

The presence of abundant foamy histiocytes is not pathognomonic of Niemann-Pick disease (sphingomyelinase deficiency). A similar morphology can be seen in conditions with lipid overload such as prolonged total parenteral nutrition (Figure 42.5) and hypercholesterolemia. In Niemann-Pick disease (Figure 42.6), the biochemical structure of the excess lipids accounts for the reactivity of the foamy histiocytes with Sudan black B and birefringence when unstained smears are examined under polarized light.

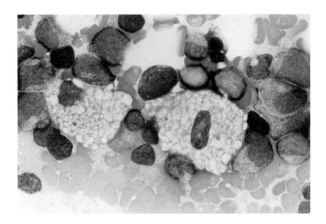

Figure 42.5 Two foamy histiocytes in a patient on prolonged total parenteral nutrition. The patient's bone marrow demonstrated numerous foamy histiocytes

42.3.2 Gaucher cells

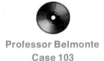

Professor Belmonte
Case 103

The identification of Gaucher cells is facilitated by the typical 'papier mâché' (wrinkled paper) appearance of their voluminous pale cytoplasm (Figure 42.7). This cytoplasmic appearance results from the accumulation of glucocerebroside in fibrils and rope-like deposits (secondary to glucocerebrosidase deficiency). Another morphologic characteristic of Gaucher cells is diastase-resistant PAS positivity. The accumulation of Gaucher cells in the bone marrow can be focal, interstitial or diffuse (Figure 42.8). Anemia and other cytopenias can result when a marked infiltrate of Gaucher cells, associated with reticulin fibrosis, is present.

Gaucher's disease is an autosomal recessive disorder resulting from mutations on both alleles of the glucocerebrosidase gene located on chromosome 1. The disease is clinically divided into three types, depending on the severity of the symptoms, especially the presence and progression of neurologic symptoms.

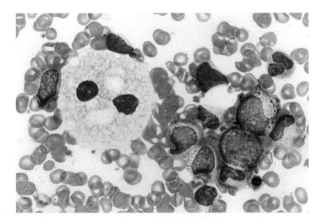

Figure 42.6 A binucleated foamy histiocyte in a child with Nieman-Pick disease

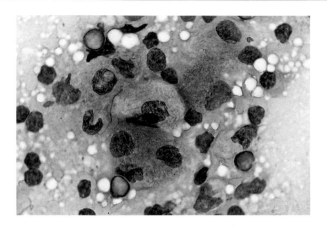

Figure 42.7 Gaucher cells: the appearance of the cytoplasm is reminiscent of wrinkled paper

The most common variant, prevalent among individuals of Ashkenazi Jewish descent, is type I Gaucher's disease. The affected patients may remain asymptomatic despite peripheral cytopenias and the disease may not be discovered until adulthood.

The determination of decreased activity of glucocerebrosidase by biochemical assay has been recommended for establishing a definitive diagnosis of Gaucher's disease. Alternatively, increased levels of the enzyme chitotriosidase can be considered as evidence of Gaucher's disease.

Sea-blue histiocytes, also referred to as Gaucher-like cells, should not be mistaken for true Gaucher cells, especially on biopsy sections. On aspirate smears the cytoplasm of sea-blue histiocytes has a waxy blue appearance (Figure 36.6). Scattered sea-blue histiocytes are a common finding in proliferative hematological disorders such as CML, multiple myeloma and hemolytic anemia. These cells are of no diagnostic significance.

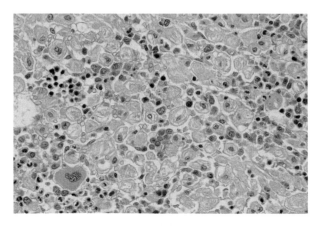

Figure 42.8 Diffuse bone marrow infiltration by Gaucher cells

42.3.3 Diffuse histiocytic proliferation with hemophagocytosis

Scattered histiocytes with evidence of hemophagocytosis are often encountered in the bone marrow in viral infections such as CMV, EBV and herpes virus (Figure 33.5). Diffuse histiocytic proliferations with hemophagocytosis are unusual, however, and are seen primarily in the context of impaired immunity, either acquired (e.g. post-transplant or an underlying lymphoid malignancy) or congenital, including familial hemophagocytic lymphohistiocytosis.

Diffuse bone marrow histiocytic proliferations cause a reduction of hematopoietic elements, resulting in peripheral cytopenias (Figure 42.9). Other organs such as the spleen (red pulp), liver (hepatic sinusoids), and lymph nodes are involved by the lymphohistiocytic proliferation. The histiocytes are morphologically benign, with abundant vacuolated cytoplasm containing phagocytized blood elements, especially RBCs. In some instances, the phagocytic activity may be subtle. Several stains, including NSE, lysozyme, and KP1 antibody, can confirm the phagocytic lineage of the cells (Figure 42.10).

Infection-associated hemophagocytic syndrome (IAHS) is an acute manifestation of severe infections in subjects with either congenital or acquired immunosuppression. Any infectious agent may induce IAHS. However, most cases are secondary to a severe viral infection. The syndrome manifests as dramatic hemophagocytosis and increased histiocytic proliferation in hematopoietic organs, resulting in hepatosplenomegaly and lymphadenopathy. Constitutional symptoms are common. The picture is indistinguishable from the intermittent manifestations of familial erythrophagocytic lymphohistiocytosis. In this rare congenital disorder, the episodes of hemophagocytosis are most likely precipitated by infections as well.

Familial hemophagocytic lymphohistiocytosis is a disorder of unknown etiology, which manifests primarily in neonates and infants. The disease presents with

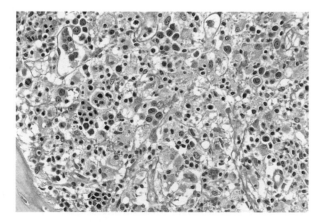

Figure 42.9 Familial hemophagocytic lymphohistiocytosis in a 14-month-old male, showing widespread histiocytic proliferation with erythrophagocytosis. The patient also had pancytopenia, hepatosplenomegaly and a reversed CD4:CD8 ratio (but no evidence of HIV infection)

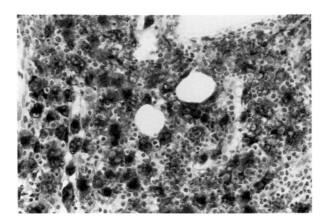

Figure 42.10 Immunostaining with KP1 antibody, highlighting the presence of abundant histiocytes in the bone marrow of the patient in Figure 42.9

hepatosplenomegaly and constitutional symptoms, such as fever and failure to thrive. The disorder is associated with numerous humoral and cellular immune defects including impaired natural killer activity, decreased T cell response to mitogens, and impaired IL-2 and interferon production. There is a close similarity between this disorder and the Chediak-Higashi syndrome.

The presence of hemophagocytosis or horseshoe-shaped nuclei in the various hemophagocytic syndromes should not be interpreted as evidence of malignant histiocytosis. If this disease exists, it is extremely rare. Before diagnosing malignant histiocytosis, other more common conditions should be excluded such as AML-M5, aggressive LGL leukemia and ALCL.

42.4 Proliferations of dendritic cells

Langerhans' cell histiocytosis (histiocytosis X) may rarely involve the bone marrow. The disease, which presents mainly in children and young adults, has been given multiple names depending on the organs involved and the resulting clinical manifestations. Multi-organ involvement correlates with severe disease and a poorer prognosis. The bony sites that may be involved include the skull, pelvis, tibia, scapulae, vertebrae, rib, and femur.

On bone marrow biopsies, the infiltration can be focal or diffuse, and is composed of bland-appearing histiocytes with ample cytoplasm, ill-defined cytoplasmic borders, and reniform nuclei with distinct nuclear grooves, admixed with a variable number of eosinophils (Figure 42.11). A similar cytology can be appreciated on air-dried preparations (Figure 42.12).

The definitive diagnosis rests on either the ultrastructural detection of Birbeck granules or S-100 positivity and the expression of CD1a. In contrast to normal Langerhans' cells, the cells of histiocytosis X express CD11c and CD14.

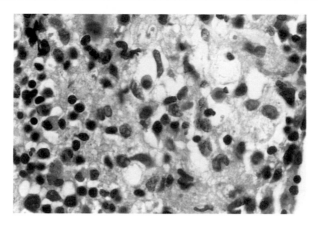

Figure 42.11 A subtle focus of Langerhans' cells on the bone marrow biopsy section (100 × oil objective)

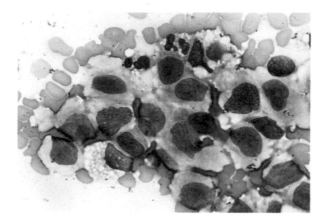

Figure 42.12 Bone marrow imprint from another case of Langerhans' cell histiocytosis. Note the deep nuclear groove in some of the cells

In some cases, the cells in histiocytosis X may assume a more spindly appearance. This should be differentiated from other cellular proliferations with spindle cell morphology, such as mast cell infiltration. The distinction can easily be achieved with a Giemsa stain on the biopsy or from the cytologic appearance on aspirates (see Section 40.3).

Suggested reading

Part One: Peripheral Blood

Bennett, J.M., Catovsky, D., Daniel, M.-T. *et al.* (1989). Proposals for the classification of chronic (mature) B and T lymphoid leukaemias. *J. Clin. Pathol.*, **42**, 567–584.

Bux, J., Behrens, G., Jaeger, G. and Welte, K. (1998). Diagnosis and clinical course of autoimmune neutropenia in infancy: analysis of 240 cases. *Blood*, **91**, 181–186.

Carmel R. (1995). Malabsorption of food cobalamin. *Bailliere's Haematol.*, **8**, 639–655.

Cazzola, M. and Ascari, E. (1986). Red cell ferritin as a diagnostic tool. *Br. J. Haematol.*, **62**, 209–213.

Diamandidou, E., Cohen, P.R. and Kurzrock, R. (1996). Mycosis fungoides and Sezary syndrome. *Blood,* **88**, 2385–2409.

Franchini, G. (1995). Molecular mechanisms of human T-cell leukemia/lymphotropic virus type I infection. *Blood*, **86**, 3619–3639.

George, J.N., Woolf, S.H., Raskob G.E. *et al.* (1996). Idiopathic thrombocytopenic purpura: a practice guideline developed by explicit methods for the American Society of Hematology. *Blood*, **88**, 3–40.

Guideline (1998). The laboratory diagnosis of haemoglobinopathies. *Br. J. Haematol.*, **101**, 783–792.

Hebbel, R.P. (1991). Beyond hemoglobin polymerization: the red blood cell membrane and sickle disease pathophysiology. *Blood*, **77**, 214–237.

Herbert, V. (1985). Megaloblastic anemias. *Lab. Invest.*, **52**, 3–18.

Lawrence, C., Fabry, M.E. and Nagel, R.L. (1991). The unique red cell heterogeneity of SC disease: crystal formation, dense reticulocytes, and unusual morphology. *Blood*, **78**, 2104–2112.

Means, R.T. Jr and Krantz, S.B. (1992). Progress in understanding the pathogenesis of the anemia of chronic disease. *Blood*, **80**, 1639–1647.

Moake, J.L. (1997). Studies on the pathophysiology of thrombotic thrombocytopenic purpura. *Sem. Hematol.*, **34**, 83–89.

Nguyen, D.T., Diamond, L.W., Priolet, G. and Sultan C. (1992). Expert system design in hematology diagnosis. *Meth. Inform. Med.*, **31**, 82–89.

Nguyen, D.T., Moskowitz, F.B. and Diamond, L.W. (1994). Potential diagnostic pitfalls caused by blood film artifacts in prolymphocytic leukaemia. Observations in two cases. *Br. J. Biomed. Sci.*, **51**, 371–374.

Nienhuis, A.W., Anagnou, N.P. and Ley, T.J. (1984). Advances in thalassemia research. *Blood*, **63**, 738–758.

NIH Conference (1982). The idiopathic hypereosinophilic syndrome. Clinical, pathophysiologic, and therapeutic considerations. *Ann. Int. Med.*, **87**, 78–92.

Pane, F., Frigeri, F., Sindona, M. *et al*. (1996). Neutrophilic-chronic myeloid leukemia: a distinct disease with a specific molecular marker (bcr/abl with C3/A2 junction). *Blood*, **88**, 2410–2414.

Rosse, W.F. and Ware, R.E. (1995). The molecular basis of paroxysmal nocturnal hemoglobinuria. *Blood*, **86**, 3277–3286.

Silvera, P., Cynober, T., Dhermy, D. *et al*. (1997). Red blood cell abnormalities in hereditary elliptocytosis and their relevance to variable clinical expression. *Am. J. Clin. Pathol*., **108**, 391–399.

Suzuki, A., Takahashi, T., Nakamura, K. *et al*. (1992). Thrombocytosis in patients with tumors producing colony-stimulating factor. *Blood*, **80**, 2052–2059.

Thein, S.L. (1992). Dominant β thalassaemia: molecular basis and pathophysiology. *Br. J. Haematol*., **80**, 273–277.

Thorley-Lawson, D.A. (1988). Basic virological aspects of Epstein-Barr virus infection. *Sem. Hematol*., **25**, 247–260.

Weatherall, D.J., Higgs, D.R. and Clegg, J.B. (1988). The molecular pathology of the α globin genes. *Br. J. Cancer*, **58** (Suppl. IX), 17–22.

Part Two: Flow Cytometry

Arnulf, B., Copie-Bergman, C., Delfau-Larue, M.-H. *et al*. (1998). Nonhepatosplenic γd T-cell lymphoma: a subset of cytotoxic lymphomas with mucosal or skin localization. *Blood*, **91**, 1723–1731.

Barlogie, B., Alexanian, R., Dixon, D. *et al*. (1985). Prognostic implications of tumor cell DNA and RNA content in multiple myeloma. *Blood*, **66**, 338–341.

Borowitz, M.J., Bray, R., Gascoyne, R. *et al*. (1997). U.S.–Canadian consensus recommendations on the immunophenotypic analysis of hematologic neoplasia by flow cytometry: data analysis and interpretation. *Cytometry (Commun. Clin. Cytometry)*, **30**, 236–244.

Bouroncle, B.A. (1994). Thirty-five years in the progress of hairy cell leukemia. *Leukemia Lymphoma*, **14** (Suppl. 1), 1–12.

Braylan, R.C. (1993). Lymphomas. In *Clinical Flow Cytometry. Principles and Application*. (Bauer, K.D., Duque, R.E. and Shankey, T.V., eds), pp. 203–234. Williams & Wilkins.

Braylan, R.C., Atwater, S.K., Diamond, L.W. *et al*. (1997). U.S.–Canadian consensus recommendations on the immunophenotypic analysis of hematologic neoplasia by flow cytometry: data reporting. *Cytometry (Commun. Clin. Cytometry)*, **30**, 245–248.

Cheson, B.D., Bennett, J.M., Grever, M. *et al*. (1996). National Cancer Institute-sponsored working group guidelines for chronic lymphocytic leukemia: revised guidelines for diagnosis and treatment. *Blood*, **87**, 4990–4997.

Christensson, B., Lindemalm, C., Johansson B. *et al*. (1989). Flow cytometric DNA analysis: a prognostic tool in non-Hodgkin's lymphoma. *Leuk. Res*., **13**, 307–314.

Davis, B.H., Foucar, K., Szczarkowski, W. *et al*. (1997). U.S.–Canadian consensus recommendations on the immunophenotypic analysis of hematologic neoplasia by flow cytometry: medical indications. *Cytometry (Commun. Clin. Cytometry)*, **30**, 249–263.

Diamond, L.W., Bearman, R.M., Berry, P.K. *et al.* (1980). Prolymphocytic leukemia: flow microfluorometric, immunologic, and cytogenetic observations. *Am. J. Hematol.*, **9**, 319–330.

Diamond, L.W., Nguyen, D.T., Andreeff, M. *et al.* (1994). A knowledge-based system for the interpretation of flow cytometry data in leukemias and lymphomas. *Cytometry*, **17**, 266–273.

Duque, R.E., Andreeff, M., Braylan, R.C. *et al.* (1993). Consensus review of the clinical utility of DNA flow cytometry in neoplastic hematopathology. *Cytometry*, **14**, 492–496.

Dworzak, M.N., Fritsch, G., Fleischer, C. *et al.* (1997). Multiparameter phenotype mapping of normal and post-chemotherapy B lymphopoiesis in pediatric bone marrow. *Leukemia*, **11**, 1266–1273.

Harada, H., Kawano, M.M., Huang, N. *et al.* (1993). Phenotypic difference of normal plasma cells from mature myeloma cells. *Blood*, **81**, 2658–2663.

Jaffe, E. S., Chan, J.K.C., Su, I.-J. *et al.* (1996). Report of the workshop on nasal and related extranodal angiocentric T/natural killer cell lymphomas. Definitions, differential diagnosis, and epidemiology. *Am. J. Surg. Pathol.*, **20**, 103–111.

Janossy, G., Coustan-Smith, E. and Campana, D. (1989). The reliability of cytoplasmic CD3 and CD22 antigen expression in the immunodiagnosis of acute leukemia: a study of 500 cases. *Leukemia*, **3**, 170–181.

Koehler, M., Behm, F.G., Shuster, J. *et al.* (1993). Transitional pre-B-cell acute lymphoblastic leukemia of childhood is associated with favorable prognostic clinical features and an excellent outcome: a Pediatric Oncology Group study. *Leukemia*, **7**, 2064–2068.

Koike, T. (1984). Megakaryoblastic leukemia: the characterization and identification of megakaryoblasts. *Blood*, **64**, 683–692.

Leclercq, G. and Plum, J. (1996). Thymic and extrathymic T cell development. *Leukemia*, **10**, 1853–1859.

Look, A.T., Roberson, P.K., Williams, D.L. *et al.* (1985). Prognostic importance of blast cell DNA content in childhood acute lymphoblastic leukemia. *Blood*, **65**, 1079–1086.

Loughran, T.P. Jr (1993). Clonal diseases of large granular lymphocytes. *Blood*, **82**, 1–14.

Macon, W.R., Williams, M.E., Greer, J.P. *et al.* (1996). Natural killer-like T-cell lymphomas: aggressive lymphomas of T large granular lymphocytes. *Blood*, **87**, 1474–1483.

Pinto, A., Gattei, V., Soligo, D. *et al.* (1994). New molecules burst at the leukocyte surface. A comprehensive review based on the 5th International Workshop on Leukocyte Differentiation Antigens, Boston, USA 3–7 November 1993. *Leukemia*, **8**, 347–358.

Robertson, M.J. and Ritz, J. (1990). Biology and clinical relevance of human natural killer cells. *Blood*, **76**, 2421–2438.

San Miguel, J.F., Martinez, A., Macedo, A. *et al.* (1997). Immunophenotyping investigation of minimal residual disease is a useful approach for predicting relapse in acute myeloid leukemia patients. *Blood*, **90**, 2465–2470.

Smets, L.A., Homan-Blok, J., Hart, A. *et al.* (1987). Prognostic implication of hyperdiploidy as based on DNA flow cytometric measurement in childhood acute lymphocytic leukemia – a multicenter study. *Leukemia*, **1**, 163–166.

Stelzer, G.T., Marti, G., Hurley, A. *et al.* (1997). U.S.–Canadian consensus recommendations on the immunophenotypic analysis of hematologic neoplasia by flow cytometry: standardization and validation of laboratory procedures. *Cytometry (Commun. Clin. Cytometry)*, **30**, 214–230.

Stewart, C.C., Behm, F.G., Carey, J.L. *et al.* (1997). U.S.–Canadian consensus recommendations on the immunophenotypic analysis of hematologic neoplasia by flow cytometry: selection of antibody combinations. *Cytometry (Commun. Clin. Cytometry)*, **30**, 231–235.

Part Three: Bone Marrow

Aerts, J.M.F.G., Boot, R.G., Renkema, G.H. *et al.* (1995). Molecular and biochemical abnormalities of Gaucher disease: chitotriosidase, a newly identified biochemical marker. *Sem. Hematol.*, **32**, 10–13.

Arnold, A. (1995). The cyclin D1/PRAD1 oncogene in human neoplasia. *J. Invest. Med.*, **43**, 543–549.

Bataille, R. (1997). New insights in the clinical biology of multiple myeloma. *Sem. Hematol.*, **34** (Suppl. 1), 23–28.

Bataille, R., Boccadoro, M., Klein, B. *et al.* (1992). C-reactive protein and β_2-microglobulin produce a simple and powerful myeloma staging system. *Blood*, **80**, 733–737.

Bennett, J.M., Catovsky, D., Daniel M.-T. *et al.* (1976). Proposals for the classification of the acute leukemias (FAB cooperative group). *Br. J. Haematol.*, **33**, 451–458.

Bennett, J.M., Catovsky, D., Daniel, M.-T. *et al.* (1982). Proposals for the classification of the myelodysplastic syndromes. *Br. J. Haematol.*, **51**, 189–199.

Boultwood, J., Lewis, S. and Wainscoat, J.S. (1994). The 5q– syndrome. *Blood*, **84**, 3253–3260.

Calligaris-Cappio, F. (1996). B-chronic lymphocytic leukemia: a malignancy of anti-self B cells. *Blood*, **87**, 2615–2620.

Callihan, T.R., Holbert, J.M. and Berard, C.W. (1983). Neoplasms of terminal B-cell differentiation: the morphologic basis of functional diversity. In *Malignant Lymphomas: A Pathology Annual Monograph*, pp. 169–268. Appleton-Century-Crofts.

Carper, E. and Kurtzman, G.L. (1996). Human parvovirus B19 infection. *Curr. Opin. Hematol.*, **3**, 111–117.

Clarkson, B.D., Strife, A., Wisniewski, D. *et al.* (1997). New understanding of the pathogenesis of CML: a prototype of early neoplasia. *Leukemia*, **11**, 1404–1428.

D'Andrea, A.D. and Grompe, M. (1997). Molecular biology of Fanconi anemia: implications for diagnosis and therapy. *Blood*, **90**, 1725–1736.

de Boer, C.J., Kluin-Nelemans, J.C., Dreef, E. *et al.* (1996). Involvement of the CCND1 gene in hairy cell leukemia. *Ann. Oncol.*, **7**, 251–256.

Delmer, A., Ajchenbaum-Cymbalista, F., Tang, R. *et al.* (1995). Over-expression of cyclin D1 in chronic B-cell malignancies with abnormality of chromosome 11q13. *Br. J. Haematol.*, **89**, 798–804.

Escribano, L., Orfao, A., Diaz-Agustin, B. *et al.* (1998). Indolent systemic mast cell disease in adults: immunophenotypic characterization of bone marrow mast cells and its diagnostic implications. *Blood*, **91**, 2731–2736.

Faderl, S., Kantarjian, H.M., Talpaz, M. and Estrov, Z. (1998). Clinical significance of cytogenetic abnormalities in adult acute lymphoblastic leukemia. *Blood*, **91**, 3995–4019.

Fenaux, P., Morel, P. and Lai, J.L. (1996). Cytogenetics of myelodysplastic syndromes. *Sem. Hematol.*, **33**, 127–138.

Filippa, D.A., Ladanyi, M., Wollner, N. *et al.* (1996). CD30 (Ki-1)-positive malignant lymphomas: clinical, immunophenotypic, histologic, and genetic characteristics and differences with Hodgkin's disease. *Blood*, **87**, 2905–2917.

Foucar, K. and Rydell, R.E. (1980). Richter's syndrome in chronic lymphocytic leukemia. *Cancer*, **46**, 118–134.

Gallagher, R.E., Willman, C.L., Slack, J.L. *et al.* (1997). Association of PML-RARα fusion mRNA type with pretreatment hematologic characteristics but not treatment outcome in acute promyelocytic leukemia: an intergroup molecular study. *Blood*, **90**, 1656–1663.

Grignani, F., Fagioli, M., Alcalay, M. *et al.* (1994). Acute promyelocytic leukemia: from genetics to treatment. *Blood*, **83**, 10–25.

Guidez, F., Ivins, S., Zhu, J. *et al.* (1998). Reduced retinoic acid sensitivities of nuclear receptor corepressor binding to PML- and PLZF-RARα underlie molecular pathogenesis and treatment of acute promyelocytic leukemia. *Blood*, **91**, 2634–2642.

Harris, N.L., Jaffe, E.S., Stein, H. *et al.* (1994). A revised European–American classification of lymphoid neoplasms: a proposal from the International Lymphoma Study Group. *Blood*, **84**, 1361–1392.

Hess, J.L., Zutter, M.M., Castleberry, R.P. and Emanuel, P.D. (1996). Juvenile chronic myelogenous leukemia. *Am. J. Clin. Pathol.*, **105**, 238–248.

Juvonen, E., Ikkala, E., Oksanen, K. and Ruutu, T. (1993). Megakaryocyte and erythroid colony formation in essential thrombocythaemia and reactive thrombocytosis: diagnostic value and correlation to complications. *Br. J. Haematol.*, **83**, 192–197.

Kantarjian, H.M., Deisseroth, A., Kurzrock, R. *et al.* (1993). Chronic myelogenous leukemia: a concise update. *Blood*, **82**, 691–703.

Lamant, L., Meggetto, F., Al Saati, T. *et al.* (1996). High incidence of the t(2;5)(p23;q35) translocation in anaplastic large cell lymphoma and its lack of detection in Hodgkin's disease. Comparison of cytogenetic analysis, reverse transcriptase-polymerase chain reaction, and P-80 immunostaining. *Blood*, **87**, 284–291.

Lambrechts, A.C., Hupkes, P.F., Dorssers, L.C.J. and van't Veer, M.B. (1993). Translocation (14;18)-positive cells are present in the circulation of the majority of patients with localized (stage I and II) follicular non-Hodgkin's lymphoma. *Blood*, **82**, 2510–2516.

Limpens, J., Stad, R., Vos, C. *et al.* (1995). Lymphoma-associated translocation t(14;18) in blood B cells of normal individuals. *Blood*, **85**, 2528–2536.

Luna-Fineman, S., Shannon, K.M. and Lange, B.J. (1995). Childhood monosomy 7: epidemiology, biology, and mechanistic implications. *Blood*, **85**, 1985–1999.

Murphy, S., Peterson, P., Iland, H. and Laszlo, J. (1997). Experience of the Polycythemia Vera Study Group with essential thrombocythemia: a final report on diagnostic criteria, survival, and leukemic transition by treatment. *Sem. Hematol.*, **34**, 29–39.

Nguyen, D., Brynes, R.K., Macaulay, L. *et al.* (1989). Acute myeloid leukemia, FAB M-1 microgranular variant: a multiparameter study. *Hematol. Pathol.*, **3**, 11–22.

Nguyen, D.T., Diamond, L.W., Cavenagh, J.D. *et al.* (1997). Haematological validation of a computer-based bone marrow reporting system. *J. Clin. Pathol.*, **50**, 375–378.

Nguyen, D.T., Diamond, L.W., Cavenagh, J.D. *et al.* (1997). Increased efficiency of bone marrow reporting with hematology knowledge-based systems. *Lab. Hematol.*, **3**, 10–18.

Nusbaum, N.J. (1991). Concise review: genetic bases for sideroblastic anemia. *Am. J. Hematol.*, **37**, 41–44.

Peterson, L.C., Kueck, B., Arthur, D.C. *et al.* (1988). Systemic polyclonal immunoblastic proliferations. *Cancer*, **61**, 1350–1358.

Raynaud, S., Cave, H., Baens, M. *et al.* (1996). The 12;21 translocation involving TEL and deletion of the other TEL allele: two frequently associated alterations found in childhood acute lymphoblastic leukemia. *Blood*, **87**, 2891–2899.

Reid, C.D.L. (1997). The dendritic cell lineage in haemopoiesis. *Br. J. Haematol.*, **96**, 217–223.

Travis, W.D., Li, C.-Y., Yam, L.T. *et al.* (1988). Significance of systemic mast cell disease with associated hematologic disorders. *Cancer*, **62**, 965–972.

Uckun, F.M., Herman-Hatten, K., Crotty, M.-L. *et al.* (1998). Clinical significance of MLL-AF4 fusion transcript expression in the absence of a cytogenetically detectable t(4;11)(q21;q23) chromosomal translocation. *Blood*, **92**, 810–821.

Yang, E. and Korsmeyer, S.J. (1996). Molecular thanaptosis: a discourse on the bcl-2 family and cell death. *Blood*, **88**, 386–401.

Young, N.S. (1992). The problem of clonality in aplastic anemia. *Blood*, **79**, 1385–1392.

Appendix: Installing and using the Knowledge-based Systems CD-ROM

Appendix contents

- Requirements
- Screen settings
- Installation
- Using the Knowledge-based systems
- Advanced settings
  — creating a database alias (TextbookDB)
  — modifying an alias
- Trouble-shooting
- Network installation and operation

This textbook is accompanied by a CD-ROM with three knowledge-based systems applied to 237 case studies. The three knowledge-based systems are:

1 **Professor Petrushka** for peripheral blood analysis.

2 **Professor Fidelio** for flow cytometry immunophenotyping.

3 **Professor Belmonte** for bone marrow interpretation.

Each system is a separate program (Petrushka.exe, Fidelio.exe, Belmonte.exe) which uses large database files. You have the choice when installing the software whether to put the database files on to your hard drive (quicker and easier) or leave them on the CD-ROM (uses much less space).

Requirements

The knowledge-based systems are designed for computers running Windows 95, Windows 98 or Windows NT.

Screen settings

The knowledge-based systems have been optimized for a screen resolution of 800×600 with 16 million colors (24-bit). They will run fine at 1024×768 resolution but the difference in screen size may cause minor differences in word spacing on some systems. Your computer must be capable of displaying at least

65,000 colors (16-bit) at the chosen resolution in order to view the photomicrographs properly.

Installation

Insert the CD-ROM and use My Computer to choose SETUP.EXE, or choose Run from the Start menu and type D:\setup.exe, where D:\ is the letter for your CD-ROM drive.

NB – Make sure that you reboot your computer at the end of the installation. If you try to run the programs when the computer has not been rebooted, they may not function correctly or at all.

There are three installation options:

1　**Typical (Recommended):** This option installs the software and databases automatically. This option requires approximately 200 MB of disk space on your hard disk drive.

2　**Compact:** This option installs the database engine only; the programs and databases will remain on the CD-ROM, and you will need to have the CD-ROM inserted in order to access them. This option requires approximately 10 MB of disk space on your hard disk drive.

   NB: You will have to manually change some settings on your computer if you choose this option (see Advanced Settings below)

3　**Custom (advanced users only):** This option allows you to choose whether or not to install the database software. If your computer already has the 32-bit version of the Borland Database Engine (BDE) installed (e.g. you are already using Paradox, version 7 for Windows 95), you can deselect (uncheck) BDE installation and install only the programs and databases to your hard disk drive.

   Note: You must create the database alias manually if you choose this option (see Advanced Settings below). If the BDE is already installed and you choose to run the programs from the CD-ROM, then you do not have to run the installation program but you must still create the database alias manually.

Using the Knowledge-based Systems

To run the programs, use the shortcut created by the installation program or use Windows Explorer or My Computer to select the appropriate file:

Belmonte.exe; Fidelio.exe; Petrushka.exe. These will be on your hard drive in the C:\Diagnostic Hematology folder, or on the CD-ROM if you selected the Compact installation.

The knowledge-based systems are very simple to use. Once the programs are running, simply choose the case study that you wish to open using the drop-down list in the tool bar at the top of the screen. The other icons in the tool bar allow you to display the photomicrographs and graphics associated with the case.

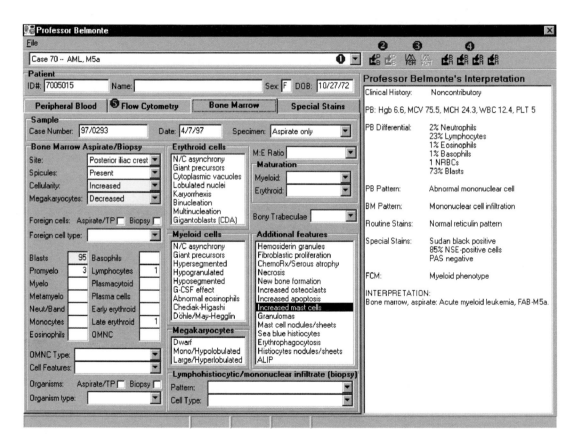

Figure A.1 Screen shot of Professor Belmonte. Each of the knowledge-based systems contains a tool bar at the top of the screen with a drop-down list for choosing cases and appropriate icons for displaying images. If an image is opened, it must be closed before proceeding. If an image icon is grey, then an image is not available for that icon.
The items numbered in red are:
❶ drop-down list of cases (choose the case that you want to view from this list);
❷ peripheral blood images (click on the icon to view the image);
❸ FCM graphics;
❹ bone marrow images;
❺ in Professor Belmonte, these tabs can be used to view the peripheral blood data, and, if appropriate, FCM immunophenotyping results and bone marrow special stains. These tabs are not present in Professors Petrushka and Fidelio.

In this educational version of the knowledge-based systems, the databases are closed. You cannot alter any of the example data.

Advanced settings

The programs require the installation of the 32-bit Borland Database Engine (BDE). In addition, a database alias 'TextbookDB' must be created. A database alias tells the BDE which directory the databases are installed in (i.e. the path). This alias is created automatically by the Typical Installation option. However, for the Compact and Custom options you will need to create and/or edit it manually.

Creating a database alias (TextbookDB)

1 When installation is complete, go to the Diagnostic Hematology group on the Start Menu, and run the BDE Administrator (BDEADMIN.EXE).

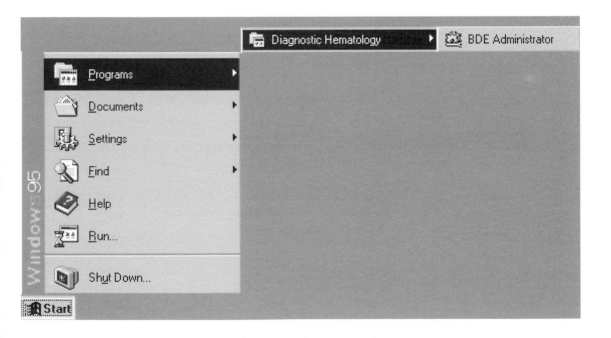

2   In the left panel make sure that the Databases tab is selected.

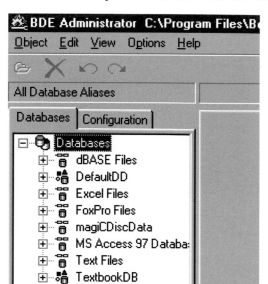

3   Check the left panel to see if the alias 'TextbookDB' exists. If it exists then skip to the section 'Modifying an alias'.

4   If the alias does not already exist then select 'New...' from the Object menu.

5   When the 'New database alias' dialog appears, leave the Database driver name as STANDARD and click OK.

6   In the left panel, change the name 'STANDARD1' to 'TextbookDB' (without the quotes) and then hit the 'Enter' key.

7   In the right panel, click on the empty field next to Path. Type in the directory where the database programs are installed. For example, if you are running the programs directly from the CD-ROM, then type 'E:\Databases' (where 'E' is the letter for your CD-ROM drive).

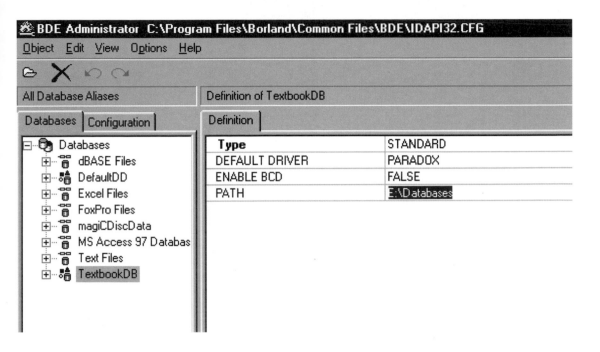

8   From the Object menu, choose 'Apply'.

9   When the confirmation dialog appears, click on OK.

10   Close the BDE Administrator.

Modifying an alias

To modify an existing TextbookDB alias using the BDE Administrator, make sure that the knowledge-based systems are closed. Follow steps 1 and 2 above and then choose TextbookDB from the databases list box in the left panel. To modify the path follow steps 7–10 above.

Trouble-shooting

To install the BDE, the install program must be able to write files to the Windows system directories. Therefore, the attributes of your system's C:\Windows and C:\Windows\System directories must NOT be 'read only'. You can check the attributes of these directories in Windows Explorer by right-clicking on the directory and choosing 'properties'.

If, when you are editing the Database Alias, the setting will not save, check to see if the Alias in the left window has a yellow box round it:

```
⊞  MQIS
⊞  MS Access 97 Dat.
⊞  Text Files
   TextbookDB
⊞  Visual FoxPro Data
⊞  Visual FoxPro Tabl
```

If it has, the database has locked the Alias and cannot be edited. Right-click on the Alias icon and select Close. This will clear the lock and allow the Alias to be edited.

Network installation and operation (advanced users only)

For network operation, the databases and programs can exist on the server. Each client workstation needs its own copy of the Borland Database Engine. To install on a network, do the following:

1 On the server: Install according to the instructions shown above but choose a 'Custom' installation and uncheck the BDE option to install only the databases and programs.

2 On each client workstation: Install according to the instructions shown above but choose a 'Compact' installation to install only the BDE on the client workstations.

3 On each client, map a drive letter to the root directory of the server (or make note of the drive letter if it already exists).

4 Using the instructions shown above to create a database alias, create an alias to 'TextbookDB' on each client workstation.

Example: If the databases and programs were installed with the default options, they exist in the directory 'C:\Diagnostic Hematology' on the server. If the server's root directory ('C:\') is mapped to drive 'K:' on the client workstation, then the path that you would enter for the 'TextbookDB' alias would be 'K:\Diagnostic Hematology'.

The BDE installation (using the default parameters) will create a 'Diagnostic Hematology' folder on each workstation. Use the 'Customize Start Menu' option in the 'Settings/Taskbar . . . /Start Menu Programs' dialog box to add shortcuts to 'Professor Petrushka', 'Professor Fidelio' and 'Professor Belmonte' (located on the server, e.g. 'K:\Diagnostic Hematology') to the 'Diagnostic Hematology' folder.

- If you experience difficulties installing or using the knowledge-based systems CD-ROM please contact Butterworth-Heinemann Customer Services on 01865 888180.

Index